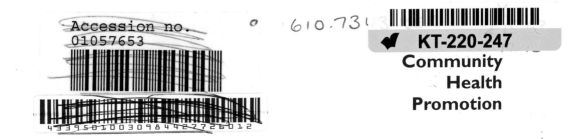

610.73

For my sons, Liam and Matthew
JK

Community Health Promotion

Challenges for Practice

Edited by

Joanne Kerr
MSc RGN RHV RNT CertEd
Fellow, Health Service Management Unit, University of Manchester, Manchester;
formerly Community Nurse Tutor, School of Nursing, Midwifery and Health Visiting,
University of Manchester, Manchester

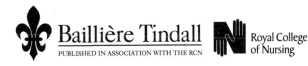

Baillière Tindall
PUBLISHED IN ASSOCIATION WITH THE RCN

Royal College
of Nursing

BAILLIÈRE TINDALL
An imprint of Harcourt Publishers Limited

© Harcourt Publishers Limited 2000

✿ is a registered trademark of Harcourt Publishers Limited

The right of Joanne Kerr to be identified as editor of this work has been asserted by her in accordance with the Copyright, Designs and Patents Act 1988

First published 2000

ISBN 07020 2284 5

British Library Cataloguing in Publication Data
A catalogue record for this book is available from the British Library

Library of Congress Cataloging in Publication Data
A catalog record for this book is available from the Library of Congress

Note
Medical knowledge is constantly changing. As new information becomes available, changes in treatment, procedures, equipment and the use of drugs become necessary. The editors, contributors and the publishers have, as far as it is possible, taken care to ensure that the information given in this text is accurate and up to date. However, readers are strongly advised to confirm that the information, especially with regard to drug usage, complies with the latest legislation and standards of practice.

The publisher's policy is to use **paper manufactured from sustainable forests**

Printed in China

Contents

Contributors vii

Introduction ix

Section One: Background to Community Health Promotion

1 Promoting the health of communities 3
 Monica Haggart

2 Community health promotion and empowerment 27
 Philip Carey

Section Two: Challenges in Practice

3 Pre-conception care 51
 Karen Dignan

4 Empowerment and childbirth 65
 Aileen McLoughlin

5 Teenage pregnancy 83
 Karen Dignan

6 Promoting child and family health through empowerment 101
 Sue Hooton

7 Youth health promotion in the community 125
 Grainne Graham

8 Homeless women and primary health care 155
 Melanie Ibbitson

9 Mental health promotion 183
 Phil Keeley

10 Men's health: concepts, criticisms and challenges 207
 Steven Pryjmachuk and Timothy Simon Faltermeyer

11 Health promotion and ethnic minority groups 229
 Abbie Paton and Julie A. Higgins

12 'Queer health': health promotion the hard way 245
 Tony Russell-Pattison

13 Health promotion for older people 263
 Gordon Evans

14 Health promotion and community care: the neighbourhood health strategy 285
 Julia Mitchell

Index 307

Contributors

Philip Carey MSc BSc(Hons)
Senior Lecturer,
Liverpool John Moores University,
Liverpool

Karen Dignan MSc RN RM ADM MTD
Midwife Teacher and Sexual Health Pathway Leader,
School of Nursing, Midwifery & Health Visiting,
University of Manchester, Manchester

Gordon Evans MSc RMN RGN RNT STD
Pathway Leader (Older Persons),
Department of Health Studies,
University of York, York

Timothy Simon Faltermeyer MIMgt MSc BA CertEd RNT RCNT RN
Lecturer in Sociology and Health,
University of Manchester, Manchester

Grainne Graham MSc MA BA
Senior Health Promotion Manager,
Salford and Trafford Health Promotion Service

Monica Haggart MSc BSc RGN RM RHV FWT RNT
Nurse Teacher, School of Nursing, Midwifery & Health Visiting,
University of Manchester, Manchester

Julie A Higgins PhD MSc
Public Health Specialist,
West Pennine Health Authority

Sue Hooton RGN RSCN CertEd
Education Officer,
English National Board for Nursing, Midwifery and Health Visiting

Melanie Ibbitson MSc BA(Hons)
Health Promotion Specialist

Phil Keeley MA BA RGN RMN CPNCert CertEd RNT
Nurse Tutor, School of Nursing, Midwifery and Health Visiting,
University of Manchester, Manchester

Aileen MP McLoughlin MSc BSc RGN RM ADM CounsellingCert
Midwife Teacher, School of Nursing, Midwifery & Health Visiting,
University of Manchester, Manchester

Julia Mitchell MSc BA(Hons) PGCE
Health Promotion Specialist,
Bolton Specialist Health Promotion Service

Abbie Paton MSc BSc
Health Promotion Specialist,
West Pennine Health Authority

Steven Pryjmachuk MSc BA(Hons) PGDipEd(Nursing) RMN RNT
Nurse Tutor, School of Nursing, Midwifery & Health Visiting,
University of Manchester, Manchester

Tony Russell-Pattison (formerly Harrison) BA RN RSCN RNT
Nurse Tutor, School of Nursing, Midwifery & Health Visiting,
University of Manchester, Manchester

Introduction

Community Health Promotion: challenges for practice is intended to encourage would-be health promoters to review their own practice and to consider how health professionals can work with imagination and enterprise to forge new health alliances. In this book, debates and dilemmas in a range of areas are discussed and examined, including discussions around how health professionals can have an active and valuable role in empowering practice, and the relevance of community development and collaboration.

Health promotion is 'everybody's business' (DHSS 1976) and interprofessional collaboration should be a priority for all health professionals. Barriers between 'lay' and 'professional' people need to be broken down and strong alliances built if we are to strive towards a healthier nation. This book is, therefore, about ways of achieving partnerships across a range of different services in an attempt to make health promotion realistic, effective and valuable.

The key theme in this book is empowerment, and this is woven into each chapter. In order to meet the needs of the consumers of health services, it is important to empower both them and the services themselves. This raises many questions regarding our health care system:

- Do services disempower users?
- Are services ready to work with empowered users?
- Is it possible to empower services to empower users?
- Can de-powered health professionals facilitate the empowerment of clients?

This book explores these issues and questions how health professionals can transform health promotion into an empowering activity. Other themes inherent in the text are community development and participation, and healthy alliances. Examples of innovative practice are highlighted to illustrate how these can, in turn, help to empower practice.

Many of the chapters contain activities, which readers are recommended to consider before progressing through the book. These are designed to enable readers to identify and develop their own values, knowledge and skills and to develop their understanding of the practical dilemmas in action. The book is clearly signposted for ease of use. Each chapter starts with an overview outlining the contents of each chapter and ends with recommendations for further reading and a comprehensive reference list.

The book is organised into two sections. In Section One (Chapters 1 and 2), the issues of community health promotion and empowerment are contextualised, thus enabling readers to explore their own ideas about them. In Chapter 1, the theory around health is examined and the debate about social versus behavioural determinants of health is considered. The notion of a public health approach to health promotion is also explored. The meaning of empowerment is explored in Chapter 2, and it is argued that the concept of empowerment has always been, and should remain, a tool for social change. The implications to health promotion of empowerment are discussed.

The chapters in Section Two relate the themes of community health promotion and empowerment in the context of practice with a particular client group. The client groups included are not intended to be comprehensive, but rather to represent the range of health promotion practice across a wide spectrum. Relevant theory and research, and useful health promotion strategies are outlined.

Pre-conception care is discussed in Chapter 3, with the aim of weaving pre-conception care into an empowerment approach to health promotion. The concept of empowerment in childbirth is considered in Chapter 4. Written from a midwifery perspective, the background to the current provision of midwifery care is reviewed and the influence of user groups on service provision is discussed.

The reasons behind the consistently high level of unintended teenage pregnancies are explored in Chapter 5, and a way forward though a multi-professional approach is offered. In Chapter 6, current approaches to child health promotion are considered. The focus is on health promotion for school children. Professional understanding of child health matters and a clearer understanding of the factors that influence children's rights to health emerge. A comprehensive overview of youth health promotion is given in Chapter 7, and the ways in which prevailing attitudes and strategies in this area are disempowering to young people are considered. The real issues for young people are identified and there is a discussion of how agencies can work together in a more empowering way.

In Chapter 8, the relationship between homelessness and ill-health is considered, focusing primarily on women. A feminist research framework is utilised in order to facilitate the empowerment of homeless women and to expand the current body of work already undertaken. The need for a strategic approach to the evaluation of mental health intervention in adults and older people is discussed in Chapter 9. Men's health from biological, sociocultural and masculinity viewpoints is the subject of Chapter 10. The challenges facing health promoters when working in the area of men's health are considered and some thoughts are given on the reduction of the mortality and morbidity statistics for men.

Approaches to health promotion with minority ethnic groups are explored in Chapter 11 and directions for the way forward, through community development and inter-agency collaboration, are suggested. In Chapter 12, the issues around HIV prevention are reviewed and questions are raised to enable readers to explore in more depth assumptions surrounding health promotion work with gay men and lesbian women.

The importance of health promotion for older people is considered in Chapter 13. Ageism and inequitable practices are highlighted and challenged, and inter-agency collaboration is suggested as a way forward.

A Neighbourhood Health Strategy is analysed in Chapter 14, very effectively illustrating multi-agency alliances within a neighbourhood/locality. A description of the project, including the strategic and operational processes, is given, and the perspectives of the health professionals working within neighbourhoods is discussed. This discussion includes consideration of the challenges faced, the strategies used to overcome problems and the issues that are inevitably raised regarding evaluation of this kind of project.

Although the contributors come from an educational or a community health promotion background, it is fair to say that each places different emphasis on the meaning and role of community health promotion and empowerment. If by observing these differences you can identify your own position within this field you will inevitably broaden your horizons with regard to empowering practice. It is hoped that readers will challenge their own health promotion practice and consider ways of being innovative in the field of health education/promotion.

Community Health Promotion: challenges for practice should appeal to students in the fields of public health, health promotion, nursing and social care. It should also appeal to busy practitioners who have little time to consult multiple texts, as it provides a wealth of information in the field of community health promotion.

Health care practitioners can attempt to empower themselves by developing the skill of reflecting on their practice. Only then can they take their profession forward and really contribute to the notion of a healthier nation.

Acknowledgement

I would like to thank my husband Eugene for his constant support and encouragement.

Joanne Kerr, 2000

Reference

Department of Health and Social Security (DHSS) (1976) *Prevention and Health: Everybody's Business.* London: HMSO

1 BACKGROUND TO COMMUNITY HEALTH PROMOTION

SECTION CONTENTS

1 **Promoting the Health of Communities**
Monica Haggart

2 **Community Health Promotion and Empowerment**
Philip Carey

Promoting the health of communities

Monica Haggart

KEY ISSUES

- Development of notions about health
- Major determinants of health
- Political dimension of health
- Social vs behavioural determinants of health
- A public health approach to health promotion

DEVELOPMENT OF NOTIONS ABOUT HEALTH

Any retrospective analysis of health improvements over the last century in Britain demonstrates declining infant mortality rates, maternal mortality rates and increased longevity. The pattern of disease dramatically changed in a comparatively short time and it is precisely this changing pattern which leads many to believe that medicine, e.g. the introduction of sulphonamides followed by antibiotics, is primarily responsible for the good health enjoyed by many people today. It is this belief that underpins the drive to find (at any cost) medical and technological developments. The historical analysis however gives a picture of concomitant social changes such as improved sanitation, cleaner water supplies, and improved housing conditions, all of which had an equally dramatic effect on people's health. So, why is there this difference in perspective? It may be useful to consider a little further back in time to the early stages of the scientific tradition.

Prior to the Renaissance period, health and well-being were intimately connected with religion. Illness was often perceived as evidence of wrongdoing or perhaps a violation of social taboos. Healers were then priests of one kind or another who used herbs, poultices, incantations or other methods of ridding the person of the evil which had beset them. The notion of viewing illness as evidence of wrongdoing may seem amusing and naïve but there could be argued to be parallels today of blaming people for the ills that befall them as a 'result' of their lifestyle over which they often have minimal choice. Skrabanek (1994) calls this process of victim blaming 'health fascism'.

An explosion of knowledge occurred during the Renaissance period. Rene Descartes (1596–1650), who was primarily a mathematician but also a philosopher, developed the idea of dualism, i.e. the mind and the body as parallel but separate entities. Descartes likened the body to a machine, capable of malfunction but also capable of being understood if broken down into its component parts in order that the malfunction of each could be discovered and corrected. The understanding of things by analysis of their smallest constituents progressed and the science of health took a different turn. Priests remained responsible for the mind and the soul, but the body was now progressively understood in scientific terms and became the domain of doctors. Later doctors started to apply scientific principles to the mind and this also became their province, hence the beginnings of psychiatry. The priests were, and still are, left with the soul which has remained of little interest to doctors up to the present time.

The scientific tradition has clearly brought many advantages but also disadvantages. What is a sociological perspective on the profession of medicine?

Many sociologists suggest that power has developed from this growth of knowledge through science. There is greater and greater knowledge about smaller and smaller aspects of the body. This knowledge is held within a small elite group and this creates a power base from which it is possible to give the impression of knowing about everything. People then lose faith in what they thought they knew and begin to depend upon the professional to tell them what is real and what is not. Consider the increase in the numbers of people consulting doctors about illnesses, e.g. coughs and colds, which need no medical expertise. Consider also the increase in people demanding prescriptions rather than relying on their inner reserves and healing processes.

Illich (1976) warns that many professionals do not stop at 'advising' but move on to monopolising the power to prescribe, i.e. they not only dictate what is bad but what is good. Additionally, because of the success of the scientific model, doctors find it hard to trust anything that is not supported by scientific research. This sometimes means that people's experiences are not valued in terms of evidence because they do not fit into the scientific model. This commonly applies to mind and body issues.

The understanding of the structure and function of living things by breaking them down into smaller and smaller components leads to the analysis of the body (and/or the mind) in terms of its anatomical, physiological and biochemical features. From this model, for disease to be 'real' it has to be organic. Where no organic malfunction is discernible, health is assumed to exist. It is easy to see how the biomedical model then leads to the view of health as the absence of disease.

The 'body as machine' account is only one of the many perceptions of health which exist and which arise from people's perceptions of the world, their experiences, their beliefs and values as well as their education.

The biomedical approach is based on a reductionist model and because of the knowledge that the scientific approach has bestowed, the biomedical approach has ascended to a powerful position over the last half-century. It is during this time that health and life in general has become increasingly medicalised. Crawford (1984), Mitchell (1982) and more recently Skrabanek (1994) argue that there is an increasingly pervasive medical way of thinking on many aspects of life where medicine has no part to play. This helps to maintain people in a position of passivity and ignorance. It is this medicalisation of all aspects of life which engenders a dependence on medicine and an expectation that the magic of medicine can overcome anything.

What ethical issues may be raised by maintaining people in this position of passivity and ignorance?

This raises the issue of autonomy and paternalism. People cannot make properly informed choices about health if information is withheld from them. A paternalistic approach to people could be argued to remove from them their confidence in their own ability to make choices and judgements.

There is a whole array of theories about the nature of health, some underpinned by a biomedical approach and others underpinned by a humanist approach, which is about personal achievement of potential.

Seedhouse (1986) and later Stainton Rogers (1991) give a comprehensive account of the differing theories of health. See Box 1.1 and Box 1.2 for a breakdown of approaches and views of health adapted from their original work.

BOX 1.1	*Theories of health*

Health as an ideal state

Principles
- Based on the biomedical principle of health as the absence of disease
- Encompasses the goal of perfect well-being in every respect
- Health is seen as an end in itself rather than a means

Examples
- The modern search to eradicate all illnesses as opposed to rectifying conditions which are damaging to health
- World Health Organisation (1946) definition of health (later updated and changed dramatically in 1984)
- The disproportionate allocation of resources to what are perceived to be 'cures' as opposed to the problems that people have to learn to live with
- Beveridge's assertions at the inception of the National Health Service (NHS) in 1948 that once all the illnesses had been eradicated, the need for the NHS would decrease

Problems
- Dubos (1959) suggests that the view of health as an ideal state is simply a mirage, i.e. ideal health doesn't exist
- People with disabilities or chronic conditions could be viewed as inferior, deviant or even repulsive
- If perfect health is seen as a possibility, it can become the cultural norm to strive towards it. Those who are seen as not cooperating in this endeavour can easily be seen as responsible for their own problems, regardless of their circumstances, i.e. victim blaming

Health as a means to functioning in society

Principles
- Also based on biomedical principles of health as absence of disease
- Health and illness are seen as polar opposites
- Health is about the possession of the physical and mental functioning necessary for them to function normally in their own society

Examples

- Parson's (1981) view of health as 'the state of optimum capacity of an individual for the effective role and tasks for which he has been socialised'
- Look at the way that in British society, illness is 'legitimised' when a doctor issues a note to say that an individual is unfit to work
- The way that individuals with mental health problems are viewed when they are absent from work, i.e. still physically able to work, therefore not legitimately ill
- When people are absent from work because of stress/depression they often give physical reasons for their absence, e.g. diarrhoea or back problems and are not expected to be out of the house because they are 'ill'.

Problems

- The theory (in keeping with all functionalist theories) implies no need for change
- The theory does not account for the possibility that a person's socialised role may be the very factor which pushes them into the 'sick' role
- This theory views health as no more than the opposite of disease/illness

Health as a commodity

Principles

- This theory is based upon a biomedical understanding
- Health from this perspective is something that can be supplied by someone else
- Health is an external phenomena that can somehow be imbued upon an individual

Examples

- Health professionals are viewed in today's professionalised society as givers or purveyors of health
- The 'magic bullet' approach of looking for a pill for every ill, i.e. when patients demonstrate a need to exit the doctor's surgery armed with a prescription
- Look at the way the 'health industry' of fitness equipment, videos, books and TV doctors is flourishing
- Some would argue that the current consultation rates for minor disorders are evidence of people viewing health as something outside of themselves to be bought or procured from a third party

Problems

- Sacks (1982) believes that by holding out the false hope of an effortless state of health, this theory 'conceals from people their wider potentials by undermining their unique metaphysical strengths'
- This theory will maintain professional (as well as commercial) power. Individuals will be led to always defer to a professional in their pursuit of health
- If health is viewed as a commodity, then spending more money would surely mean guaranteeing a greater level of health

Humanist theories of health

Principles
- Health is seen as an ability to adapt positively and strive for growth in all of life's circumstances
- These abilities can be encouraged but they can also be lost or undermined
- Health is viewed as a means for personal growth rather than an end in itself
- Disease or illness have little bearing on this view of health. The determinant is how the person responds

Examples
- Sacks provides examples in his experiential account 'Awakenings' where patients showed positive adaptations to life after years of existing in a semi-comatose state. Sacks was also anxious to demonstrate that the person and their spiritual health were present even when unable to be communicated or expressed in socially acceptable ways
- The old/new holistic approach to health in nursing where the spirit is a legitimate focus for nursing care as much as the body (Haggart, 1996)

Problems
- Argued by many that these strengths and abilities are too nebulous or vague
- This view of health is so vague that it gives people who wish to work for health nothing to aim at
- Positive adaptation is something that may be perceived differently by different people

(Adapted from *Health. The Foundation for Achievement*, Seedhouse, D., 1986 with kind permission from J. Wiley & Sons.)

BOX 1.2	*Explanations of health*

'Body as machine' account
- Operates within the world view of science where illness is regarded as naturally occurring and 'real,' and modern biomedicine is seen as the only valid source of effective treatment for serious illness

'Body under siege' account
- The individual is viewed as under threat and attack from germs and diseases, interpersonal conflicts and the 'stress' of modern life acting upon the body through the agency of the mind

'Inequality of access' account
- People who held this perception were convinced of the benefits of modern medicine, but were concerned about the unfair allocation of those benefits and their lack of availability to those who need them most

'Cultural critique of medicine' account
- This perception was based upon a 'dominance' sociological world view of exploitation and oppression and an analysis of knowledge as socially constructed

'Health promotion' account

- An institutionally promoted and popularised account which recognises both collective and personal responsibility for ill health, but stresses the wisdom of living a 'healthy lifestyle' in order for good health to be achieved

'Robust individualism' account

- Based on human rights principles of people having the right to do whatever they will and the denial of the right of the state to interfere with what they choose to do

'God's power' account

- Health is viewed here as a product of 'right living' and spiritual well-being. Recovery from illness is viewed as regaining a spiritual wholeness through intercession to a spiritual power

'Will-power' account

- This perception views the individual as in control and stresses the moral responsibility of the individual to use their 'will' to maintain health

(Reproduced from *Explaining Health and Illness. An Exploration of Diversity*, Stainton Rogers, W., 1991, with kind permission from Harvester Wheatsheaf.)

Seedhouse (1986) sees a common thread to all of these theories and that is that they all view the removal of obstacles as important in the achievement of human potential. The difference between them is in the theory of what human potential should be (aimed for) and the nature of the obstacles.

Stainton Rogers' (1991) cultural analysis adds another dimension to this. Her results seem to demonstrate two poles of thinking which affect people's views of health, i.e. the individual as helpless or the individual in total control. The 'body as machine', the 'body under siege' and the 'inequality of access' accounts tend to view the individual as helpless. These accounts view the medical service as dominant and individuals as passive recipients of whatever (at times inadequate) health care is available from professionals. Health care is viewed as treating the manifestations of disease.

The 'cultural critique' account also, to some degree, views the individual as helpless in the current dominant medical paradigm. However, it is this very helplessness that this account views as the problem or obstacle to health.

The 'God's power', 'will-power' and 'robust individualism' accounts tend to view the individual as in some form of control and have commonalities with the humanist theories as described by Seedhouse. These accounts are similarly about 'metaphysical strength' whether that comes from within or via intercessions to God; it is up to the individual to marshal their reserves and internal power to maintain health. Much of the 'mind over matter,' psycho-dynamic and complementary therapy theories can also be viewed from this perspective.

The health promotion account tends to straddle the two poles in that, depending upon the way it is used, it can either be seen to empower and emancipate individuals to plan and make sense of their own actions or, alternatively, it can be used to 'blame the victim', denying in the process the structural problems faced by many in their attempts to maintain health as they define it.

The polarisation then is between control and helplessness but overlaying that is the polarisation between health as the absence of disease and health as a broader state of well-being. From the preceding accounts it seems that those who view health as the absence of disease are more likely to view the individual as helpless. This is an important consideration when moving on to look at how to promote the health of people within a community.

MAJOR DETERMINANTS OF HEALTH

Health promotion emerged as a concept against the backdrop of changing health needs, where infectious disease was thought to be a diminishing threat and the major diseases affecting people could be attributed to external factors. If the promotion of health is about the removal of barriers to health, the barriers must first be identified. Perception of the barriers is dependent upon an individual's view of their health, their values and beliefs about the nature of the person and, to some degree, their political persuasion. The barriers can generally be categorised into individual/behavioural and social/environmental (structural). MacDonald and Bunton (1992) recognise these two themes as the twin pillars underpinning health promotion activity, with emphasis on one area or the other being dependent upon ideology, goals, target population as well as focus and type of intervention.

Individual/behavioural factors

The theory that most illnesses which currently affect Western populations are essentially preventable, leads many people to believe that health is in the hands of each individual who may choose health damaging or health enhancing behaviour. Health promotion, from this perspective, is very simple. It involves mostly an educational approach to inform people of the effects of certain behaviours, e.g. smoking, lack of exercise, alcohol consumption. The theory is that once people understand the problems, they will change their behaviour.

This theory is based on the notion that knowledge, attitude and behaviours are congruent and, that once an individual has the required knowledge, they will change their attitude which will ultimately lead to a change in their behaviour. Most health promotion theorists now recognise this simplistic connection as naïve. Successive governments however can be seen to have favoured the knowledge–attitude–behaviour (KAB) approach. Note the many mass media campaigns which are used to 'heighten public awareness' but which have questionable impact on people's everyday lives and decision making.

However, even if the simplistic behaviour model is accepted, it is more complex than simply the notion that 'knowledge changes attitude which in turn alters behaviour'. Bandura (1977) for example suggests that behaviour is guided by the value which an individual places on the perceived outcome for the behaviour (incentives), the level to which the individual believes that a certain action will result in the desired outcome (outcome expectancy) and the confidence that the individual feels in their own ability to change (efficacy expectancy). Rotter (1954) described the theory of locus of control, which suggests that people who feel that they are in control of their lives (internal locus of control) are more likely to be able to undertake changes (including health-promoting changes) than people who feel powerless (external locus of control). Even the much-criticised Health Belief Model (Rosenstock, 1966; Becker, 1974) demonstrates that behaviour change is based on much more than simply receipt of information. They suggest that an individual's willingness to take preventive action is dependent upon how 'at risk' they perceive them-selves to be, how serious they view the consequences of the condition, how effective they believe the preventative measures to be and the physical, psycho-logical and financial barriers to change.

The concentration on individual behaviours is initially difficult to refute. Smoking, alcohol consumption, high fat diets at first glance are tempting explanations for many health problems. *The Health of the Nation* (DoH, 1992) document compounded this attitude in identifying undeniably serious health problems affecting England today (separate documents for Scotland, Wales and Northern Ireland) and then concentrated upon the identification of individual risk factors whilst giving scant attention to the structural risk factors. The structural risk factors are however given more attention in the recent Green Paper *Our Healthier Nation* (DoH, 1998a). The document outlines a role for everyone in health improvement. This includes government, health authorities, local authorities, voluntary organisations and businesses as well as individuals. For the ideals in this document to be realised however will take time and a level of commitment which could be viewed as naïvely optimistic. Disease targets are still the cornerstone of the document and it may be that the organisations outlined will find it easier to concentrate on the obvious individual behaviours rather than the structural and social difficulties which lead people into these behaviours.

Clearly if stress were identified as a factor in heart disease for example, it would lead to demands for radical restructuring measures to society to make it less stressful. This would involve changes in work practices, changes in expectations of individuals and families, for example in supporting others in the community. These are likely to be unpopular options to the government of a society where success is measured by economic growth. It is much easier and politically more popular to tell an individual that it is their smoking behaviour which is the cause of so many problems.

People's behaviour does not occur in a vacuum – it has a context which includes an individual's beliefs and values which arise from their upbringing as well as their experiences and expectations in life. The context is also social and this social context includes the level of access that individuals have to alterna-tives. Mitchell (1982) for example disputes the concept of people making 'unhealthy choices'. She asserts that one reason that people 'choose' unhealthy luxuries is because they cannot afford healthy ones, for example living in the suburbs where it is cleaner and safer to go outside, or holidays abroad, or a car to take them to the shops where they can shop more cheaply.

It is perhaps this issue of 'free choice' which is at the heart of the individualist argument. This assumption is a myth in a society where choices can clearly be seen to be limited by environmental and social factors but also by vested commercial interests such as the powerful food, tobacco and alcohol lobbies which help to shape government policies and legislation through funding and sponsorship. These policies and legislative measures provide a framework of pressures, mixed messages, lack of access to untainted information and limited availability of products from which the individual makes her/his 'free choice'.

Whilst recognising that individual lifestyles have a bearing on their health status, to consider the behaviour of individuals as of prime importance would be to see only the symptoms. To treat the cause would involve looking beneath the behaviour at the social conditions which create it.

Social/environmental (structural) factors

In the nineteenth century, death and disease were common features of larger cities. An analysis of measures taken then demonstrate that it was the public health measures such as ensuring clean water supplies, improving sanitation and sewage disposal systems as well as improving working conditions which had the greatest impact on health. A similar analysis of today's health problems would demonstrate similarly that poor living conditions predispose people to poorer levels of health than people who enjoy good living conditions. This kind of analysis is not universally popular, possibly because it requires a collective rather than an individual response, whereas, as already discussed, the general political trend since the 1980s has been more toward individual responsibility.

The Black Report (DHSS, 1980) demonstrated major socio-economic differences in health and Sir Douglas Black was quite clear in his analysis when he suggested that the root cause of these inequalities in health was poverty. Working on this premise, the determinants of health can be identified in social terms.

Initially, for example, determinants may be identified amongst those that precipitate poverty such as unemployment or low paying work. Unemployment has distinct effects on health that are well-documented, e.g. elevated blood pressure, colds, ulcers and arthritis (Cobb and Kasl, 1977). Low paying employment may also lead to material deprivation but add to this the possibility of employment-related illness or injury, which is more likely in unskilled, low paying work. It is then interesting to analyse one step further and look at who may be more likely to be unemployed or in low paying employment and this gives further social determinants of health.

Which groups in British society are more likely to be unemployed or in low paying employment?

Women and people from ethnic minority groups (especially young people) are more likely to be in lower paying work, part-time work or unemployed.
Unskilled work is lower paying than skilled work and is often more transient in nature and therefore less secure. These individuals are then more likely to be made unemployed.

Other factors may then be identified which may be seen to be a result of an impoverished lifestyle, e.g. poor housing or poor nutrition. Housing which is occupied by families with inadequate money is less likely to be heated adequately. Damp weather means that clothes often have to be dried indoors but if a window is opened to aid drying, needed heat will be lost. This leads to inefficient ventilation and a greater probability of dampness, which is more likely to precipitate asthma, rhinitis, alveolitis, headaches, aches and pains, diarrhoea and vomiting. The Regional Unit in Health & Behavioural Change (RUHBC, 1986) also point out how people belonging to deprived groups disproportionately occupy housing in poorer areas of the inner cities or peripheral housing estates. The problems that arise from this are noise and pollution from the inner city and lack of amenities, and higher food prices in the housing estates.

The lack of amenities and higher food prices make the maintenance of a healthy food intake more difficult for people living in poor circumstances. Add to this the possibility of inadequate cooking facilities, long hours of working or even homeworking (for example sewing at home or envelope addressing etc. – all traditionally jobs occupied by women with children), which is notoriously low paying work. Also, with a low income, a parent's first priority is that their children should feel full and satisfied and this may involve a high-fat, high-carbohydrate intake of food with little fresh fruit or vegetables.

In addition to these social determinants of health resulting from disadvantage, there is the possibility of disenfranchisement that can result from generation upon generation of people maintained in poverty. This disenfranchisement has its own results on education, attitudes to others, levels of crime and use of and access to, health services.

Is most crime committed by people living in poverty?

Not at all. It may even be argued that it is the way that 'crime' is defined that means it involves the deviant activities of the poor rather than the rich. However, sociological research seems to demonstrate that sometimes people with few material resources may be pushed into activities that are against the law. They are more likely to be caught, then taken to court and given a custodial sentence than someone from a more affluent background. Sociological research also seems to suggest that people who feel disenfranchised are less likely to value education and so are less likely to succeed in academic terms with concomitant effects upon employment prospects.

Sir Kenneth Calman (DoH, 1998b) alludes to this in his interim report on the 'Project to Strengthen Public Health Function'. Calman identifies five major themes (or needs) underpinning his far reaching proposals, i.e.

1. A wider understanding of health
2. Better coordination
3. An increase in capacity and capabilities
4. Sustained development
5. Effective joint working.

The report clearly recognises the cost down the generations of social policies which disenfranchise people. The wide ranging short- and medium-term outlines for action in the report demonstrate a commitment to developing policies which work towards improvements in health and well-being.

People's behaviour does not occur in a vacuum and concentrating on behaviour to the exclusion of other issues is akin to treating only the symptoms of an illness. People's behaviour happens within the context of the social conditions which contribute to its creation. Health promotion work should aim to change the social conditions from health damaging to conditions which enable and empower people and which gives them a belief in themselves and others as valuable human beings with the confidence, self-esteem and power to be able to act as change agents.

Additionally many policies which are formulated in the interests of economic growth are in fact responsible for creating the social conditions which lead to ill health as well as supporting the inequalities of access mentioned previously. An example of this would be an economic policy which creates unemployment as an 'inevitable' consequence of tackling inflation and then makes it more difficult to obtain welfare benefits. Health promotion work must also involve lobbying and working with people to change health-damaging policies and, at a local level, to encourage groups and committees to consider health first before formulating policies. This involves putting health on everyone's agenda and, using a systems approach, everyone involved in working with people recognising their potential effect on the health of the people they serve.

PROMOTING HEALTH IN THE COMMUNITY

The original public health movement of the nineteenth century with its emphasis on health improvement via environmental change gave way to the more individualistic approach based on the biomedical belief in the potential for conquering disease (rather than preventing it). Even when concentrating on terms of prevention, the biomedical approach is one of conquering the disease or the potential for disease within the individual (e.g. with immunisation/screening) rather than changing the circumstances within which the disease flourishes (e.g. by improving housing conditions).

The new public health movement, spearheaded in this country to some extent by Ashton (Ashton and Seymour, 1988), recognises the need for, and works to create, health-supporting environments whilst at the same time assisting people and enabling them to reclaim power and control over their lives, i.e. empowerment. The goals of the protagonists of *The new public health* are closely aligned to those of the World Health Organization in their *Health for All by the Year 2000* initiative (WHO 1981), which represents a collective approach to health in contrast, and possibly as a challenge to, the recent popular emphasis on personal responsibility.

The new public health initiative offers a strategy which works towards changing damaging public policies, working with communities to identify and meet health needs as well as building a more enabling, rather than a disabling, health care system. This matches neatly the strategy of *Health for All*, which views primary health care as central to the attainment of the *Health for All* goals and it is recognised that this strategy has three main pillars:

1. Inter-sectoral collaboration
2. Community participation
3. Equity.

Intersectoral collaboration

Intersectoral collaboration is something that can be operationalised at each level of policy and/or decision making. At the most local level it is about individuals from health, social, voluntary and private bodies working together to seamlessly meet the varied needs of their client groups. This mode of working is also something which can be operationalised at the highest policy-making level. This would involve coordinating policies and priorities across agencies and, in this context, considering health consequences of potential policy-making decisions.

It is collaboration at all levels that is the underpinning philosophy of *Our Healthier Nation* (DoH, 1998a). The document envisages a collaborative approach which, whilst still retaining a disease focus, identifies national, local and individual actions which can be taken at a social/economic, environmental, lifestyle and service level. Calman (DoH, 1998b) also identifies intersectoral collaboration as a key theme of his proposals when he talks of 'better coordination' and 'effective joint working'. In order to achieve this however there first needs to be some kind of shared philosophy and/or ideology. This must be a starting point for professionals to work together with each other and the public. It is this to which Calman refers when he talks about the need to develop a wider understanding of health.

What sort of social policies might affect people's health?

Social policy is generally agreed to be those policies which are designed to harmonise society in some way. They are concerned with collective interventions to promote the welfare of individuals. So, examples of policies which may affect health could be education policy. Consider for example the effects on individuals of the national curriculum, local management of schools and the policy for university students to support their grant with the use of loans as well as the policy for students to pay tuition fees for university previously paid as part of their local authority grant. Housing policy, transport policy, welfare benefits policy, employment policy and many other factors could also be viewed in this way.

It is through various policies that people's 'choices' are dictated and limited by their life circumstances and the environment in which they live. These choice limitations are brought about by government and business decisions at a local, national and global level and it is the process of this decision making which can be influenced if people, departments, organisations and statutory bodies were to collaborate.

Getting different professional interests to work together is not an easy challenge and if it were to be considered as an individual worker's task, they would most likely throw up their hands in despair. Intersectoral collaboration must work at all levels with each individual recognising their part in it as important but not exclusively so.

Over years of building bigger bureaucracies, sophisticated societies develop cumbersome decision-making structures which are often sheltered from recognising the effects that the decision may have on ordinary people. This occurs not just between different organisations but even separate departments within the same organisation. Decisions made in these kinds of structures are more likely to reflect the needs of the bureaucracy rather than the needs of the people it serves.

Intersectoral collaboration is about each person seeing the important part they play in working for health and working together to offer the same, rather than conflicting messages. Look for example at the potential for intersectoral collaboration in a small northern town:

> A local factory was identified as producing noxious fumes which were considered to be causing the local community increasing incidences of asthma and other respiratory problems. Just a few years before, this same company had been allowed to expand and build a bigger chimney because of the increasing output (economic growth). The local council agreed to the expansion by only considering the extra jobs (health promoting) but without considering the health effects of the chimney (health damaging) or the environmental damage which has not yet been measured (health damaging). Had there been any kind of collaboration between councillors, health authority representatives and environmental health departments, this decision may have been modified. Instead permission was given, expansion occurred and many people suffered respiratory diseases until pressure from the local community and local health workers brought about a legal requirement on the company to install equipment which reduced the pollution. This, after a great deal of pressure, but no loss of jobs, the company eventually complied with.

There are many examples large and small, up and down the country of how intersectoral collaboration is being taken seriously as a vital structural approach to promoting people's health. Thoms (1992) for example describes how Sheffield has established collaborative working arrangements between health authority and local authority departments. Liverpool took a similar interesectoral approach to health planning based on *Health for All* targets (Ashton and Seymour, 1988; Ashton, 1992).

Stockport, a town on the outskirts of the city of Manchester have also put into operation a localised system of intersectoral collaboration. The directors of public health, the department of health promotion and the community nursing directorate together developed a system which involves the employment of public health nurses who work to profile local communities and identify health needs. Coordinators for each area then work to draw together an impact group of local interested parties (including health, social, commercial, church, lay people) to work together in trying to meet these identified health needs. The coordinators have an annual recurring budget which is used to support the various projects which develop as a result.

It could be argued in health promotion terms that intersectoral collaboration is all about a top-down approach, i.e. professionals or workers still making and imposing decisions upon communities. This is a valid argument and, if this were all there was to the *Health for All* strategy, would be valid in its criticism. However, intersectoral collaboration is one element of the strategy and should be viewed as occurring at the same time as the other elements, not in hierarchical order. Without the participation of the community, expressing its own needs and how they should be met, these needs will only be viewed from the professionals' perspective and the status quo of universal and too often inappropriate information and services will be maintained.

Community participation

There is clearly a need for a rational framework for measuring and prioritising competing claims and interests within any community. 'Top-down' approaches can work synergistically with 'bottom-up' approaches to health promotion. Indeed strength can be derived from this synergy. An empowered, participating community is more likely to be able to enter into partnership with 'top-down' initiatives (Barr, 1995) and participation in such initiatives could be seen to contribute to empowerment (Tones and Tilford, 1994).

Community participation entails enabling all people to have a more influential voice in defining factors which they feel to be important in determining their community's health. Community participation also challenges traditional notions of professionalisation and promotes new democratic ways of working within statutory organisations.

There is a large proportion of work for health already going on in communities which is sometimes considered less significant because it doesn't have a 'professional' label. The health work of women in caring for family and significant others is an example, as are the many self-help groups, social groups and pressure groups which exist in many communities.

What is 'hidden health work'?
This is work that is carried out by individuals within a community which has a positive effect on health. For example, people who care for others, mothers' care of their children, self-help groups and social organisations. As this kind of work is carried out free of charge and the people working in this way are unqualified, it is often viewed as less valid or at least inconsequential in the biomedical model.

The nature of the community participation approach is to harness and utilise all work for health by the members of community themselves and draw in all members of the community in identifying health needs and making decisions about the nature of health care delivery.

The White Paper *The New NHS Modern, Dependable* (DoH, 1997) identifies potential opportunities for communities participating in meeting their own health needs. Health authorities are exhorted to work with the public in developing health improvement programmes and health action zones. The public are also expected to lend their voice to the development of healthy living centres. Calman (DoH, 1998b) similarly identifies the need for public participation and advises 'strong incentives' for health authorities and local authorities to involve the public in their strategic planning. It seems clear however that the incentives will go to the authorities rather than to the public. This could be viewed as giving incentives to professionals to achieve what should be considered good practice anyway. It may be time to consider giving the incentives to community groups to encourage and enable their participation in policy making so that they become a means to their own ends rather than a means to someone else's.

The World Health Organization (1981) conceives community participation as a goal in its own right as well as something that will work towards overcoming some of the barriers to health. However, most health authorities work on the principle of outcome measurement as a way of evaluating effectiveness. In this kind of community health work, outcomes that can be measured against mortality and morbidity statistics are very much in the long term if indeed possible or even desirable. This does not mean that the value of community participation is unmeasurable. Local workers can work with local people to identify their own positive indicators, an evaluation of which can be used to lobby for further resources or support or to prevent the removal of current resources and support. This kind of work is intrinsic to community participation and is a way of helping individuals and groups to become more self-advocating and powerful by beginning to set their own agenda for health.

Gaining the involvement of *all* people and not just a vocal minority is a difficult task. The difficulty of the task may lead to a form of 'tokenism' in that the only people to be consulted are those who are most vocal and who for the most part, genuinely believe that they represent a silent majority, and who may have become 'professional participators'. Bracht and Tsouros (1990) identify this phenomenon of a 'community elite' who may in reality be promoting themselves into positions of power.

Tokenism comes in other forms, Brager and Specht (1973) for example demonstrate the different perceptions and subsequent manifestations of 'participation' (see Box 1.3). Arnstein (1969) (see Box 1.4) saw it more politically when talking not simply of 'non-participation' but 'manipulation' and 'therapy'. In other words, not only not having any power to make change but also having power wielded over you to ensure that you comply or perhaps don't actively disagree.

BOX 1.3	*Spectrum of community participation in planning policies of activities*

From
No participation
to
Information given
to
Community agreement with plans
to
Consultation
to
Joint planning
to
Delegated authority
to
Control

(Adapted from *Community Organising*, Brager, C. and Specht, H., 1973, with kind permission from Columbia University Press.)

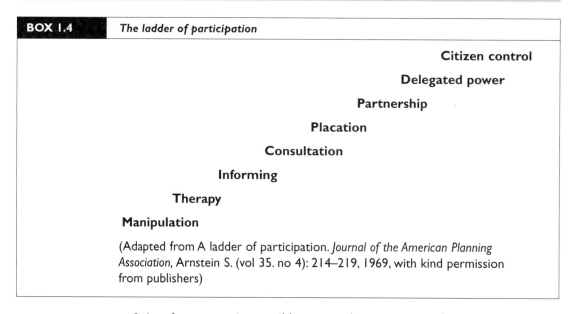

BOX 1.4   *The ladder of participation*

Citizen control

Delegated power

Partnership

Placation

Consultation

Informing

Therapy

Manipulation

(Adapted from A ladder of participation. *Journal of the American Planning Association,* Arnstein S. (vol 35. no 4): 214–219, 1969, with kind permission from publishers)

It is, of course, quite possible to give the impression of participation whilst continuing to control and oppress; efforts towards community participation must include a true commitment from organisations, professionals and the people themselves, otherwise it may act counterproductively as tokenism. The groundwork that must be done to move in this direction is often hidden because it is in the form of early work in building up trust and rapport with individuals in the community. Work that is interpersonal to build up people's self-esteem and ability to self-advocate is work that will not produce short-term measurable outcomes within the current popular mortality and morbidity statistics. However, there is much to be learned from qualitative research and techniques such as 'fourth generation evaluation' (Koch, 1994; Beattie, 1995) and this could provide direction for health and community workers to highlight both the depth and the value of this work.

Equity and community development

Inequalities in health could be argued to be, to some extent, inevitable in terms of biological and genetic differences. Total equality in health and health outcomes is not possible. Equity however is different, in that it has a generally accepted moral dimension; equity is about justice.

The Alma Ata declaration (WHO, 1978) proposes equity as one of the three pillars of promoting health through a primary care approach. The conference decries the level of inequality which exists and also recognises the role of social conditions and their contribution to the high level of health inequality which exists both between and within nations.

In Britain, the Black Report (DHSS, 1980) followed by the Health Divide (Whitehead, 1987) were two reports which clearly demonstrated the disparities in health existing between the 'haves' and the 'have nots'. Clearly the debate is not quite this simple and some would argue that inequalities are simply the unintended consequences of success in expanding the advantages of the upper socio-economic groups (Charlton, 1994). Others proffer biological explanations associated with random variation in the population distribution of health (St Leger, 1994). However, Beaglehole and Bonita (1997) point out that inequalities are less in countries where income distribution is relatively equal compared to those countries where gross disparities occur. It appears that it is relative deprivation which is a key factor and health inequalities are an outcome of social policies which neglect the needs of poorer groups in a society.

Inequalities in health have now been accepted as a phenomenon and the need to tackle the phenomenon is identified in successive government documents. Creating a just, inclusive health service can be identified as a theme within *The New NHS. Modern, Dependable* (DoH, 1997). Similarly issues of inclusion, justice and participation are featured as essential underpinnings to responsibility within *Our Healthier Nation* (DoH, 1998a) and Sir Kenneth Calman's interim report (DoH, 1998b). This represents a change of government attitude and may yet work towards reversing the trend of individual responsibility and even blame, which were the hallmarks of previous years.

To aim for equity in health means an acceptance of the severe yet avoidable imbalances between people and groups in communities. Working to redress these injustices or imbalances is work for improving equity in health and this is inevitably a highly political activity.

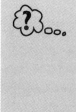

What may notions of justice be based upon?

What a person considers to be equitable or fair may be based upon their perspective and political ideology. For example, they may feel that justice is about every person being given an equal share, or that distribution should be decided according to need, or perhaps according to effort, or possibly according to an individual's contribution or what they merit according to some criteria of achievement. Alternatively, a person may view justice as distribution according to free market exchanges (i.e. according to what each can afford).

Community development is a way of working in and with communities to redress some of the imbalances and to promote a climate and culture which enables participation to occur. It has a chequered history, arising as it did from the paternalistic charitable organisations and strategies used during Britain's colonisation of other countries where community development was used as a way of maintaining political and economic power. However, history also shows another side to community development in the emergence of people-led organisations such as trade unions and the suffragette movement.

The concept of change occurring from *within* communities was given greater recognition and in 1953 the United Nations described community dev

'... a movement to promote better living for the whole commu
active participation and, if possible, on the initiative of the cc
but if this is not forthcoming, by the use of techniques for a
stimulating it'. (UN, 1953)

This still of course has overtones of paternalism and manipulation but through the next 40 years of growing recognition of the struggle and oppression that existed because of race, class or gender, community development work evolved into the more politically charged consciousness-raising role that is seen today.

What must be learned from history is that all work can be used for good or ill, for liberation or oppression and all work can be used cynically to meet the desires and ends of the dominant group rather than the people whom the work is intended to benefit. For this reason, workers for health should constantly question what they are doing, how they are doing it and essentially *why* they are doing it.

Community development is a type of work which is being encouraged in different professional groups. More recently health workers are being employed with this remit and, it is anticipated, they will use a community development approach in pursuit of health in its broadest sense by working with communities on an agenda devised by the people.

Paid community development workers cover a geographical patch (usually within what is considered to be a disadvantaged community) and work with people in that community in identifying their own needs and interests and in organising themselves to get their needs met. In this way, community development should be seen as a process, not as an outcome. It is a way of working which helps people to develop, to gain confidence, self-esteem and knowledge of the power systems which, in turn, enables them to regain control over their lives and consequently their health, i.e. empowerment.

The notion of empowerment is used in different ways, but does it have more than one meaning?

Empowerment is a concept so, like all concepts, it can have different connotations depending upon who is using the term. In some government documents the term 'empowerment' is used as a way of suggesting 'responsibility for' rather than 'power to'. If the former definition is ascribed, then the work which ensued could not be described as community development and would be more like the 'manipulation' described by Arnstein (1969).

Community development work clearly involves a level of conflict and this may raise a dilemma for the community development worker if he/she is working with a community and is brought into conflict with the organisation who is her/his employer.

Community development can be described as a more 'bottom-up' approach than the intersectoral collaboration section described earlier. However, the power of this overall strategy of the new public health is in the use of the approaches together as a single strategy; one cannot select either intersectoral collaboration *or* participation *or* community development – they will only work effectively as part of an overall strategy.

Community development for health is clearly a political process as it involves raising people's consciousness and helping them to voice their needs. It is also a tool which potentially could be used as a weapon. For example, where disadvantaged people are setting up projects and working to improve their situation within an unfair system, the powerful groups could:

1. see the area as no longer in need of redevelopment, improvement or subsidies to encourage commercial input, and so leave people literally doing it themselves
2. value the self-help principle, so reinforcing their perception about personal responsibility for health
3. ignore the fact that people in disadvantaged areas are having to work many times as hard as people in advantaged areas simply to maintain these basic amenities.

An analysis of the nature of power in social welfare demonstrates how people with no power have to work harder to maintain basic needs and also the way political power is used to shape opinion which maintains people in their situation. This is the reason that community development is also recognised as political consciousness raising, not party politics but the politics of power of one group over another.

A final point in this section is that taking *control of* one's health is different to taking *responsibility for* one's health. Watt and Rodmell (1993) point out that taking responsibility negates societal responsibility for ill health, whereas taking control places health firmly in the political arena of limited resources. Community development is about bringing a level of equity to health by helping people to take control.

Primary health care

The World Health Organisation (1978) sees the three principles of intersectoral collaboration, community participation, equity and community development as being delivered through a vehicle of primary health care. However, their view of primary health care may be influenced by their global view. Laura and Heaney (1990) suggest that what we call primary health care in Britain is actually secondary care because, for the most part, the service is involved with individuals only when a disease process has presented. Macdonald (1992) takes account of the preventive work but suggests that, far from a primary health service, what we have in Britain is a primary medical service.

The Alma Ata declaration (WHO, 1978) presents primary health care in the context of social justice, recognising the issues of social, economic, cultural and political development as foundations for health. This vision of primary health care is what the World Health Organisation mean when they suggest that health can (and should) be promoted through primary health care. This concept of primary health care will necessarily involve a shift in emphasis from the current medical concept of primary care to a much wider concept of health for populations as well as individuals, involving a range of people other than trained health workers. It is interesting to set this changing emphasis from the World Health Organisation into the current context of the NHS changes since 1990 but also the current changes since *The New NHS. Modern, Dependable* (DoH, 1997). Both systems have as a linchpin, general practices, which are essentially small businesses used as an agency to deal with ill health. Primary care groups are to have nurse, social services and other representation in order to commission to meet health needs. However the prediction is that there will be a majority of general practitioners (GPs) on these groups.

GPs can be seen to be highly effective in what they do in terms of being the first port of call for meeting people's needs in the event of sickness. However, to return almost full circle to the original discussions in this chapter, health is more than the absence of disease and therefore in order to maintain health, broader group membership and more flexible strategies of health needs assessment are needed. This will contribute towards diffusing the power base of medicine and fully exploiting the expertise of all other key players including the public.

Surely epidemiological data helps us to prioritise health needs?

A criticism of much of our epidemiological data in Britain today is that it is disease focused. Tannahill (1992) warns against using simplistic epidemiological data as the primary feeder for health promotion. This, he suggests, results in oversimplified, outmoded model of health education 'campaigns' for a confusing 'hotchpotch' of disease and risk factor-based initiatives. Tannahill suggests the adoption of health profiling methods which study the community's health-related beliefs, attitudes and behaviours in order to provide an expanded health database upon which meaningful health promotion strategies can be built.

Many of GPs' health promotion activities whilst laudable still remain within the narrow focus of the medical rather than the health service. They also retain a practice focus which does not consider the needs of the community outside the given practice. This inevitably revolves around individuals, their behaviour and given risk factors rather than working to alleviate some of the wider social and environmental conditions leading to those behaviours and risk factors.

Of course medical care is a vital part of health care but it is only a part. When the Alma Ata declaration stated that the primary health care system was central to the promotion of health, it was not referring to the small business of primary medical care which operates in Britain – rather it refers to a service which works to promote health and prevent disease as well as treating the conditions of ill health. This vision of primary health care must involve more than simply medical personnel. It must be conducted within the context of a planned systematic strategy towards changing health-damaging policies and creating health-enhancing policies. This should be a collective response to the diverse influences on health and should not be led by any one group.

This would seem to be the direction and intention of current health and health service policy in the creation of primary care groups, health action zones and health improvement programmes. This policy seems to recognise the diverse nature of health and the inclusive and flexible approach required in order to improve. people's health experiences. It remains to be seen whether the measures are sufficient to develop a truly primary *health* care-led NHS.

CONCLUSION

Health is a dynamic process and an individual concept and individuals and groups must interact with their environment if health promotion is ever to achieve its aims. The educational arm of health promotion in recent years has been conducted in such a way .that it concentrates mostly on individual behaviours, leaving unattended the underlying social, political and environmental issues which profoundly affect health.

This chapter highlights a tension between personal responsibility for health and structural/societal responsibility for health. This tension may mean that professionals and non-professionals will view one or other pole as the only one of importance, leading to a fragmented and piecemeal approach to health and its promotion. The New Public Health approach which reflects the World Health Organization approach to achieving *Health for All by the Year 2000* can be seen as an approach that can bring both poles together, recognising and promoting the positive aspects of each. This approach is about working with communities in pursuit of health, working in a collaborative way with different organisations to change health-damaging public policies and building and strengthening a primary health care system which is available, accessible, acceptable and appropriate to all people.

There is evidence of some move forward from the bioreductionist approach in the most recent documents to emerge from the Department of Health (DoH) and it will be interesting over the next decade to analyse how this works in practice and outcome. Collaboration is to replace competition and a multi-agency approach to health improvement is recommended. These recommendations would seem to heartily espouse the new public health approach.

The public health approach to health improvement will require honesty and power sharing between professionals to enable them to work in a power-sharing way with the individuals and communities they work with. Empowerment is becoming an overused and often ill-used word in that it is used at times as a way of giving responsibility without power whether within professional or public life. Rissel (1994) warns of this misuse, as does Doyal (1993), suggesting that workers in this field must exercise vigilance to avoid using empowerment strategies in disempowering ways. They refer to the work of Freire (1973) and Buber (1965) in recognising that responsibility comes only with the freedom to exercise it.

Workers can help to break the cycle of increasing medicalisation of everyday life and increasing development of responsibility for things over which people have no control, by sharing the power of information and working with individuals and groups to help raise consciousness, working towards personal development and assisting in social action for health. In this way the dependence created by years of medical dominance will also be recognised and questioned, placing people into a position where they can truly make decisions for themselves, supported by a health-enhancing environment.

REFERENCES

Arnstein, S. (1969) A ladder of participation. *Journal of the American Planning Association*, (vol 35, no 4), 214–219.

Ashton, J. (1992) *Healthy Cities*. Milton Keynes: Open University.

Ashton, J. & Seymour, J. (1988) *The New Public Health*. Milton Keynes: Open University.

Bandura, A. (1977) *A Social Learning Theory*. Englewood Cliffs. N.J.: Prentice Hall.

Barr, A. (1995) Empowering communities – beyond fashionable rhetoric? Some reflections on Scottish experience. *Community Development Journal*, 30(2): 121–132.

Beaglehole, R. & Bonita, R. (1997) *Public Health at the Crossroads*. Cambridge: Cambridge University.

Beattie, A. (1995) Evaluation in community development for health: an opportunity for dialogue. *Health Education Journal*, 54, 465–472.

Becker, M.H. (1974) The Health Belief Model and personal health behaviour, *Health Education Monographs*, 2: 324-508

Bracht, N. & Tsouros, A. (1990) Principles and strategies of effective community participation. *Health Promotion International*, 5(3): 1991–208.

Brager, C. & Specht, H. (1973) *Community Organising*. New York: Columbia University.

Buber, M. (1965) *Between Man and Man*. New York: Macmillan.

Charlton, B.G. (1994) Is inequality bad for the national health? *Lancet*, 343, 221–222.

Cobb, S. & Kasl, S. (1977) In Regional Unit in Health & Behavioural Change (RUHBC) (1986) *Changing the Public Health*. Chichester: J. Wiley.

Crawford, R. (1984) In *Issues in the Political Economy of Health Care*, McKinlay, J.B. ed. London: Tavistock.

Department of Health & Social Security (DHSS) (1980) *Inequalities in Health. Report of the working group chaired by Sir Douglas Black*. London: DHSS.

Department of Health (DoH) (1992) *The Health of the Nation. A strategy for health in England*. London: HMSO.

Department of Health (DoH) (1997) *The New NHS. Modern, Dependable*. London: HMSO.

Department of Health (DoH) (1998a) *Our Healthier Nation. A contract for health. A consultation paper*. London: HMSO.

Department of Health (DoH) (1998b) *An interim report of a project to strengthen the public health function in England*.

London: HMSO.

Doyal, L. (1993) In *Community Care. A Reader*, eds Bornat, J., Pereira, C., Pilgrim, D. & Williams, F. Milton Keynes: Open University.

Dubos, R. (1959) *The Mirage of Health*. New York: Harper & Row.

Freire, P. (1973) *Pedagogy of the Oppressed*. London: Penguin.

Haggart, M. (1996) Nursing the soul. *Complementary Therapies in Nursing and Midwifery*, 2, 17–20.

Illich, I. (1976) *Medical Nemesis. Limits to Medicine*. London: Marion Boyars.

Koch, T. (1994) Beyond measurement: Fourth generation evaluation in nursing. *Journal of Advanced Nursing*, 20, 1148–1155.

Laura, R.S. & Heaney, S. (1990) *Philosophical Foundations of Health Education*. London: Routledge.

Macdonald, J. (1992) *Primary Health Care*. London: Earthscan.

Macdonald, G. & Bunton, R. (1992) *Health Promotion. Disciplines and Diversity*. London: Routledge.

Mitchell, J. (1982) Looking after ourselves, an individual responsibility? *Journal of the Royal Society of Health*, 4, 169–173.

Parsons, T. (1981) Definitions of health and illness in the light of American values and social structure. In: *Concepts of health and disease: interdisciplinary perspectives*. Caplan, A.L., Englehardt, H.T. & McCartney, J.J. Menlo Park, CA: Addison Wesley.

Regional Unit of Health & Behavioural Change (RUHBC) (1986) *Changing the Public Health*. Chichester: J. Wiley.

Rissel, C. (1994) Empowerment: The holy grail of health promotion. *Health Promotion International*, 9(1): 39–7.

Rosenstock, I.M. (1966) Why people use health services. *Millbank Memorial Fund Quarterly*, 44, 94–124.

Rotter, J.B. (1954) *Social Learning and Clinical Psychology*. Englewood Cliffs. N.J.: Prentice Hall.

Sacks, O. (1982) *Awakenings*. London: Picador.

St Leger, A.S. (1994) Inequalities in health. *Lancet*, 343, 538.

Seedhouse, D. (1986) *Health. The Foundation for Achievement*. Chichester: J. Wiley.

Skrabanek, P. (1994) *The Death of Humane Medicine and the Rise of Coercive Healthism*. London: Social Affairs Unit.

Stainton Rogers, W. (1991) *Explaining Health and Illness. An Exploration of Diversity*. London: Harvester Wheatsheaf.

Tannahill, A. (1992) In *Health Promotion. Disciplines and Diversity.* eds Bunton, R. & Macdonald G. London: Routledge.

Thoms, G. (1992) In *Healthy Cities.* Ashton, J. ed. Milton Keynes: Open University.

Tones, K. & Tilford, S. (1994) *Health Education. Effectiveness, efficiency and equity.* London: Chapman & Hall.

United Nations (1953) *Report of the Mission on Rural Community, Community Organisation and Development in the Caribbean and Mexico.* New York: United Nations.

Watt, A. & Rodmell S. (1993) In *Health & Wellbeing.A Reader.* eds Beattie, A., Gott, M., Jones, L. & Siddell, M. Milton Keynes: Open University.

Whitehead, M. (1987) *The Health Divide.* London: Health Education Council.

World Health Organization (1946) *Constitution.* Geneva: WHO.

World Health Organization Alma Ata (1978) *Primary Health Care. Report of the International Conference on Primary Health Care.* Geneva: WHO.

World Health Organization (1981) *Regional strategy for attaining Health for All by the year 2000* Copenhagen: WHO.

FURTHER READING

Illich, I. (1976) *Medical Nemesis. Limits to Medicine.* London: Marion Boyars.

Gillon, (1987) *Philosophical Biomedical Ethics.* Chichester: J. Wiley.

Beauchamp, T.L. & Childress, J.F. (1989) *Principles of Biomedical Ethics* 3rd edn. Oxford: Oxford University.

Brewin, T.B. (1995) In *Health & Disease: A Reader*, eds Davey, B., Gray, A. & Seale, C. Milton Keynes: Open University.

Strachan, D. & Elton, R. (1986) Respiratory morbidity in children in the home environment. *Family Practitioner* **92**, 137–142.·

Martin, C.J., Platt, S.D. & Hunt, S.M. (1987) Housing conditions and ill health. *British Medical Journal* **294**, 1125–1127.

Ackers, L. & Abbott, P. (1996) *Social Policy for Nurses and the Caring Professions.* Buckingham: Open University.

Watt, A. & Rodmell, S. (1993) In *Health & Wellbeing. A Reader*, Beattie, A., Gott, M., Jones, L. & Sidell, M. Milton Keynes: Open University.

2 Community health and empowerment

Philip Carey

'Talkin' 'bout a revolution? A critical exploration of the concept of empowerment within health promotion theory and practice.'

KEY ISSUES

- Meaning of empowerment
- Use of the term 'empowerment' in modern health promotion rhetoric
- Whether empowering health-promoting practice is actually possible
- Implications of empowerment for health promotion

INTRODUCTION

The purpose of this chapter is to explore the meaning of empowerment and its relevance to present day health promotion. The author will argue that the concept of empowerment has always been, and should remain, a tool for radical social change. The agenda for this change is the evolution of a fairer and more equitable society. This, in itself, is wholly consistent with the ideals expounded in much health promotion rhetoric. These principles provide the ideological backbone to, for example, the World Health Organization's *Health for All by the Year 2000* (WHO, 1981) and the Ottawa Charter for Health Promotion (WHO, 1986). These two policy documents have been highly influential in shaping the direction of health promotion theory in the 1980s and 1990s. It is the author's belief that there are major philosophical and structural obstacles to any notions of empowering practice in health promotion. In practice, awkward questions arise around how the health promoter can encourage empowerment. More fundamentally, however, there appears to be an inevitable conflict between the notions of liberty and autonomy (as implied in empowerment theory) and the assumption of behaviour change (often seen as the *raison d'être* of health promotion). Indeed, much health promotional activity is criticised for being more concerned with promoting conformity rather than promoting equality (Petersen and Lupton, 1996). Fundamentally, therefore, health promoters need to consider critically the philosophy behind their practice if they are to adopt an empowering approach.

Power is the central theme of emPOWERment. Theoretical perspectives on power have shifted from the Marxist sense where power is held over subordinate groups by an economically dominant elite. The present view is that power is dispersed and disguised. Turner (1997) provides a useful metaphor to illustrate this: '... power is rather like a colour dye which is diffused throughout the entire social structure and is embedded in daily practices.' (pxii). It shapes, and is shaped by our every interaction in the world(s) in which we live. Foucault said: 'nothing is more material, physical, corporeal than the exercise of power' (1980). If we accept this, it follows that power will fundamentally affect health. We need only to consider the well-acknowledged and often ignored links between socio-economic status and health to see this. Perhaps more pertinently, Richard Wilkinson's research indicating that health is most significantly influenced by position and hierarchy is telling evidence of the relationship between power and health (Wilkinson, 1996).

To overlook the implications of power relationships between people and institutions is to undermine the whole concept of empowerment. Traditionally, theorists have seen empowerment as a challenge to established power dynamics. It was originally related to concepts of liberation and equality (Friere, 1972). Indeed, Fahlberg et al (1991) defines empowerment as: '... an ongoing process of liberation.' The agenda is clearly the promotion of autonomy, embracing concepts of resistance and change. Yet, in much of the recent discourse around empowerment, this agenda seems to have shifted dramatically. Health promoters are not alone in their adoption of the vocabulary of empowerment – the word has become a fashionable term in the 1990s. It seems that everyone is jumping on the empowerment bandwagon. Manufacturers seek to 'empower' their employees, with the aim being a more committed workforce, increased 'shop floor' innovation and the production of better goods and services (Bernoth, 1994). Advertisements for shops and banks speak of 'empowered' customers, the agenda here presumably being for them to spend more and show 'customer loyalty'. There have even been claims that television programmes can 'empower' their viewers (Squire, 1994). At any time it would seem somewhere, someone is claiming to 'empower' someone else. A review of many and varied uses of empowerment would suggest that it is a universal cure-all for the ills of the postindustrial age. It seems that the only common element between these is that they show no real endeavour to foster individual or community autonomy. Instead there are a multiplicity of opposing agendas and assumptions. As a result, the notion of empowerment is in danger of becoming no more than a trashy piece of consumerist jargon.

Empowerment has its roots in liberatory pedagogy; a concept which effectively refers to freedom through education. To understand empowerment, it is worth bearing in mind the work of Paulo Friere. Friere was a Brazilian educator who believed that education (in this case basic literacy) was the means by which subordinate groups could challenge the systems behind their oppression, and so improve their position in life. He claimed that colonisation had denied many Brazilians their historical roots and so marginalised them in Brazilian society. They were exposed to 'cultural invasion' from the colonisers, who had become the elite in Brazilian society, and in doing so had imposed their language and cultural perspectives upon the indigenous population. As a result, these people were effectively denied the tools of self-expression. This contributed to the maintenance of their powerlessness. To challenge this successfully, Friere argued that they must be able to critically assess and respond to the world in which they live (Friere, 1972). This requires a form of learning that simultaneously equips learners with the traditional means of articulation, whilst encouraging them to fundamentally question their world. By doing this, the theory goes, people will question experiences from their own context and perspective, and so set their own agenda for action. The reader might be doubtful of the relevance that techniques used in Brazil in the 1950s and 1960s have for modern day Britain. The connection is the recognition of not 'having a voice' and the accompanying reality of powerlessness. This is as common for many groups in Britain today as it was for the Brazilian underclasses in the 1960s. The route to redressing the power imbalance through empowerment will be similar, even if the setting is radically different.

Empowerment should be a dialogue and an active experience for all involved in the process (Friere, 1972). It involves authentic communication and partnership and abandons the traditional power relationship that exists in education. Part of Friere's rationale for this was his view that traditional education exists to maintain the status quo:

> 'It is society which, having formed itself in a certain way, establishes the education to fit the values which guide the society – the society which structures education to meet the needs of those who hold power finds in education a fundamental factor for the preservation of this power.'
>
> *(Friere, 1975 p16)*

The aim of empowerment is to challenge that power base. This will only occur if there is a process of *conscientisation*, or critical consciousness raising. Friere draws a distinction between three forms of human consciousness. He describes these as 'magic', 'naive' and 'critical' (Friere, 1972). Magic consciousness refers to the attribution of the cause of events to superior powers such as a deity. This state is essentially fatalistic and implies that the individual has no authority over her or his circumstances. Naive consciousness constitutes an acknowledgement of the cause of events, but these are accepted uncritically. The individual has some sense of the situation, but no understanding of *why* it should be challenged, never mind *how* it could be challenged. The process of conscientisation moves us from magic or naive thinking into a more critical mode of exploring our existence, which involves reflection upon reality. The outcome of this process is the identification of the causes of this reality, consideration of their implications and the development of plans to transform reality. The next step from conscientisation, and the ultimate aim of empowerment, is *praxis*. This embraces a constant interaction between action for change and reflection upon this action. As a result, the change process is continually subjected to critical reflection. This will ensure that people will embark upon change in an open, honest and discriminating manner.

The twin processes of conscientisation and praxis have enormous implications for the meaning and outcome of empowerment. First, it is clear that empowerment is an continuous phenomena as reflection upon action will lead to the development of further plans for change. The second implication is that the personal and the political cannot be separated. Notions of critical consciousness raising require acknowledgement and exploration of, and challenges to, systems of oppression. The theory is that this will lead to eventual transformation of society into a more equitable system. As Friere puts it, into:

> '... a democracy which does not fear the people, which suppresses privilege, which can plan without becoming rigid, which defends itself without hate, which is nourished by a critical spirit rather than irrationality.'
>
> *(Friere, 1973 cited in Tight, 1988)*

Friere is rare in that he is one of the few theorists from outside Europe and North America whose accomplishments have gained international recognition. The reason could be that his work has coincided with the growth and acceptance of postmodernist thought. His notion that people are both actors and acted upon, that they are influenced by their subjective understanding of the world and that this in turn can influence the world, is congruent with these ideas. As a result, empowerment 'theory' can go beyond modernist discourses such as feminism or Marxism to better explain the distribution of power (Carley, 1991). Ironically, commentators have criticised his work for overemphasising the influence of socio-economic factors and, in particular, for ignoring gender issues. However, the spirit of Frierian philosophy can easily accommodate these criticisms and to focus on them is to miss the value of his philosophy (hooks, 1993). Any factors that influence our identity will inevitably affect the process of empowerment. The important issue is not what is relevant, but who identifies relevance and the process by which it is identified.

It is clear from the above that empowerment is intrinsically tied to ongoing political activity in which ordinary people are political actors. Empowerment inevitably confronts any political system where professional politicians and powerful lobby groups shape the political landscape. Empowerment cannot succeed while decisions are made centrally and the public's only involvement is passive, for example observing political activity, or paltry, such as voting once a year (Tones, 1994). In addition to the strong political dimension to empowerment, it requires self-reflection, dialogue, action and a commitment to change. Because of this, it can easily be dismissed as idealistic daydreaming and filed alongside communism under the heading: 'Nice idea ... but people just aren't like that' However, the evidence suggests that it may be premature to condemn empowerment to the ideological dustbin. Consider, for example, the achievements of women, black people, lesbians and gay men in their respective challenges to inequality and gradual acquisition of human rights. One could argue that these have come from a process of empowerment. The relevant factor in all these cases is that a benevolent elite did not give these rights. Rather, they were taken by groups of people who felt that they deserved equality and, more importantly still, that they could act to achieve equality. These examples also illustrate that empowerment is an ongoing and continuous process (Schuftan, 1996). None of the aforementioned groups have attained full equality – the battle continues and its main focus remains to challenge the political system. However, despite the centrality of the political dimension of empowerment, many theorists have de-politicised the concept. Jeanne Brady has slated much modern empowerment theory as an 'insipid and dreary list of methodologies dressed up in progressive labels that belie the truncated nature of the ideology that informs them' (Brady, 1994, p144).

Health Promotion and Empowerment

The radical and political nature of empowerment sits comfortably within the rhetoric of a movement that sees its function as one of '... enabling people to increase control over, and to improve, their health' (Ottawa Charter for Health Promotion, WHO, 1986). The effect of these aspirations is that '... as a concept in health promotion, it [empowerment] signifies possibly the most important trend in the latter part of the 1980s, namely that of people – not just institutions, bureaucrats, professionals and technology – holding power in health matters' (Green and Raeburn, 1988 p155). Whether this shift in rhetoric is matched by a shift in practice is a moot point. In reality, health promoters may be equally as guilty as anyone else of blindly jumping on the empowerment bandwagon. The word has become ubiquitous in modern health promotion discourse, seemingly applied with casual abandon to many health promotional activities regardless of their nature and function. So, why has empowerment captured so many health promoters' imaginations, when the agenda for much health promotion remains the change of individual behaviour?

It is worth considering that health promotion essentially grew from notions of public health and medicine. Consequently, it retains a strong biomedical foundation and is open to the accompanying implications that this will have for power dynamics within health promotional activity (Gastaldo, 1997). The medico-scientific establishment exercises power over the body. This creates power relationships by using elitist knowledge–based constructs such as 'disease' and 'health' or 'deviant' and 'normal' behaviour (Petersen and Lupton, 1996). The information base for this is garnered from the 'traditional' reductionist methods of clinical observation and epidemiology. Therefore, experts in these fields determine the suitability of data sources and also control data collection and analysis. Furthermore, peers usually judge the standard of such work, and so it is rarely subjected to criticism from outside this elite. In consequence, a small, but exceptionally powerful group set the agenda for what is regarded as 'healthy' or 'normal'. The reductionist nature of such work means that concepts such as disease causation and risk are viewed from a highly individualistic orientation. This is because the inter-relationship between health and social, cultural, economic or political factors is often too complex for accurate epidemiological analysis (Krieger, 1994). In addition, 'lay' knowledge has no direct bearing upon epidemiology. The required mathematical framework cannot be imposed upon what are essentially subjective accounts of the experience of health (Lupton, 1995). As a result of this, the epidemiological perspective provides an account of health that is often removed from the everyday experiences of people.

Epidemiology strongly influences health promotion (Nettleton, 1997). In consequence, it tends to see epidemiological data as objective and pure. Meanwhile, the qualitative data that relates to people's personal experiences may be discounted as 'unscientific' and anecdotal. As a consequence, the latter is often overlooked in the development of health promotional interventions. This has implications for prioritisation of health promotion services.

> '... community concerns with such health determinants as racism and poor housing have been derailed by epidemiological risk factor surveys that 'prove' that heart disease and smoking are 'objectively' the major health problems.'
>
> *(Labonte, 1995, p166)*

One can argue, therefore, that health promotion serves the objectives of an established elite. It does this by emphasising the relationship between risk and 'lifestyle' or health-related behaviour. In consequence, it has created and uses a vocabulary of 'good' and 'bad' or 'healthy' and 'unhealthy' behaviour, which reinforces existing power relationships and encourages surveillance. In effect, such activity results in health promotion becoming an agency charged with regulation of behaviour and encouraging self-regulation (Lupton, 1995). Clearly, health promotional activities based on such assumptions will impact upon the authority of the individual regarding their own health. O'Brien (1994) argues that the result of this is that health promotion has become an activity which curbs people's understanding and control over their own health and suppresses collective action.

Yet, literature and policy often emphasise the importance of health promotion challenging the authority of the elite. The Ottawa Charter for Health Promotion (WHO, 1986), for example, states one of its goals to be '... to reorient health services and their resources towards the promotion of health, and to share power with other sectors, other disciplines and most importantly with people themselves'. There would appear to be a disparity between the stated aims of health promotion and what it actually does. The dilemma for health promoters is stark and can be summed up in the following question: 'can the two separate intentions – allowing self-determination and seeking health improvement – be reconciled?' (Duncan and Cribb, 1996, p341). Nowhere, it would seem, is this tension more evident than in the relationship between health promotion and empowerment.

This is markedly the case for health promotion in the UK as it has become tied to predetermined health targets as a consequence of national health policy. This policy does not lend itself to innovation and has restricted the range of health promotional activity (Yen, 1995). Certainly, the promotion of autonomy did not fit with the demands of *The Health of the Nation* (DoH, 1992). The emphasis of the present Blair administration on general practice-led commissioning and 'patient care' (DoH, 1997) does not herald a shift away from established disease/risk orientation and individualism. Indeed, Ranade (1997) has argued that the present government's apparent faith in medical experts may strengthen the domination of biomedicine in health policy. This will undermine the potential for health-focused public health and health promotion in the UK. *Our Healthy Nation* (DoH, 1998) more neatly compliments the rhetoric of *Health for All* than its predecessor did. The notion of *health impact assessment* throughout government policy, for example, recognises that responsibility for health is universal and goes far beyond the medical establishment (Thompson, 1998). Yet, the Green Paper's confidence in disease-based targets suggests the reality will be the maintenance of health policy based around notions of sickness and treatment delivery. More worryingly, although there is an acknowledgement of the influence of social exclusion on health, there are no solid commitments to challenging the inequalities that cause ill health (Chadda and Limb, 1998). However, the rhetoric of the document does provide scope for health promoters to legitimately broaden their range of activities and offer innovative practice within nationally defined health policy. Increased emphasis on the community, for instance, offers a potential route for empowering activity through community development. Encouragement of local partnerships through health action zones could provide a further impetus for empowering health promotion. Although the notions of success being judged through the meeting of '*milestones*' and evidence of '*concrete gains*' does leave the worrying impression that this will mean appraisal by traditional health indices. This would rule out immeasurable concepts such as empowerment.

That health policy has encouraged health promotion to adopt an individualist, behaviour change stance is a reasonable and well-debated criticism (Petersen and Lupton, 1996). When health promoters attempt to move away from this, often the best they can achieve is enablement, not empowerment. One reason for this, and a major concern for those interested in empowering health promotional activity, is that health promotion is often guilty of '*cultural invasion*'. Just as, for Friere, the Brazilian underclasses were victims of colonisation, so too are many people in the UK. The colonisation may, or may not, have much to do with race, but there is nevertheless, a phenomenon of health promoters attempting to impose their culture onto their client groups. An example of this is the promotion of the idea of negotiating safer sex. At face value this appears to be a sensible and appropriate response to sexual health promotion. Yet, for people who are powerless in their sexual relationships, it is at best meaningless and, at worst could reinforce any existing sense of inadequacy.

One possibility for the primacy of empowerment within health promotion rhetoric is that it is seen as an antidote to the rampant individualism of the 1980s. It appears that empowerment is now the preferred rhetoric for areas of health promotion where the ideals of individualism once dominated. Examples include: substance abuse (Wallerstein and Sanchez-Merki, 1994); accident prevention (Crew and Fletcher, 1995); infant mortality (Plough and Olafson, 1994) and treatment choice (McDougall, 1997). Although these areas still presume individual changes in behaviour, the 1980s crude 'do-this-or-be-damned' approach has lost favour. The feeling now appears to be that people need support and enablement to adapt their behaviour. However, the common theme in much of the 1990s 'empowerment' rhetoric is disturbingly similar to 1980s individualism. With the empowerment technique, however, rather than using clumsy coercive techniques, people are given an illusion of choice. The danger is that the rhetoric of empowerment can serve as a useful front for the most typical of health promotion agendas, getting people to do what we want them to do. Duncan and Cribb (1996) argue that there is an ambiguity in some uses of empowerment and pose the question: '... do advocates of empowerment want to help people or do they want to change people?' (p340).

There seems to be a presumption in health promotion that people will want to change, that change will be voluntary and therefore the approach is inherently good. The key, it appears, to maximising and maintaining health is to encourage behaviour change through empowerment. Given the apparently uncritical usage of the term, this ignores the damage done by inequalities and discrimination. The use of term 'empowerment' salves calls for greater accountability and community control and undermines the drive for equality. Meanwhile, practice retains its traditional top-down, authority-based approach. Empowerment in the 1990s may well become another element of that great health promotion tradition – victim blaming.

Victoria Grace (1991) voices concern over use of the term 'empowerment' in health promotion, with all its associated notions of autonomy, control and equity. She argues that it provides a façade behind which health promotion agencies can persuade groups of people to develop the skills of self-regulation with regard to supposed deviant behaviour. In these terms, the notion of empowerment becomes little more than an instrument for social control. This bears no relation to its original purpose of encouraging radical social change.

This poses a fundamental challenge to health promoters seeking to adopt 'empowering practice'. Unfortunately, all too often this challenge appears to be approached with a lack of critical insight into the real meaning of the term 'empowerment'. Rissel (1994) sees this as the continuation of long-time failing throughout health promotion. The field tends to be practice based and does not have a strong theoretical foundation. Therefore, there is a tendency for health promotion to borrow from other disciplines without the necessary understanding of the theoretical implications. In light of this, health promotion has been called the 'magpie profession' (Seedhouse, 1997). This describes how it often justifies taking bits and pieces of other disciplines' theoretical perspectives as a rationale for its own activity. The implications of this are neatly summed up in the words of David Seedhouse: '... haphazard acquisitiveness can no more furnish a theoretical basis for coherent practice than a magpie can be a discriminating collector of fine art' (Seedhouse, 1997, p29). Lupton (1995) suggests that this divergence of theoretical approaches can be overcome if health promotion focuses on autonomy and control. From this perspective, empowerment could become the philosophical backbone to the profession.

A sound basis in empowerment will require going back to basics and reconsidering the origins of the concept and its development within health promotion theory. First, how we use the term has implications for practice. Some health promotion literature implies that health promoters can empower others. This suggests that the 'other' can be a passive recipient of power, that empowerment is something done to the individual on her or his behalf. Not only does this contradict the Frierian concept of people actively involved in the reconstruction of their worlds, it also suggests a paternalistic response to the position of others:

'To empower someone else implies something which is granted by someone more powerful to someone who is less powerful: a gift of power, made from a position of power.'

(Gomm, 1993, p137)

As this quotation illustrates, there is a contradiction in this image of a 'gift of power' – such a gift will inevitably result in the maintenance of the 'position of power'. It draws upon notions of altruism and philanthropy, but leaves the impression of the maintenance of professional control.

An aligned notion that often appears in health promotion is 'self-empowerment'. In light of the above, 'self-empowerment' appears to be a tautology – if one person cannot empower another, empowerment necessarily comes from within and so the 'self-' is redundant. Challenging such usage is more than petty semantics – how we use language shapes how we think. Reinforcing the relationship between the personal and the political will serve to remind health promoters that empowerment requires a specific approach to health promotion. To effect empowering practice, health promotional activity must look beyond the individual and embrace collective action.

So what sort of health promotion can facilitate empowerment? Some commentators see a divergence between personal psychological empowerment and the more collective and political empowerment. The implication of this is that the health promoter can attend to one or other of these. Hopson and Scally's *Lifeskills* approach to health education (1988) presents an individually focused view of empowerment. It can be criticised for actually being more concerned with helping people to cope with, rather than challenge the problems posed by a rapidly changing society. This is the danger of any approach that seeks to achieve personal empowerment, without attention to the broader political environment. Keith Tones' early work also focused on the notion of personal empowerment, but since the late 1980s, he had become increasingly interested in the area of community empowerment (Tones, 1994). He is criticised for still using the language of individualism, in terms of attempting to encourage responsible and informed decision making in an environment shaped by health education (Lupton, 1995). The impact of traditional health education could consistently undermine the empowerment process. The reason for this is that notions of risk reduction shape health education and leave it open to domination by the medical elite. Nevertheless, Tones describes a political role for empowerment in health promotion, by discussing the need for *critical consciousness raising*, which is strongly aligned to the Frierian notion of *conscientisation*.

With empowerment approaches to health promotion seemingly requiring a combination of collective action and 'bottom-up' approaches, it is unsurprising that there is a history of reference to empowerment in community development. Beattie's classic model of health promotion identified community development as a collective and negotiated form of health promotion (Beattie, 1992).

Empowerment, community development and health promotion

The community is the focus for a wide variety of health promotion initiatives. Many individually focused behaviour change programmes have a community setting, but they remain strongly associated with medical services through health promotion in general practice or community nursing. At the other end of the spectrum, the community is linked to sustainable development as seen in Local Agenda 21 and its mantra of 'Think globally, act locally'. However, empowerment does not necessarily follow from a community setting. The key is the extent to which communities are involved in the whole health promotion process. Considering the previous examples, it seems unlikely that general practitioner (GP) or community nursing health promotional activity will be empowering. This is not to say that these are necessarily ineffective, but acknowledges the influence of biomedicine in determining the agenda for action. However, sustainable development will require a commitment a dialogue between people and policy makers. Consequently, such programmes could have a high 'empowerment potential' (Gamble and Weil, 1997).

In 1986, the Ottawa Charter placed empowerment at the heart of health promotion through community action. The community has become a prime focus in health promotion policy documentation:

> 'Health promotion works through concrete and effective community action in setting priorities, making decisions, planning strategies, and implementing them to achieve better health. At the heart of this is the process of empowerment of communities, their ownership and control of their destinies.'

> (WHO, 1986)

One of the tenets of community action is for members of the community to be involved in the process and involved from the outset. This includes encouraging people not only express their own problem(s), but to also develop the processes that will enable them to identify their problem(s). This requires a dialogue between the health promoter and the community to explore and utilise needs assessment procedures that serve the agenda of the community and not that of the health promotion agency. Unfortunately, this adds an element of uncertainty to the procedure that is at odds with the normal contracting process within the health service. It would be inappropriate, for example, for a health promotion team to seek funding to reduce coronary heart disease in a local south Asian community using an 'empowerment approach', without that community identifying this as a priority of its own. Whatever intervention is developed will be contingent on what the community wants and not the plans of the fundholders.

Although community development should have a bottom-up focus for health promotion activity, many such interventions are often top-down in nature (Douglas, 1995). The advantages of top-down approaches are that they can provide easier access to expertise and resources through planning and can be part of broad and balanced health promotion policy. They also enable simpler evaluation. This is a result of the imposition of projected outcomes against which success can be measured. In view of these, one can argue that top-down programmes have value in the health promotion repertoire. It is beyond the scope of this chapter to explore this, but health promoters need to be aware that they do not stem from or result in 'empowering' practice. Such programmes can be depowering as a result of their bureaucratic and undemocratic foundation. They effectively express the power of professionals over their 'clients' (even the use of terms such as 'client' imply some form of power imbalance). They may also encourage dependence on service providers that undermines the authority of the user.

The need for a bottom-up approach in community development strategies in health promotion is well documented in the literature. Yet, the reality of much community-based activity is that it is effectively top-down, with the agenda firmly set by the health promotion agency or imposed by a funding authority. Tones and Tilford (1994) consider this a form of colonisation, with the health promoter using community mobilisation to meet existing health goals.

Taking health promotion activities aimed at black communities as a case study, Jenny Douglas (1995) reviewed a series of such health promotion programmes in the USA. She found that while these were often grounded in the rhetoric of community development, they tended to be fairly traditional health persuasion programmes. The community element was that the community was the setting for the activity. She found few occasions where there were attempts to encourage, or even invite members of the community to participate in the planning and implementation of these programmes. The implication was very much that these communities should be transformed in line with dominant (white) ideals. The solution to this is for members of the community to be able to participate fully in all stages of the health promotion process. This in itself presents some unique problems which challenge health promotion practice.

Participation in community development

Participation is a crucial factor in community development approaches to health promotion. This is not to say that participation has no relevance for other forms of health promotion. All health promotion interventions require some level of participation. Encouraging individual changes in behaviour, for example, presupposes that the individual will act to change. In other words, that she or he will participate in the programme. Clearly, in this case, the level and nature of participation is determined by the health promoter who has set the agenda for the intervention. In consequence, the individual has very little power over the programme, except to refuse involvement. Indeed, in any form of health promotion, assumptions of the nature of participation will have implications for empowering practice and participation. There is a reasonable case for arguing that health promotion does not have to be participatory to have value. Few, for example, would argue that public health legislation should have no place in health promotion. Yet, people are often no more than passive recipients of the benefits of health-related social and environmental policy. However, this should not be confused with empowering practice. To be empowering, the focus of community development should be maximum participation.

The meaning and implications of participation are usefully clarified by considering the concept of a 'spectrum of participation' (Brager and Specht, 1973 cited in Tones and Tilford, 1994). This suggests a continuum of control, with diminishing professional influence correlated with increasing participation (Table 2.1).

The spectrum of participation offers a valuable perspective on the relationship between participation and power. It is clear from this that programmes requiring minimal participation, rely on individual compliance. They subjugate

TABLE 2.1	Spectrum of participation by member of a community
Level of participaton	Action by participant
Low	None - the community is told nothing; therefore participation is impossible Receives information - the community is told what is planned and compliance is expected Is consulted - compliance is sought through developing support for the plan Advises - the nature of the intervention is still top down, but there is sufficient flexibility to allow for the community to suggest changes Involved in planning - there is a greater expectation of change from the organisers Has authority - the community are involved in the planning process from the outset, but there's still a top-down element
High	Has control - the community both identify the problems and seek the solutions

(Adapted from Brager & Specht, 1973, cited in Tones & Tilford, 1994).

the needs of the people to the wishes of the authorising agency. As participation increases there is a growing sense of negotiation and dialogue in the processes of planning and implementation. Maximum participation implies that the agency becomes a resource to enable the community to operationalise its own programmes.

In community-based practice, health promoters can perform the vital task of encouraging community participation by acting as a resource for communities. How they respond to this role will influence the empowerment potential of the programme. The first stage in this is to assess the needs of the community in question. Often, health promoters base interventions on assumed need and, as a result, these may fail to target real needs. This, in itself, is sufficient reason for involving people in assessing their own needs. Furthermore, as these assumptions are often based on community profiling and epidemiological data sources, they will inevitably reflect the dominance of the medical elite. Hence, not involving the community amounts to the imposition of a biomedical narrative upon the lives of that group. This reinforces, rather than challenges, traditional power relationships. Thus, in community development, the involvement of the community at this stage is imperative (Poland, 1996). Effective and participatory needs assessment strategies are required to encourage communities to see the programme as relevant to their needs and priorities. Failure to do this will inevitably, and understandably, result in low participation (Marti-Costa and Serrano Garcia, 1983).

This highlights what is perhaps the fundamental question in empowerment: Who sets the agenda for action? Of prime importance is whether the 'client' group sets the agenda for health promotion. Agenda setting is an important stage in empowerment and is possibly the most problematic. It requires that professionals should allow people to express their needs and preferences. As Ronald Labonte says '... the most important act of power is naming one's experience and having that name heard and legitimised by others' (1994, p257). The notion of legitimisation leaves a disturbing impression of authority. However, the implication here is that this 'act of power' provides an important experience of powerfulness. Positive experience may be the key to the continuation of community empowerment programmes. This can link in with the individual's perceptions of control. Research by Schulz et al (1995) identified this as a significant factor in determining continued involvement in community initiatives. Hence, community empowerment becomes less of a linear transition from personal empowerment to community action (Rissel, 1994), and more of an holistic interaction between personal, group and community factors (Labonte, 1994).

The nature of participation raises some important issues. The participation process often depends upon key players; these include particularly active members of the community, community leaders or community groups. There are understandable concerns over such reliance. A vital question for the health promoter to address is ... do these individuals reflect the needs or concerns of the whole community or just their own? Puddifoot (1996) argues that, while there is some evidence that community groups can represent the views of the wider community, the extent to which this is the case is difficult to establish. An aligned issue is appropriateness of interventions for cultural minorities within the community, who may not share the dominant value system of the rest of this community. On a macro level, this begs the question: How much can participation occur for communities that do not subscribe mainstream discourses? Becker (1967, cited in Phillimore and Moffatt, 1994) identified a 'hierarchy of credibility' that enables society to recognise the views of some groups and ignore those of others. It will come as no shock that those groups whose voices are often ignored by representatives of dominant society are those who do not subscribe to the dominant norms and values (Petersen and Lupton, 1996).

Health promotion faces a number of problems if it is to overcome this. Responding to the needs and preferences of the group may be difficult due to the perceived unpopularity of that group. This will be confounded if the activities of the group involved are illegal. The encouragement of self-reliance among drug users, for example, will hardly seduce health service managers obsessed with political expediency. Finally, the health promoter may find the practices and/or desires of a group of people unpalatable. While we may strive to be forward thinking libertarians, prejudice will prejudice practice. Critical self-reflection will help keep prejudices in check, and may even overcome them. It is not the role of health promotion to pass judgement on participants. To do so not only makes participation unlikely, but undermines any hope for equality and amounts to the imposition of the health promoter's perspective. In other words, it is not conducive to empowerment.

Involvement in needs assessment is integral to the community development planning process. Acting upon them also assumes community involvement in the process of development of interventions and their implementation. Central to this is appropriate community organisation to enable effective functioning. So, another role for the health promoter is to facilitate community groups. This may incorporate help in agenda setting, group maintenance, overseeing action and the provision of adequate resources – in other words, to enable community groups to function properly. Booth (1997) describes the role of the community development worker as 'oiling the wheels of participation'. Involving the community in planning raises unique problems for the health promoter. Labonte (1994) argues that communities may respond to issues from a differing position to health promotion. He suggests that health promoters tend to view a situation from a behavioural perspective and therefore will view the best response as those that relate to behaviour. Community groups, on the other hand, might see the same situation as related to social and environmental conditions. The health promoter would therefore have to be prepared to abandon their assumption of what people need and take on board the community's perspective.

Community participation in planning may lead to proposals that seem unattainable to the health promotion worker from a cash-starved health service, local authority or voluntary group. This may lead to a sense of inadequacy, as Blaxter (1996, p33) questions: '... what is a public health department to do if a community insists on defining its most important health problems as vandalism, or loneliness, or poverty?' An aligned problem is that many of the communities in most need of action, are in the worst position for action. Poor and deprived communities may not be in a position to take control. Whilst it may be patronising to suggest that such groups have no potential for autonomy, it is an abdication of responsibility not to acknowledge that taking this will be an uphill struggle. In many communities there are high levels of drug abuse and associated crime. The response towards these is often that the community needs to take responsibility for this and address the activities of those members of the community who are 'causing' the problem. The implication is that these communities have created their own problems situation and therefore need to act to solve them. Yet, as the following quotation from a speech given at the US National Medical Association assembly on the epidemic of violence graphically illustrates, this response is ignorant of the broader social determinants of community problems. It effectively amounts to victim blaming on a community scale:

> 'Violence is a product of social dysfunction ... You begin in a black community with a baseline of alienation that is higher than that in the (sic) white community. We know that the withdrawal of resources has weakened the infrastructure of our community. In the period between 1980–1990, the Federal government withdrew $261 billion from direct support of inner city communities. You add to that the withdrawal of the tax base (caused by) individuals moving out of the inner city, add to that the withdrawal of hundreds of thousands of jobs in the same period and you have a scenario which says that the drug trade can walk in, sit down, and become the industry of choice for many of our children'
>
> *(Walters, 1993 cited in Wallerstein and Bernstein, 1994, p143)*

Clearly, the solutions to the sorts of problems identified here require more than a community-based programme. Health promoters should not overestimate the potential outcome of community development approaches. They can provide solutions to some problems, but will have limited impact on the macro-economic environment. Inevitably, policy aimed at the regeneration of communities, through the provision of adequate resources and the development of real economic opportunities, requires a commitment from both central and local government that the health promoter cannot rely upon. The urban regeneration schemes of the 1990s have gone some way to alleviating some of the nation's worst housing problems. Yet, without adequate education, meaningful occupations and appropriate wage or benefit rates, the efficacy of these is questionable.

The effects of material disadvantage will not be ameliorated by money alone. One problem facing the health promoter is that the cosy picture of the community depicted in much of the literature is a stark contrast to the reality of many people's lives. Commenting on the implications of *Our Healthier Nation* for the socially excluded, Bobbie Jacobson (Director of Public Health for East London) said: '... the neighbourhood for immigrant groups is very often an alienating and isolating experience' (cited in Gould, 1998, p14). Furthermore, within underprivileged areas, there is often an understandable antipathy towards authority figures. This may be a result of negative experiences in education, health and social services; in the workplace; long-term unemployment; unfair representation in the media or discriminatory encounters with the judicial system. Whichever of these factors, it reinforces the assumption that some groups are society's outcasts. As a representative of authority, the health promoter may have to overcome these feelings. This will take time, commitment and resources. In addition, disadvantage encourages a vicious circle of failure and hopelessness; breaking this to provide some experience of efficacy could also be an important step in encouraging participation (Tones, 1994).

However, by its very nature, community participation will require responding to these challenges. It may also result in a wide and sometimes disparate range of solutions being suggested. But, as Rappaport (1981) says: '... that a variety of contradictory solutions will necessarily emerge and that we ought not only to expect them, but to welcome them, the more different solutions to the same social problem the better' (p9).

Participation will also be influenced by the availability of suitable supportive resources. These can range from the provision of suitable child-minding facilities to encourage attendance to skills development for group management (Mayo, 1997). Information is another resource for effective community participation. This provides a significant philosophical stumbling block to empowering health promotional activity. Namely, that the nature of the information supplied will profoundly influence the process. The principle of empowerment requires that the participants request information, but health promoters need to take care that the information provided meets the agenda of the community and not that of themselves. Mayo (1997) argues that communities have the right to access independent information and advice from a range of perspectives, and not just that of the funding body. This is wholly in tune with the objective of 'healthy alliances', and therefore complements both health promotion theory and health policy. However, interagency work can lead to tensions between agencies, uncertain role definition and conflicting messages (Beattie, 1994). A further problem is that power structure of professional alliances is such that the dominant group often have disproportionate influence over the process. An additional and perhaps more intractable problem is that many disadvantaged groups may be unaware of the range of options open to them. Clearly, informing them of these could inevitably be met with concern over the imposition of a particular set of values onto the community in question.

The function of information giving always needs to be approached with caution. Ideally, of course, the role of the health promoter should be to encourage individuals to access information for themselves. This is not only less paternalistic, but acknowledges the importance of lay knowledge. The role of the health promoter therefore becomes one of acting as a support to established groups. This may involve advocacy work or networking with similar groups to encourage sharing of resources and mutual support. The literature suggests that many community development workers feel isolated and unsupported in their role (Booth, 1997). A potential function of health promotion could be to provide official support for such workers in a more supervisionary capacity. Yet, although their work is clearly health promotional, many of these workers are not officially designated as health promotion specialists. Hence, the fact that the health promoter and community development worker may be employed by different divisions of the public sector is likely to render such a role unworkable, at least in a formal sense.

Increasingly, community development is 'health promotion speak', but rarely translates into practice. There appear to be too many barriers to community development and overcoming these is problematic. Practical problems centred on encouraging and maintaining participation throughout programme development and implementation cannot be overlooked. Despite this, possibly the predominant barrier to community development approaches to health promotion is that they do not complement the present ideology of health service provision in the UK. Health promotion suffers from limited funding and health service policy prioritises GP-based interventions. Programmes that seek to encourage communities to take control rarely easily conform to the traditional framework of health services in the UK. Consequently, community development projects are a low funding priority. As a community development worker is quoted as saying: '... the vast majority of pioneering projects continue to be under-resourced, time limited, peripheral to mainstream services and existing on a knife edge' (Farrant, 1991, p425). Furthermore, many authors (e.g. Breitenbach, 1997) have pointed out that community programmes are dependent on funding, and no matter how effective these programmes may be, continued support is contingent on political will. This leads to the more intractable problem that true community development, with its emphasis on social action and change, is unlikely to win support from the very institutions that it will inevitably challenge. Research by Flick et al (1994) shows how, in one community development initiative, institutional concerns over the financing of overt political action lead to a threat of withdrawal of funding. This effectively polarised the workers and the ensuing conflict undermined the effectiveness of the programme.

There is also a need to clarify the distinction between the provision of resources appropriate to such work and the transfer of responsibility to unpaid workers in the community. Community development is not a cost-reducing exercise, but an effective means of promoting health if given the appropriate resources. Failure to adequately resource community programmes will result in exploitation rather than empowerment (Barnes, 1997). Kenny (1996) suggests that this complements the New Right agenda of reinforcing the notions of individual responsibility and 'family values'. Without attention to this, community development approaches to health promotion would fail to address power imbalances and possibly exacerbate the situation, by encouraging victim blaming where the victim is a whole community. There is a real danger that such approaches to health promotion could maintain the status quo, while presenting a façade of accountability and liberalism. Furthermore, Smith (1996) argues that community mobilisation generally focuses on immediate issues and self-interest and that these may be in a source of conflict with other groups. One could argue that this could undermine the potential for political action on a broad level.

The ideals of community development and participation seem far from the reality of practice. Indeed, as empowerment is so tied to the concept, it is worth just reviewing that:

> '... the term 'empowerment', which in its fullest sense is a liberating grass roots concept involving confrontation, has now been so sterilised and depoliticised by the health and development establishment that it has become more pacifying than liberating. We have all but forgot its political roots in *power by the people*.'
>
> *(Werner, cited in Farrant, 1991, p452)*

This leads us to the inevitable paradox of any participatory form of health promotion. No participation process can be truly liberatory because engagement requires the participant to develop the discipline associated with the process. Petersen (1997) argues that community participation is seen to be at once radical and liberatory, whilst simultaneously demands the participants' commitment to the whole process. Gastaldo (1997) has identified a shift in health promotion from subjugation to liberation, but argues that both rely on ingrained power relationships. In the latter, however, normal behaviour is determined by participation, but still relies on notions of rewards and punishment and thus constitutes an exercise of power. This relates to professional dominance, as professionals set priorities from their own medically dominated perspective. Therefore, a pertinent question is whether community participation is no more than a sophisticated form of community manipulation. Kelly and Charlton (1995) identify this as a source of contradiction in health promotion: '[e]xperts still appear to be in control ... Communities remain marginalised and invisible – other than in the rhetoric' (p81).

Part of the reason for this is the tendency for health workers to attempt to provide the answers, and not help the community seek solutions for themselves. A potential reason for this is professional education and training that suggests that failure to provide the answer equals a failure to do the job, even though we intuitively know that we cannot answer anyone else's questions. Traditional views of expert-dominated practices form the basis for much of this. Abandoning these ideas is difficult. Williams et al (1995) maintain that practitioners need some experience of the empowerment process to enable them to participate in appropriate health promotional activities. The rationale behind this is clear – experience will encourage a deeper and more critical theoretical understanding (D'Onofrio, 1992) and an empathic response to participants. Nevertheless, it does pose some conceptual problems. Not least among these is the fact that low morale and underfunding are characteristics of many of the professions charged with health promotion work. This is not an environment that is immediately conducive to empowerment. Simons-Morton and Davis Crump (1996) argue that empowerment education is in its infancy in health promotion. Consequently, there is insufficient understanding of the processes that encourage empowerment. Therefore, those involved in empowering practice should be less concerned with whether radical social change actually occurs than developing a sound comprehension of the processes that will lead eventually to these changes.

A lack of 'adequate' research to support community development is another possible barrier to practice. The philosophy behind community development and empowerment does not lend itself to reductionist research methods and evaluation procedures. It is almost impossible to impose a quantitative framework on to empowerment related data because the process acknowledges the uniqueness of each participant's responses. Furthermore, establishing cause and effect relationships is problematic. Yet, it is precisely these methods that fundholders require as evidence of effective practice (Smithies and Adams, 1993). In addition, the timeframe required by funding bodies may be too short to enable proper evaluation of what is inevitably a long-term and ongoing process. Therefore, in a health system captivated by 'short-termism' and the provision of simple, positivistic evidence as a basis for funding, under-resourcing of community development initiatives seems an inevitability. Burrows et al (1995) caution against hegemony of modernist discourses such as health economics in health promotion evaluation and call for a pluralistic response to evaluation. Indeed, with an increasing understanding of the value of qualitative work, appropriate evidence upon which to base funding bids might be not only available, but accepted. Unfortunately, though, much community development work does not appear to be rigorously evaluated, or if it is, the findings are not published. As a result, examples of good practice may disappear when funding runs out or staff leave. Those involved in developing and supporting effective community development work may not have the time, the resources or the skills to collect sufficient data, analyse it and then write it up in a format suitable for publication in respected journals. The reliance of the journal system on traditional forms of presentation and inquiry reflects traditional academic norms. In itself this is elitist and helps to maintain establishment perspectives. This may result in the advancement of more individually focused health promotion at the cost of potentially empowering community programmes.

CONCLUSION

Empowerment in the first instance appears to be a very simple concept to grasp, but with increasing critical analysis becomes more obtuse and problematic. An important concept in empowerment is to grasp what the outcome of power is. Friere (1972) makes it clear that this refers to challenging oppression, not changing it. In other words, the process of empowerment should provide people with the '*power to ...*' and not '*power over ...*'. Therefore, one can view the purpose of empowerment as '... to enhance the possibility for people to control their own lives' (Rappaport, 1981 p15). The following quotation unpacks this concept and indicates areas that need action:

> 'In modern health promotion parlance, empowerment has come to represent efforts to foster bottom-up social change through consciousness raising, self-help, capacity development and political action. Through empowerment education, theoretically, individuals within groups can develop motivation and skills enabling them to advocate for social reforms to better the lot of the group or broader community'
>
> *(Simons-Morton and Davis Crump, 1996 p291)*

The implication is clearly that 'Empowerment is more likely to evolve than suddenly occur' (Simons-Morton and Davis Crump, 1996 p292).

To some, the challenge of empowering health promotion may appear too severe. It seems to contradict typical responses to health issues. How, for example, can the principles of empowerment thrive in a system that appears to regard workers' smoking habits as a greater evil than the fact that an employer can legally pay them less than £4/hour? Similarly, is there any hope for empowerment when young people's drug taking causes more outrage than the existence of an education system which denies many of them hope and opportunity?

There are undoubtedly enormous obstacles against empowering practice – the real challenge facing practitioners is how we can overcome these. Indeed, some fundamental questions must be asked before going down the road of empowering health promotion as listed in Box 2.1.

The complexities of the responses to these, and other relevant questions, may leave the health promoter paralysed with despair at the seeming impossibility of the tasks facing them. Indeed, the changes demanded by empowerment require a revolution in policy and practice at all levels. Yet, for others this will be a goal worth aiming for, as long as it is entered into with a critical spirit. As Whitelaw and Whitelaw (1996) contend: '... the main concern ... is not whether

BOX 2.1	*Essential questions to empowering health promotion*

- How will present society deal with empowered citizens?
- To what extent can empowerment occur in a social and health system that is inherently based in status and hierarchy?
- What implications will the dominance of traditional biomedical philosophies within the health services (where health promotion is usually situated) have for empowerment?
- What are the national policy implications for empowerment, and to what extent can we expect policy to change accordingly?
- How can depowered health professionals facilitate the empowerment of their clients?

empowerment is or is not of universal importance, but the consequences of believing that it is, or is not' (p353). Practitioners should place the principles of empowerment at the heart of their practice, and use these principles as a critical lens through which they can view their own activities. Doing this will go some way to transforming health promotion into an empowering activity and continue revolution that will enable us to challenge the wasted human potential caused by material and social disadvantage.

REFERENCES

Barnes, M. (1997) *Care, Communities and Citizens.* London: Longman.

Beattie, A. (1992) In *The Sociology of the Health Service.* eds Gabe, J., Calnan, M. & Bury, M. London: Routledge.

Beattie, A. (1994) In *Going Inter-professional: Working Together for Health and Welfare* ed. Leathard, A. London: Routledge.

Becker, H. (1967) Whose side are we on? *Social Problems* 14:239-247.

Bernoth, A. (1994) Mindbender explores the future at Mercury. *The Sunday Times*, 24 April.

Blaxter, M. (1996) In *Health & Social Organisation.* eds Blane, D., Brunner, E. & Wilkinson, R. London: Routledge.

Booth, M. (1997) Community development: oiling the wheels of participation? *Community Development Journal*, **32**(2): 151–158.

Brady, J. (1994) In *Politics of Liberation: Paths from Friere.* eds McLaren, P.L. & Lankshear, C. London: Routledge.

Breitenbach, E. (1997) Participation in an anti-poverty project. *Community Development Journal* 32(2): 159–168

Burrows, R., Bunton, R., Muncer, S. & Gillen, K. (1995) The efficacy of health promotion, health economics and late modernism.

Health Education Research: Theory and Practice, **10**(2): 241–249.

Carley, J. (1991) In *Roots and Branches: Papers From Open University/HEA Winter School on Community Development and Health.* London: HEA.

Chadda, D. & Limb, M. (1998) Anger as green paper falls short on inequalities and funding pledges. *Health Service Journal*, 12 February 1998.

Crew, K. & Fletcher, J. (1995) Empowering parents to prevent childhood accidents. *Health Visitor*, **68**(7): 191

Department of Health (DoH) (1992) *The Health of the Nation.* London: HMSO.

Department of Health (DoH) (1997) *The New NHS: Modern, Dependable.* London: HMSO.

Department of Health (DoH) (1998) *Our Healthy Nation.* London: HMSO.

D'Onofrio, C. (1992) Theory and the empowerment of health education practitioners. *Health Education Quarterly,* 19(3): 385–403

Douglas, J. (1995) Developing anti-racist health promotion strategies. In *the sociology of health promotion.* eds Bunton, R., Nettleton, S. & Burrows, R. London:

Routledge.

Duncan, A. & Cribb, A. (1996) Helping people change: an ethical approach. *Health Education Research: Theory & Practice*, **11**(3), 339–348.

Fahlberg, L.L., Poulin, A.L., Girdano, D.A. & Dusek, D.E. (1991) Empowerment as an emerging approach in health education. *Journal of Health Education*, **22**(3): 185–193.

Farrant, W. (1991) Addressing the contradictions: health promotion and community health action in the UK. *International Journal of Health Services*, **21**(3): 423–439.

Flick, L.H., Given Reese, C., Rogers, G., Fletcher, P. & Sonn, J. (1994) Building community for health: lessons from a seven-year-old neighbourhood/university partnership. *Health Education Quarterly*, **21**(3): 369–380.

Foucault, M. (1980)

Friere, P. (1972) *Pedagogy of the Oppressed*. London: Penguin.

Friere, P. (1975) Pilgrims of the obvious. *Risk*, **11**: 12–17.

Gamble, D.N. & Weil, M.O. (1997) Sustainable development: the challenge for community development. *Community Development Journal*, **32**(3): 210–222.

Gastaldo, D. (1997) Health education and the concept of bio-power. In *Foucault, Health and Medicine* eds Petersen, A. & Bunton, R. London: Routledge.

Gomm, R. (1993) In *Health, Welfare & Practice* eds Walmsey, J., Reynolds, J., Shakespeare, P. & Woolfe, R. London: Sage.

Gould, M. (1998) Up against the odds. *The Health Service Journal*, 26 February 1998.

Grace, V. (1991) The marketing of empowerment and the construction of the health consumer: a critique of health promotion. *International Journal of the Health Services*, **21**: 329–343.

Green, L. & Raeburn, R. (1988) Health promotion: what is it? What will it become? *Health Promotion*, **3**: 151–159.

hooks b (1993) bell hooks speaking about Paulo Friere – the man, his work. In *Paulo Friere: A Critical Encounter*. McLaren, P. & Leonard, P. London: Routledge.

Hopson, M.P. & Scally, B.E. (1988) *Lifeskills Teaching Programme Number 4*. Leeds: Lifeskills Associates.

Kelly, & Charlton, (1995) In *The sociology of health promotion*, eds Bunton, R., Nettleton, S. & Burrows, R. London: Routledge.

Kenny, S. (1996) Contestations of community development in Australia. *Community Development Journal*, **31**(2): 104–113.

Krieger, N. (1994) Epidemiology and the web of causation: who has seen the spider? *Social Science and Medicine*, **39**(7): 887–903.

Labonte, R. (1994) Health promotion and empowerment: reflections on professional practice. *Health Education Quarterly*, **22**: 253–268.

Labonte, R. (1995) Population health and health promotion: what do they have to say for each other? *Canadian Journal of Public Health*, **86**(3): 165–168.

Lupton, D. (1995) *The imperative of health: Public Health and the Regulated Body*. London: Sage.

McDougall, T. (1997) Patient empowerment: fact or fiction? *Mental Health Nursing*, **17**(1): 4–5.

Marti-Costa, S. & Serrano Garcia, I. (1983) Needs assessment and community development: an ideological perspective. *Prevention in human services*, **2**(4): 75–88.

Mayo, M. (1997) Partnerships for regeneration and community development. *Critical Social Policy*, **17**(3): 3–26.

Nettleton, S. (1997) In *Foucault, Health and Medicine*, eds Petersen, A. & Bunton, R. London: Routledge.

O'Brien, M. (1994) The managed heart revisited: health and social control. *Sociological Review*, **42**(3): 393–413.

Petersen, A. (1997) In *Foucault, Health and Medicine*. eds Petersen, A. & Bunton, R. (1997) London: Routledge.

Petersen, A. & Lupton, D. (1996) *The New Public Health: Health and Self in the Age of Risk*. London: Sage.

Phillimore, P. & Moffat, S. (1994) Discounted knowledge: local experience, environmental pollution and health. In Researching the People's Health eds Popay, J. & Williams, G. London: Routledge.

Plough, A. & Olafson, F. (1994) Implementing the Boston Healthy Start Initiative: a case study of community empowerment and public health. *Health Education Quarterly*, **21**(2): 221–234.

Poland, B.D. (1996) Knowledge development and evaluation in, of and for healthy community initiatives. Part 1: guiding principles. *Health Promotion International*, **11**(3): 237–247.

Puddifoot, J. (1996) Are community campaign groups representative? *Community Development Journal*, **31**(4): 351–353.

Ranade, W. (1997) *A Future for the NHS? Healthcare for the Millennium 2nd edn*. London: Longman.

Rappaport, J. (1981) In praise of paradox: a social policy of empowerment over prevention. *American Journal of Community Psychology*, **9**: 1–25.

Rissel, C. (1994) Empowerment: the holy grail of health promotion. *Health Promotion International*, **9**(1): 39–47.

Schuftan, C. (1996) The community development dilemma: what is really empowering? *Community Development Journal*, **31**(3): 260–264.

Schulz, A.J., Israel, B.A., Zimmerman, M.A. & Checkoway, B.N. (1995) Empowerment as a multi-level construct: perceived control at the individual, organisational and community levels. *Health Education Research: Theory and Practice*, **10**(3): 309–327.

Seedhouse, D. (1997) *Health Promotion: Philosophy, Prejudice and Practice*. London: Wiley.

Simons-Morton, B.G. & Davis Crump, A. (1996) Empowerment: the process and the outcome. *Health Education Quarterly*, **23**(3): 290–292.

Smith, G. (1996) Ties, nets and an elastic band: community in the postmodern city. *Community Development Journal*, **31**(3): 250–259.

Smithies, J. & Adams, L. (1993) Walking the tightrope: issues in evaluation and community participation for Health for All. In *Healthy Cities: Research and Practice* eds. Davies, J.K. & Kelly, M.P. London: Routledge.

Squire, C. (1994) Empowering women? The Oprah Winfrey Show. *Feminism and Psychology*, **4**(10): 63–79.

Thompson, E. (1998) New green shoots in old ground. *Health Service Journal*, 26 February 1998.

Tight, M. (1988) Education for Adults, Volume 1. Audit Learning and Education. Buckingham: Open University Press.

Tones, K. (1994) In *Action & Action Competence as Key Concepts in Critical Pedagogy*. Studies in Educational Theory and Curriculum Vol 12, Royal Danish School of Educational Studies. eds Jensan B.B. & Schnack K.

Tones, K. & Tilford, S. (1994) *Health Education: Effectiveness, Efficiency & Equity (2nd Ed)* London: Longman.

Turner, B. (1997) From governmentality to risk: some reflections on Foucault's contribution to medical sociology. In *Foucault, Health and Medicine*. eds Petersen, A. & Bunton, R. London: Routledge.

Wallerstein, N. & Bernstein, E. (1994) Introduction to community empowerment participatory education, and health. *Health Education Quarterly*, **21**(2): 141–148

Wallerstein, N. & Sanchez-Merki, V. (1994) Frierian praxis in health education: research results from an adolescent prevention programme. *Health Education Research: Theory & Practice*, **9**(1): 105–118.

Whitelaw, S. & Whitelaw, A. (1996) What do we expect from ethics in health promotion and where does Foucault fit in? *Health Education Research: Theory & Practice*, **11**(3): 349–354.

Wilkinson, R. (1996) *Unhealthy Societies: Afflications of Inequality* London: Routledge.

Williams, J., Carey, P., Graham, G. et al (1995) Education for empowerment: implications for professional development and training in health promotion. *Health Education Journal*, **54**: 37–47

World Health Organisation (WHO) (1981) *Regional strategy for attaining Health for All by 2000*. Copenhagen: WHO.

World Health Organisation (WHO) (1986) *Ottawa Charter for Health Promotion: An international Conference on Health promotion: the move towards a new public health*. Ottawa: WHO.

Yen, L. (1995) From Alma Ata to Asda – and beyond: a commentary on the transition in health promotion services in primary care from commodity to control. In *The sociology of health promotion*. eds Bunton, R., Nettleton, S. & Burrows, R. London: Routledge.

2 CHALLENGES IN PRACTICE

SECTION CONTENTS

3 **Pre-conception care**
Karen Dignan

4 **Empowerment and childbirth**
Aileen McLoughlin

5 **Teenage pregnancy**
Karen Dignan

6 **Promoting child and family health through empowerment**
Sue Hooton

7 **Youth health promotion in the community**
Grainne Graham

8 **Homeless women and primary health care**
Melanie Ibbitson

9 **Mental health promotion**
Phil Keeley

10 **Men's health: concepts, criticisms and challenges**
Steven Pryjmachuk and Timothy Simon Faltermeyer

11 **Health promotion and ethnic minority groups**
Abbie Paton and Julie A. Higgins

12 **'Queer health': health promotion the hard way**
Tony Russell-Pattison

13 **Health promotion for older people**
Gordon Evans

14 **Health promotion and community care: the neighbourhood health strategy**
Julia Mitchell

3 Pre-conception care

Karen Dignan

KEY ISSUES

- Multidisciplinary team collaboration
- Holistic health achievement
- Prevention of ill health complications
- Education with regard to lifestyle issues and screening

CHAPTER AIM

The aim of this chapter is to present a broad overview of the factors which may affect conception and the normal development of that conception to a full-term infant. The author will offer evidence in support of information and research which can reduce the risk of delivering an unhealthy or handicapped infant. It is also intended to present a strategy for implementing pre-conception care into a health-promoting model in a way that will raise the profile of pre-conception care to a level it deserves. Finally, it is proposed to suggest an alternative view of the subject in a way that those in power to allocate resources, both in terms of finances and specialised staff, may consider pre-conception care as a priority worth investing in.

INTRODUCTION

Pre-conception care is an area of health care provision that is sadly lacking within the majority of health service provider units. It is an aspect of care, intervention and management that can have significant positive effects upon the outcome of a pregnancy and therefore the future health of the nation as a whole. It is not the responsibility of one health professional but one that invites integration and cooperation between a multidisciplinary team. Members of the multidisciplinary team may include midwives, nurses, doctors, health visitors and geneticists. Within today's health care system it would be unwise to omit lay organisations from an arena such as pre-conception care. Organisations such as the National Childbirth Trust or parents' groups play a very important role within this type of health care sphere. The knowledge and skills of those professionals and laypeople mentioned is diverse and wide, which further supports the fact that pre-conception care should be a multidisciplinary approach.

It seems an absurdity to discuss the value of pre-conception care when the majority of pregnancies are not planned, however the notion of pre-conception care is by far not a new one but has only in fairly recent years received any notable attention. There have been many definitions of what pre-conception care is, however the one which the author likes and which is put most succinctly is by Chamberlain (Chamberlain and Lumley, 1986): 'The physical and mental preparation for childbearing of both parents before pregnancy.'

This definition encompasses the external factors which affect physical and mental well-being of both partners such as nutrition, social class, poverty, employment/unemployment and environmental factors. Pre-conception care is such a wide area of preventative health in which very positive strides in terms of health achievements can be made that it is perhaps a sad reflection of how much value is placed upon health promotion when areas such as this are left underdeveloped and under-resourced. It is worth considering the factors relevant to pre-conception care in more depth in order to give a greater understanding of the importance of each element.

CONTEXT

Factors affecting healthy embryo to fetal development

Nutritional status

There is evidence around (Lloyd, 1983) to suggest that the first acknowledgement of the link between nutrition and normal healthy development of the fetus was made by Hippocrates. Since those early times there has been other more up-to-date evidence to support Hippocrates' theory. The Dutch hunger winter of 1944–1945 is perhaps the most often quoted. During this period of time there was an increase in amenorrhoea among women of reproductive age, and those that conceived and delivered during that time had an increase in morbidity and mortality rates of the infants delivered. The main causes of increased morbidity and mortality were due to congenital abnormalities and the delivery of infants of low birth weight (Stein et al, 1975). There is now strong evidence to suggest (Doyle, 1992), that birth weight is perhaps the most important factor in predicting the health of the nation, as it is the strongest indicator of morbidity and mortality. Although this statement may appear simple it is quite a strong statement to make. Doyle is suggesting that the healthier babies are the ones that are delivered at full-term and are a higher of weight, and these infants suffer less ill health during their developmental years and grow to become healthy adults. This would support the fact that pre-conception care should be the beginning of this process.

Ideal weight for height

The weight of the woman prior to conception, at the time of conception and beyond is also of significance and this applies to whether she is underweight or overweight. A woman who is constantly on reducing diets may maintain low levels of progesterone, which ultimately results in a suppression of ovulation (Wynn and Wynn, (1994). These women will have increased difficulties in conceiving and also once conception has been achieved there is an increased risk of delivering an infant of low birth weight (Brown et al, 1981). The woman who is overweight at the time of conception and beyond is more at risk from obstetric complications during pregnancy, such as diabetes and hypertension

(Levitt, 1993). Pre-conception care would benefit these categories of women in providing dietary advice in order to achieve optimum weight for height, which would improve their chances of conception. It is important that this advice is started early when a couple embark on the path to parenthood because eating habits may need to alter and this requires a change in behaviour (Dimperio, 1990). It is also of vital importance that the diet not only addresses the woman's target weight but that it is also well balanced and healthy (Ford et al, 1994).

Folic acid supplementation

The value of folic acid supplementation prior to and during the first trimester of pregnancy can not now be ignored after all the hard evidence supplied by Smithells et al (1976, 1980 and 1983). Folic acid is the most common nutrient of deficiency in the woman and it is perhaps one, if not the one, that is most important at the time of conception and in the first trimester. During the first 28 days of pregnancy, there is rapid cell division, which is termed 'organogenesis, and requires the correct level of folic acid to be achieved in order for normal development to be accomplished. The neural tube is formed during the first 21 days after conception and complete closure of the neural tube occurs by the 28th day. Should complete closure not take place then one of two abnormalities occur: either anecephaly, where the cerebral hemispheres and cranial vault do not develop or spina bifida, where the spinal column fails to close completely. Both of these conditions are distressing and the former is not compatible with life. It is now known that in the majority of cases prevention may be possible. In studies by Smithells et al (1983), the Medical Research Council Vitamin Study Group (1991) and Czeizel and Dudas (1992), women who had previously given birth to a baby with a neural tube defect were prescribed multivitamin supplements which included folic acid, prior to pregnancy and for the first trimester. The incidence rate of the aforementioned abnormalities was significantly reduced. The most significant nutrient in reducing the incidence was folic acid because of its involvement in nuclear acid synthesis. All women who are planning a pregnancy are advised to take additional folic acid supplementation of 400 mcg/day and to continue for the first trimester of pregnancy (DoH, 1992). There is no evidence to show that additional supplementation has any adverse effects upon the woman or the developing embryo. Due to the media coverage, not just in professional journals but in the better lay health journals, a significant proportion of women who conceive are aware of the value of folic acid supplementation. There has been an extensive health promotion campaign in this area backed by the Department of Health (DoH), which has given its support to this health promotion venture. Every health professional who counsels women who wish to embark upon a pregnancy should now be advocating folic acid supplementation. It is hoped that through this tripartite approach, that is the professionals, the media and the Government, that all women embarking upon a pregnancy will be fully aware of the need and health value of taking folic acid supplementation.

Social class and poverty

The social class a person belongs to plays a very important role in the health stakes, but unfortunately this is not always a positive one and is often a negative one, particularly in the lower socio-economic groups. There is medical evidence by Scambler (1993) that the lower social classes are likely to smoke more and drink increased quantities of alcohol than those in the higher social classes. Both of these have a damaging and detrimental effect upon the ability to conceive and the continued development of the embryo to a full-term healthy baby. Poverty and social class are often interlinked as people in the lower socio-economic classes are those most likely to be living in poverty (Townsend, Davidson and Whitehead, 1992). Poverty in this special group of women may lead to poor maternal nutritional status, of which the consequences may be delivery of a premature and/or low birth weight infant (Scambler, 1993). Women who fall into this socio-economic group are on the whole the ones who begin having sexual intercourse at an early age, have multiple partners, become mothers at a young age, have repeated pregnancies with little time lapse between them and often may end up alone and unsupported (Fullerton, 1997). These women deserve special attention and it is important not to adopt the 'victim blaming' approach, but the reasons behind such unhealthy behaviours should be explored. The benefits of health promotion strategies within this group of women would reap enormous benefits in terms of improving their own health and the future health of their infants. Health promotion strategies such as smoking cessation groups, stress management sessions and healthy eating advice would be valuable in beginning to break the cycle of unhealthy behaviours through education. It must be realised that these women do value their pregnancy and obviously want a healthy baby but other factors which are beyond their ability to change, such as social and environmental influences need to be tackled on the macro level of health promotion rather than on the micro level.

Education

Education plays an important role in pre-conception care and again is often linked to social class. The higher the social class a person belongs to the better educated they are and therefore more aware of the need to plan for a healthy baby. If a person belongs to one of the higher social classes then they are more likely to have continued into further and higher education, which delays conception and brings more self-awareness and self-confidence on the wider issues which affect health (Wellings et al, 1996; Kiernan, 1995). Whereas, if a person belongs to one of the lower social classes, there is more likelihood that they will leave school early and not continue education, which often results in poor employment opportunities, low self-esteem and young unplanned parenthood. Again, it can be seen that the lower socio-economic groups are the ones that are most disadvantaged in the health stakes.

This area opens up good opportunities for a collaborative health care team with laypeople included where appropriate, to take education on matters pertinent to pre-conception care into schools and plant the seeds for future health developments. In order to attempt to break the 'cycle of depravation' education must begin early, preferably in the young adolescent years. It is hoped that through educating these young people that healthier behaviours will be adopted and their own self-esteem and self-confidence will grow. If this improvement takes place; this vulnerable group should be in a more positive position to adopt and assert themselves when it comes to health and lifestyle options.

Lifestyle factors

There can be no doubt that the way people live their lives can have a positive or negative effect upon their health. There is no doubt whatsoever that smoking causes cancer and yet there are a great proportion of people, especially the young, who still continue to smoke cigarettes while knowing the dangers. Hilary Graham's research into the smoking habits of young mothers concluded that although the adverse effects of smoking were known to the study participants, the habit enabled them to cope with the daily stresses of motherhood and improved their self-esteem because it was the sole activity that they undertook by themselves for themselves (Graham, 1988). One has to accept that it is the choice of the individual to smoke or not to. However, when the quest for parenthood is embarked upon then the growth and development of the fetus should be afforded some consideration because of the potentially harmful effects of nicotine upon pregnancy outcome. There is firm correlation between tobacco use and infertility, menstrual disorders, spontaneous abortions, ectopic pregnancies, low birth weight infants, placental abnormalities and infant mortality and morbidity (Cefalo and Moos, 1995). Smoking in pregnancy increases the risk that the baby will be born premature, growth retarded or of low birth weight and smoking also increases the peri-natal mortality rate by an estimated 28% (Dines and Cribb, 1993; Davis, 1996). There is evidence to suggest that men who smoke may have altered spermatogenesis, sperm mobility and sperm morphology (Summers and Price, 1993). This may have consequences for the couple who are experiencing difficulties in conceiving.

Health professionals must be careful when advising against the dangers of smoking and the effects that it can have upon the ability to conceive and the developing conception. It may be frightening for the woman/couple to realise the harmful effects of nicotine not only to their own health but perhaps more importantly to them, the health of their future infant. It is important that health promotion activities aimed at helping to reduce and/or stop smoking are offered. The success of health promotion advice lies in the ability to offer supportive strategies in a non-judgmental way.

Another of the lifestyle factors which can have a significant effect upon the ability to conceive, and for that conception to grow and develop normally is the consumption of alcohol. This substance is perceived as being far more socially acceptable than smoking. Unlike smoking it does not carry a Government health warning on the label. However, there is information readily available as to the number of units of alcohol which is within the safe limits for both females and males. Margaret and Arthur Wynn, who are strong supporters of pre-conception care, believe that the consumption of alcohol during the pre-conception period and during pregnancy should be avoided by both parties. Alcohol has been linked to repeated abortions, particularly mid-trimester abortions, and in the quantity and quality of the sperm produced (Summers and Price, 1993). It would seem sensible then that a couple embarking on a much wanted and desired pregnancy should abstain from consuming any amount of alcohol. There are others (Balen and Challis, 1993), who take a more liberal view and suggest that a small amount of alcohol is not harmful providing it is limited to no more than 6 units per week. What is perhaps more damaging is binge drinking, where large amounts of alcohol are consumed in a single drinking session. It is suggested by the Health Education Authority (1993) that once pregnant, the woman should not consume alcohol at all. It is evident that there is no firm conclusive evidence on this aspect of pre-conception care but that perhaps there needs to be the adoption of a sensible approach to the consumption of alcohol.

The abuse of other substances, such as heroin and cocaine, can have serious and far reaching consequences for both the mother and the developing fetus. Withdrawal from heroin can be fatal to the developing fetus so a more positive and supportive approach in terms of pre-conception care counselling should be employed. This should preferably take place prior to conception although realistically if counselling support is taken up it will no doubt be during the pregnancy because this special group of women on the whole have unplanned pregnancies. Cocaine withdrawal can be achieved in early pregnancy and is associated with improved birth outcome, however the continued use during pregnancy is associated with spontaneous abortion, premature delivery, abruptio placenta, intrauterine growth retardation and congenital abnormalities (Hollingworth, 1988). A study by Chasnoff, Chisum and Kaplan (1988) on the effects of cocaine use during pregnancy correlated a positive link between cocaine use and abnormalities, particularly of the genitourinary tract. There is also an unfounded belief that the long-term consequences of cocaine use can cause the infant/child to suffer from neurodevelopmental inadequacies and eventually find it difficult to socialise into normal society. Before this *unfounded belief* is accepted as firm evidence this aspect needs to be fully researched and investigated.

Environmental factors

The environment that people live and work in can also have a detrimental effect upon their health and well-being. The type of occupation that people are employed in may have a damaging effect upon their physical health in terms of their ability to conceive (Caulfied, 1988). This is particularly true of people who work in the chemical industry as certain chemicals may reduce sperm morphology (Cefalo and Moos, 1995). The physical environment that people live in may also make conception difficult. A couple must feel relaxed and happy in order to achieve the optimum conceptus, but in some situations this desired environment may not be attained for several reasons. A couple who are in a difficult financial situation will exhibit signs of stress; a couple who are desperate to conceive and therefore their lovemaking sessions are governed by the most optimum time to conceive will also be stressed and stress is an inhibiting factor to conception. These factors may not seem to be very significant in playing such a vital role in conception, however if the couple have low fertility then this may make the situation that much more difficult.

Maternal age

The age of the woman is particularly important when embarking upon parenthood because of the increased risk of mortality and morbidity to both the mother and the infant. It must be stressed here that due to healthier lifestyles that people on the whole are leading (and this appears to apply throughout the range of social classes), many women are purposely delaying motherhood until they are into their 30s, when they have an established career and are stable in their home life. This means that many women are more socially, psychologically and physiologically ready for the demands of childbirth and motherhood. The older woman was always deemed to be an obstetric risk, in terms of increased fetal abnormalities, hypertensive disorders, placenta praevia and postpartum haemorrhage to mention a few, but due to the improvements made in lifestyle on the whole, these risks are now minimal. There has been vast improvement in obstetric care in such fields as screening procedures (both maternal and fetal), and the management of obstetric complication that the risk of having a baby in the latter part of a woman's reproductive life has also been minimised.

The other end of the age range, that is the woman who bears children at an early age, may be socially, psychologically and physiologically disadvantaged for several reasons. A young woman will not have fully established a career, which brings with it financial instability. She may not be psychologically ready to accept and cope with the demands that being a mother places upon her and physiologically she may not be in the best optimum state of health for conception and pregnancy to be achieved. There is evidence around to support the fact that adolescent childbearing is linked with social and economic problems (McAnarney and Hendee, 1989; Capitulo and Maffia, 1992).

It is within this field that help and advice by all the agencies involved can go some way to addressing the problems, however there are some factors which are beyond the scope of individual organisations and need to be addressed at government level.

What should the health professionals and the health service offer in the field of pre-conception care?

There are many factors which contribute to the conception and healthy growth and development of a baby as many health professionals will know. However, it is the responsibility of every health professional working within this field to inform those people who are embarking upon the road to parenthood of the value of achieving optimum health prior to conception. What should a pre-conception care clinic offer these people in order for them to avail themselves of the information and the professional help available, in order that a healthy infant may be conceived? The essential requirements for are listed in Box 3.1

One of the main functions, if not the main function, of a pre-conception care clinic is the screening services offered. Screening comes under the auspice of preventative health care and within the field of pre-conception care the value

---

BOX 3.1	*Necessary requirements for the pre-conception care clinic*

The clinics should:

- be staffed by health professionals who have a passionate interest in the health and future welfare of the next and subsequent generation
- be organised in such a way as to meet the needs of the individuals attending them, for example time and venue of the clinic sessions and the needs of the ethnic minorities addressed
- make it the responsibility of the staff to provide up-to-date information on a variety of topics relevant to the field of pre-conception care and importantly they should be understanding and approachable as this is a very sensitive issue.

placed upon screening procedure undertaken can be extremely important. The value in terms of health protection and health promotion may be priceless. The importance and value placed upon the correct and in-depth taking of a full history from the couple seeking pre-conception care advice cannot be overemphasised. A fundamental aspect of pre-conception care is the screening procedures that are performed on both parties, and these will be dependent on the areas highlighted from the histories obtained. These screening procedures will form the basis for the individualised planned care of management for that particular couple, and as can be appreciated, each couples' needs will differ according to the specific areas highlighted. The screening procedures undertaken will link into the areas already addressed earlier in the chapter, such as lifestyle issues, weight and ideal weight for conception, the taking of blood for rubella status, full blood profile, screening for sexually transmitted infections and the taking of a cervical smear and perhaps semen analysis. As can be appreciated these tests and investigations may cause some degree of distress and embarrassment due to their sensitive nature and it is the skills of the health professionals involved in this field that can do much to minimise any undue anguish.

Another important aspect of pre-conception care screening is that of genetic counselling. The issue in this particular area may not necessarily be that of planning a pregnancy but may be more concerned with knowing risk factors to specific inherited diseases, such as sickle-cell anaemia or Tay-Sachs. A couple facing this particular dilemma, when given their estimated risk factor to conceiving a child with the acquired disorder may choose to remain childless, or may equally decide that the estimated risk is worth taking and therefore embark upon a pregnancy with informed choice and the support of all the health professionals involved in their care.

Health-promoting strategy

The value of pre-conception care cannot be over stressed. By informing the couple of their health risks and providing them with choices in order to minimise those risks and maximise health potential, then great strides will have been made in planning for, conceiving and hopefully delivering a healthy infant, whilst at the same time achieving the optimum health for the couple. The most appropriate way of utilising a health promotion model in the field of pre-conception care is by incorporating a preventative model approach that also allows for self-empowerment to be the underpinning force. Adopting this type of approach will develop within the individual/couple the behaviour change, particularly with respect to lifestyle issues that may be required. This approach also places the ownership for their health back to the individuals concerned therefore giving them self-confidence in their ability to improve upon their own health. Prevention may come on three levels: (1) primary, (2) secondary and (3) tertiary (Leavell and Clarke, 1965; Tones and Tilford, 1995). This seems the most appropriate model to use because of the three levels of intervention.

Primary prevention

Primary prevention is concerned with averting a disease before it starts. Shamansky and Clausen (1980) identified primary prevention as including generalised health promotion as well as specific protection against disease.

This is also supported by Ewles and Simnett (1995), who also view primary prevention as being the prevention of ill health before disease arises and acknowledge that this is directed at healthy individuals. One could argue that the Ewles and Simnett definition does not fit so well into the pre-conception care arena, however the author would dispute that. Couples who actively seek pre-conception care advice may see themselves as being relatively healthy and not in a state of illness. Therefore, these two statements fit nicely into the area of pre-conception care because not only are health professionals attempting to promote healthy pregnancies, they are also looking more widely into facilitating a fuller healthy lifestyle change for the promotion of general health. This bears a lot of relevance when considering factors such as the lifestyle issues that may be influential in preventing the conception and healthy development of the embryo. Primary prevention allows such factors to be highlighted and positive steps taken in order to facilitate change.

Secondary prevention

Secondary prevention is concerned with intervention when a health deficit has been identified. The purpose of secondary prevention is to minimise the complication once the problem has been identified. Secondary prevention leading to intervention still slots nicely into pre-conception care if one looks at it from a slightly different viewpoint. For example, a woman seeking pre-conception care advice who has a medical problem identified will benefit from this approach. Medical conditions such as diabetes or a heart conditions should be managed by all the specialists involved in caring for that woman. Medical intervention and supervision along with obstetric and midwifery care during the pre-pregnancy period will enable the woman to be in optimum health for conception, and for the pregnancy to progress and develop to its fullest potential with the hopeful outcome of a healthy infant. Identification and appropriate early management of the woman with an existing condition will cause minimal effect upon her general health and hopefully the optimum health gain in terms of the pregnancy outcome. This type of tripartite care is to the best advantage in promoting optimum health and minimal complications in both the woman and the fetus.

Tertiary prevention

Tertiary prevention is concerned with maximising potential once the disease process has stabilised. This, the author would agree may seem very difficult to comprehend as to how this may fit into a model for promoting pre-conception care. It is every parent's wish to have a normal healthy infant, but sadly that is not always possible. There are couples who are at a greater risk of having a baby with affected conditions such as sickle-cell anaemia or neural tube defects, who still wish to conceive and continue with the pregnancy once this condition has been identified. Health maximisation does not only refer to the physical health but to viewing the couple holistically and incorporating other aspects of health, such as the social and psychological influences. Coping with a baby who has a disability, no matter what that disability may be, is made easier by the support and experience of other couples who have a child with the same disability. This type of support network also allows the couple to see that they are not the only couple to bear a child with this type of disability, and therefore they do not feel alone and isolated.

A thread which weaves throughout each of these levels of health promotion is that of empowerment and choice. Tones (1994) defined empowerment as 'a state in which an individual actually possesses a relatively high degree of power: that is having the resources which enable that individual to make genuinely free choices'. Tones also states that 'individual empowerment is associated with certain beneficial psychological characteristics of which the most significant are: beliefs about personal control'. In order for people to be empowered they have to be given information on which to make a choice. In the primary level of health promotion, information with regard to lifestyle issues and risk factors are given for the individual couples and on the basis of that information they are then able to make an informed choice as to what if any lifestyle changes to make or what for them may be an acceptable level of risk to take.

The secondary level of health promotion is concerned with limiting the degree of complication or disability. The choice may be harder to make here. The giving of information on which to make an informed choice may in this situation be in relation to the identification of an unexpected abnormality. This poses moral, ethical and religious dilemmas for some couples who may have to decide whether to continue with a pregnancy knowing that the baby will have an abnormality, which may or may not be correctable, or whether to request a termination of that pregnancy. Whichever decision that couple arrives at will be perhaps the hardest decision that they will have had to make in their entire lives and one in which the support of the multidisciplinary team is required.

The tertiary level of health promotion involves the giving of information relevant to the specific complication identified and the support of the health professionals and other relevant bodies, such as The Downs Syndrome Society or Still Birth and Neonatal Death Society. It is with all these organisations working in cooperation that the maximum health care benefit can be provided.

It may seem to some that pre-conception care and the degree of input from the health professionals, in terms of the skilled knowledge and care required and the amount of resources needed, may make pre-conception care an expensive luxury. The author would dispute this because if money and resources were to be ploughed into this field of preventative medicine then the long-term gains, not just in monetary terms but perhaps more importantly in terms of more successful pregnancy outcome for mother and baby would be immeasurable. Improved physical health when there is an existing medical condition will result in less medical and obstetric intervention and an improved childbirth experience for the couple. The better emotionally and psychologically prepared parents are for childbirth and particularly when the baby is known to have a degree of disability, the more favourable the adaptation to parenthood will be. To the purchasers and providers of health care, these may be less important factors when faced with other health care dilemmas. In order to have a realistic and holistic view of the situation, it is necessary to have an insight into how the purchasers and providers of health care have to make their decisions.

Purchasers and providers of health care

In order to provide a service which fits the needs of the consumers, there has to be a method of assessing the health needs of the population that the hospital and community serve. It is therefore appropriate that a framework of service provision is implemented in order that a full and complete range of services may be provided to meet that specific population's health needs. The National Health Service (NHS) and Community Care Act (1990) was the beginning of a new way of meeting the health needs of the population by in essence giving the people choice (Kroll, 1996). This change in the organisation of the way health care was purchased and provided in theory meant that the needs of the population were met in relation to specific needs and that the purchasers were able to shop around for the best possible providers of those services. One important feature was that in many instances health promotion was often written into the service contracts (Scriven and Orme, 1996). This occurred in three ways. First, the NHS had an obligation to promote the health of the staff and patients, and a good example of this is in making hospitals a smoke-free environment. Second, health promotion was made a requirement in specific specialism, such as maternity care. A good example of this would be in implementing a smoking cessation intervention group. Third, and one that bears the most importance to pre-conception care was the provision of specialist health promotion services. The value of pre-conception care can be further augmented by providing an organised and structured service of which its availability is known about by the people who may require it. Within this service should be the ability to provide information and care for people on an individualised basis which is in keeping with their own culture. Often the luxury of pre-conception care counselling is only accessible by the predominantly white middle classes and does not reach the groups in most need, that is the lower socio-economic groups and ethnic minorities. These are the groups that experience greater morbidity and mortality in relation to childbirth (Scambler, 1993).

There is no doubt that in today's climate of health care provision that all services must justify their value to the purchasers. Services that do not provide good quality care and value for money will not be subscribed to by the purchasers of health care in the future. So how can we convince the purchasers of pre-conception care services that they are of value? It may seem a harsh fact but one has to begin by looking at what happens if pre-conception care advice is not available, that is looking at the outcomes of pregnancies that do not end in a full-term healthy infant. By viewing the peri-natal and neonatal mortality and morbidity statistics with particular reference to cause may be the starting block. In line with that course of action, it may also be relevant to collate the late spontaneous abortion rates because of the lifestyle factors involved. The final strand that brings the three approaches together is to analyse the number of couples that are attending a recognised specialist unit for infertility treatment. This as stated earlier seems a very harsh approach to take because it could be construed as being a victim-blaming approach. This is far from the intention of the author but it does seem the most appropriate way to tackle this issue. It is only by first viewing the outcomes or failed outcomes to intended pregnancies that one is able to then back track in order to determine, if possible, the causative factors. Now in some cases these may be multifarious and therefore it may be difficult to decide on the exact cause. However, in a larger proportion of cases it may be possible to form direct links between known causative agents and conception/birth outcomes. Having the ability to make definite links between lifestyle factors, environmental agents and biological make-up, and conception failure or poor outcome that perhaps purchasers and providers of health care will sit up and take notice. It is only then through multidisciplinary collaboration that this health arena can begin to move forward.

Health needs assessment is a tool which is used to achieve a needs-led approach to planning, purchasing and providing health care needs. Health needs assessment also involves the preventive health care facilities, such as screening services. There is a need to predict future health needs as well as to address the present day needs. From this stance it can be seen that factors known to affect health, for example, social, environmental and geographical factors also need to be taken into account as the literature referred to would suggest. In the author's opinion, there is not a more important and needy area within health care provision and management that is affected by or has an effect upon, than pre-conception care. There is a need for those resources already available both on a personal and community level to be assessed.

CONCLUSION

The whole area of pre-conception care should be of interest to every individual because of the profound effect that pre-conception care advice can have upon the present and future generations. In order to achieve maximum health there is a need to measure health status and health resources in order to maximise health gains. This would not be difficult to assess in relation to the field of pre-conception care because as evident from the literature reviewed, the future health of the nation begins prior to conception with two healthy individuals, who then go on to produce a healthy infant. One of the most positive ways forward in achieving health gains may be to increase health resources in the field of family care because the family in its broadest sense should be the cornerstone of society and one which provides the country with the future generation.

Pre-conception care should be of importance not just on a personal level but also on a local and governmental level. It is a sphere where involvement from many parties, such as health professional, school educators, environmentalists and governmental agencies all collaborating together will be instrumental in promoting a future healthy nation.

REFERENCES

Balen, A.H. & Challis, J.D. (1993) Dietary Advice for Women Wishing to Conceive. *British Journal of Midwifery*, 1(5): 238–241

Brown, J.E., Jacobson, H.N., Askue, L.H. et al (1981) Influence of pregnancy weight gain on the size of infants born to underweight women. *Obstetrics and Gynaecology*, 57, 13–17. Cited in *Preconception Evaluation and Intervention* Olsen, M.E. (1994). Department of Obstetrics and Gynaecology, East Tennessee State University. Johnson City, TN, USA.

Capitulo, K.L. & Maffia, A.J. (1992) *Adolescent Pregnancy. Series 4 Nursing issues for the 21st Century; module 2.* White Plains, New York: March of Dimes Birth Defects Foundation. Cited in *Preconceptional Health Care: A Practical Guide*. 2nd edn. Cefalo, R.C. & Moos, M.K. (1995). St Louis: Mosby.

Caulfield, C. (1988) *Multiple Exposures: Chronicles of the Radiation Age*. Toronto: Stoddart.

Cefalo, R.C. & Moos, M.K. (1995) *Preconceptional Health Care: A Practical Guide*. 2nd edn. St Louis: Mosby.

Czeizel, A.E. & Dudas, I. (1992) Prevention of the first occurrence of neural tube defects by periconceptual vitamin supplementation. *New England Journal of Medicine*, 327, 1832–1835.

Chamberlain, G. & Lumley, J. (1986) *Pregnancy Care, A Manual for Practice*. London: John Wiley.

Davis, B.H. (1996) *Public Health, Preventive Medicine and Social Services*. 6th edn. Edward Arnold.

Department of Health (DoH) (1992) *Folic Acid and the Prevention of Neural Tube Defects* (Report from an Expert Advisory Group). London: HMSO.

Dimperio, D. (1990) Preconceptional Nutrition. *Journal of Paediatric and Perinatal Nutrition*, 2(2): 65–78.

Dines, A. & Cribb, A. (1993) *Health Promotion Concepts and Practice*. London: Blackwell.

Doyle, W. (1992) Preconceptional Care – Who Needs It? *Modern Midwife*, January/February, 18–22.

Ewles, L. & Simnett, I. (1995) *Promoting Health: A Practical Guide*. London: Scutari.

Ford, F., Fraser, R. & Diamond, H. (1994) *Healthy Eating for You and Your Baby*. Basingstoke: Macmillan.

Fullerton, D. (1997) A Review of Approaching Teenage Pregnancy. *Nursing Times*, 93(13): 48–49.

Graham, H. (1988) Women and Smoking in the United Kingdom: Implications for health promotion. *Health Promotion*, 3(4): 371–382.

Health Education Authority (HEA) (1993) *New Pregnancy Book*. London: HEA.

Hollingworth, D.R. (1988) Drugs and Reproduction: Maternal and fetal risk. Cited in Levitt, C. (1993) Preconception health Promotion. *Primary Care* 20(3): 537–549.

Kiernan, K. (1995) Transition to Parenthood: Young Mother, Young Fathers – Associated Factors and Later Life Experiences. Welfare State Programme Discussion Paper 113. London Family Planning Association, cited in *Effective Health Care*, Preventing and Reducing the Adverse Effects of Unintended Teenage Pregnancies.

Kroll, D. (1996) *Midwifery Care for the Future: Meeting the Challenge*. London: Baillière Tindall.

Leavell, H.R. & Clarke, E.G. (1965) *Preventative Medicine for the Doctor in His Community*. New York: McGraw-Hill. Cited in King, P.M. (1994) Health Promotion: the emerging frontier in nursing. *Journal of Advanced Nursing*, 20, 209–218.

Levitt, C. (1993) Preconception Health Promotion. *Obstetrics* 20(3): 537–547.

Lloyd, G.R. (1983) *The Nature of the Child in Hippocratic Writing*. London: Penguin.

McAnarney, E.R. & Hendee, W.R. (1989) Adolescent Pregnancy and its Consequences. *Journal of the American Medical Association*, 262, 74–77

Medical Research Council Vitamin Study Research Group (1991) Prevention of neural tube defects: results of the Medical Research Council Vitamin Study. *Lancet* 338: 131–137

Scambler, G. (1993) *Sociology as Applied to Medicine*. 3rd edn London: Baillière Tindall.

Schorah, C.J. & Smithless, R.W. (1991) Maternal Vitamin Nutrition and Malformations of the Neural Tube. *Nutrition Research Review* 33–49. Cited in Dickerson, J. (1995) Good Preconception Care Starts in School. *Modern Midwife*, November, 15–18

Scriven, A. & Orme, J. (1996) *Health Promotion: Professional Perspectives*. London: Macmillan.

Shamansky, S.L. & Clausen, C.L. (1980) Levels of Prevention: Examination of a concept. *Nursing Outlook*, **28**, 104–108.

Smithells, R.W., Sheppard, S. & Schorah, C.J. (1976) Vitamin Deficiences and Neural Tube Defects. *Archives of Disease in Childhood*, **51**, 944–950.

Smithells R.W., et al (1980) Possible prevention of neural tube defects by peri-conceptual vitamin supplementation. *Lancet* **I**, 339–340.

Smithells, R.W., Nevin, N.C., Seller, M.J., et al. (1983) Further experience of vitamin supplementation for prevention of neural tube defect recurrences. *Lancet*, **I**, 1027–1031.

Stein, Z. et al (1975) *Famine and Human Development*. Oxford: Oxford University. Cited in Roberts, P. (1989) Preconceptual care. *The British Journal of Family Planning*, **15**, 41–43.

Summers, L. & Price, R.A. (1993) An Opportunity to Maximize Health in Pregnancy. *Journal of Nurse/Midwife*, 38(4): 188–198.

Tones, K. & Tilford, S. (1995) *Health Education, Effectiveness, Efficiency and Equity*. 2nd edn London: Chapman & Hall.

Townsend, P., Davidson, N. & Whitehead, M. (1992) *Inequalities in Health: The Health Divide*. Revised ed. London: Penguin.

Wellings, K., Wadsworth, J., Johnson, A., et al (1996) *Teenage Sexuality, Fertility and Life Chances*. A Report for the Department of Health Using data from the National Survey of Sexual Attitudes and Lifestyles. London School of Hygiene & Tropical Medicine, cited in *Effective Health Care*, Preventing and Reducing the Adverse Effects of Unintended Teenage Pregnancies, February (1997).

Wynn, M. & Wynn, A. (1994) Slimming and Fertility. *Modern Midwife*, **June**, 17–20.

FURTHER READING

Niven, C.A. & Walker, A. (1996) *Reproductive Potential and Fertility Control*. Butterworth-Heinemann.

Cefalo, R.C. & Moss M.K. (1995) *Pre-Conceptional Health Care: A Practical Guide*. London: Mosby.

Barnes, B. & Bradly S.G. (1990) *Planning for a Healthy Baby*. London: Ebury.

Empowerment and childbirth

Aileen McLoughlin

- Midwifery/midwife's role
- Childbirth
- Concept of choice
- Communication skills
- User groups and childbirth

INTRODUCTION

Empowerment and childbirth are inextricably linked. Who could fail to be impressed while witnessing the emotional and physical reserves of power upon which every woman draws as she undergoes this life-changing experience? Power and change would appear to be issues at the heart of the modern childbirth experience for women and midwives alike and so the opportunity to explore some of the issues surrounding empowerment and childbirth is timely. Written from a midwifery perspective, this chapter seeks to review some of the background to the current provision of midwifery care, discuss the influence of user groups within service provision and offer a personal viewpoint on the discussion.

BACKGROUND

Traditionally midwifery care has been linked with the drive to empower women. Generations of midwives, allied at the beginning of the twentieth century to the struggles of the women's movement, fought to provide qualified, supervised midwifery care for all childbearing women. The modern education and practice of midwives was founded upon the belief that all childbearing women had a right to the care of a qualified, licensed practising midwife as opposed to the local source of assistance: the 'handy woman'. This drive was initially manifested in the work of the Midwives Institute and their considerable influence upon the First Midwives Act of 1902 (Leap and Hunter, 1993). There developed a link between the education of the 'handy women' as midwives, enhanced care for women and the birth of midwifery as a profession rather than a craft to be applied.

   At first glance this appears to be at odds with the notion of empowerment and caring within the community. How much more empowered could a woman in childbirth be than to select from her own community a trusted birth attendant?

Theoretically the woman could exercise choice as to when she called for help, whether labour take place at home in her own environment and payment negotiated in the manner most suited to them both, often payment in kind. This is a dangerous and rather rosy assumption to make for two reasons.

First, reforms were called for by the Midwives Institute out of concern for poor standards of hygiene, deprivation and high rates of infection and maternal and infant mortality. Mortality rates for all other subgroups except mothers and infants had fallen from the mid- to late-nineteenth century (Tew, 1990), and so it was understandable that the work of the handy woman would come under public scrutiny. There is no doubt that there was a need to recognise and value those good 'handy women' and to educate or withdraw from practice those who applied their craft in a dangerous manner.

Second, the idealistic notion of an empowered woman, in charge of her own destiny and childbirth experience is called into question by Leap and Hunter (1993). The women who called upon neighbourly help were those who could not afford any other means of assistance such as treatment by a doctor and hospital delivery. It was a time perhaps when women were truly disempowered in relation to their reproductive lives. Houldsworth (1988) depicts a time when women were largely ignorant about reproduction and had no reliable means of contraception. Frequent pregnancy and its associated risks coupled with poorer levels of health and hygiene resulted in childbirth becoming an accepted trial and tribulation rather than an empowering manifestation of womanhood.

At a time when the role of women in society was deemed to be less than useful, the Midwives Institute appears to have paralleled the work of the liberal feminist movement (Tong, 1989). As Leap and Hunter (1993) imply, this group of pioneering women saw themselves in an extremely paternalistic way as saviours of the poor. Unfortunately, whilst the feminist movement sought to emancipate women from the bonds of a restrictive patriarchal system, the founders of the profession of midwifery inadvertently sowed the seeds for an equally oppressive regime in relation to childbirth. Midwifery care became bounded by statute and the remit of the midwife as a practitioner of 'the normal' was defined. A gradual shift in the emphasis of care from community centredness to hospital centredness took place, along with an increasing sense of professional rivalry between midwives, general practitioners (GPs) and obstetricians which has coloured debates, policies and government reports ever since. Thus, the reforms called for by the Midwives Institute were motivated by a latter day sense of health promotion in order to improve outcomes for mothers and babies but were grounded in a paternalistic medical model of care. The positivistic drive to improve outcomes was further highlighted during the 1980s and 1990s. There appeared at that time a number of reports advocating that all women be cared for in hospital including attending hospital for their antenatal care and some postnatal care as well as care in labour (Ministry of Health, 1959; DHSS, 1970; Social Services Committee, 1980). This focus upon hospitalisation was rooted in the concerns for maternal and infant health at the time of the First Midwives Act of 1902 and this concern gained impetus and strength throughout the following decades. Weight was added to the argument by the predominantly powerful medical profession, and apparently impressive improvements in maternal, fetal and infant health indicators (Tew, 1990).

Much has been made of the professional rivalry between midwives and their obstetric colleagues, and its history has been ably and eloquently documented

(Donnisson, 1977; Abbott and Wallace, 1990; Oakley, 1980). Midwifery remained for the most part dominated and controlled by obstetric policies, practices and procedures. As Abbott and Wallace (1990) highlight, most women throughout their antenatal, intrapartum and postnatal periods are attended by a midwife, having booked for their maternity care under the controlling eye of an obstetrician or GP. Even those systems which declare themselves to be midwife led may often have the parameters of normality defined by the obstetrician, who determines what constitutes normal and therefore who the midwife should see.

However, notwithstanding our professional struggles undoubtedly it is the midwife who remains the key person during the majority of a woman's visits throughout her care, and as such is best placed to empower her and to act as a health promoter. Such empowerment, as outlined in Chapter 2, requires a major shift in the balance of power between the midwife and client. It is part of the midwife's role to be a health educator and health promoter, in order to ensure as far as possible a healthy and happy outcome to the pregnancy. This educational role is linked throughout the whole of childbirth ranging from conception to postdelivery. Education on such aspects as diet, screening tests, analgesia in labour and baby care skills theoretically enables a family to make informed decisions, encouraging involvement and participation and increasing the family's sense of autonomy and responsibility. This requirement to provide support, information and care is laid down within the Midwife's Code of Practice (UKCC, 1994) and the Midwives Rules (UKCC, 1993). However it is apparent that in everyday practice at the midwife client interface, the system within which the midwife operates does not allow this to be done in the most effective way. Whilst some may consider these regulations to give freedom to practice, the policies and procedures within most midwives' terms of employment may serve to harness that freedom (Silverton, 1995).

Rothman (1996) eloquently illustrates some of the reasons why this may be so. Although when comparing the American model of childbirth with that of the Netherlands, parallels can be drawn with the British experience. Rothman highlights an argument that has long been voiced by user groups. The medicalisation of childbirth, where delivery of the baby is viewed as something to be purged from the body, does nothing to empower women. Whilst acknowledging that providers of care may be well meaning, nurturing in approach and kindly, Rothman argues that we nurture women's weakness rather than their strength. For example rapid technological advances allow us to provide diagnoses and solutions to problems, and inform women of what is happening to them. The emphasis moves therefore from women listening to and being guided by their own bodies and telling us how they feel, towards women acting as receptacles for information from and listeners to the perceived experts. This she takes pains to point out is done with the best of intent, and that most midwives are caring individuals anxious to do the best they can for their clients. Perhaps this is part of the problem? Doing one's best whilst not disrupting the status quo are values inherent in the National Health Service (NHS) (MacKay, 1990) and are characteristics equally valued in its employees as well as in the clients who use the system. Thankfully, the user groups of the maternity services, are vociferous and strong and have done much to improve the status of the client within the service. Some of the ways they have achieved this will now be explored.

USER GROUPS: INFLUENCE UPON POLICY AND PRACTICE

Had it not been for the strong and persistent voice of the consumer movement in the 1970s and 1980s, the current climate of change might never have taken place. Care became more centralised, less personalised and resulted in decreased satisfaction for both women and midwives. Both felt an increasing sense of powerlessness and pressure groups formed demanding change and a swing back towards continuity and choice.

It is interesting to note that at this time, since the introduction of the oral contraceptive pill giving women more power over their fertility and allowing them to choose when to achieve a pregnancy, consumer groups were stating that women felt disempowered by the maternity services provided for them once that pregnancy was achieved. Perhaps as Kroll (1996) suggests, with time and an improvement in health outcomes, attention moves towards the quality of service provided as opposed to the provision of the service alone. It has also been suggested that in terms of measuring the outcome of a pregnancy, women and professionals have very different yardsticks. Whilst both aim to produce a healthy baby, the conflict between them results in women feeling disempowered, losing control over their bodies and midwives at a loss as to how best to help them (Churchill, 1995).

The following text will outline perhaps two of the most influential user groups: the National Childbirth Trust (NCT) and the Association for Improvements in the Maternity Service (AIMS), and will also consider one of the newest user groups: Action on Pre-Eclampsia (APEC).

The NCT developed from the Natural Childbirth Association, originally founded in the 1950s to provide education and information to childbearing women in the hope of reducing the fear and ignorance surrounding birth. It has gone from strength to strength conducting research, educating lay childbirth teachers, breastfeeding counsellors and providing a network of postnatal support (Kitzinger, 1990). The promotion of choice and communication were key issues and despite early conflicts with professionals, the contribution of the NCT in questioning practice and informing the consumer has gained the respect it deserves. NCT representatives formed part of the advisory body the Expert Maternity Group.

AIMS also emerged at a similar time and has campaigned mainly in relation to the provision of service facilities, technological advances and the right to choose the place of birth, be it hospital or home. Interestingly, Durward and Evans (1990) note that part of the inspiration for the Association's formation was from women seeking the right to give birth in hospital.

The strength of both the NCT and AIMS is their ability to keep up with the pace of change via direct contact with consumer opinion at grass roots level. They have an ability to encompass new ideas and plan for the future, a lesson which we all could learn from as professionals. This willingness to learn has been demonstrated by the uptake of research information undertaken by user groups and appearing in midwifery journals and texts, the liaison between mid-wives and volunteers, and the formal representation upon advisory bodies such as the Maternity Services Liaison Committees and the most recent Expert Maternity Group (DoH, 1993). From personal experiences as a midwife teacher, the pre-registration programme of midwifery education has also given representatives from such user groups the opportunity to embark upon a career in midwifery, formalising their interest, bringing their expertise and superimposing midwifery skills upon an often longstanding experience in the voluntary sector. But what of the newer user groups? One of the most recently formed and potentially influential is the rapidly successful APEC, based in Middlesex and formed by Isobel Walker in conjunction with Dr Chris Redman in 1991, as a result of her own experience of the disease. Having produced study days for professionals highlighting good practice and research-based evidence, APEC has also produced a series of client- and midwife-friendly information leaflets on the subject. So far the uptake of study days has been greater on behalf of midwives than doctors. APEC's philosophy is slightly and justifiably different to that of the previous two user groups. It emphasises the dangers to women of potential problems going unrecognised in the drive to stress the normality of the childbirth experience; it also stresses the need for specialist intervention in such instances. Perhaps in light of her own personal experience, Ms Walker feels that women are currently sold a myth of normality and control by those who care for them during pregnancy. Women are taught that pregnancy is normal and can largely be controlled; the same teachers can then offer little comfort when mother nature proves them wrong (Walker I, 1996). Could this be the first indication that the pendulum of opinion is beginning to swing in the other direction just as it has taken decades of campaigning to review the place of intervention within obstetrics? This trend would also seem to be reflected in the growing number of positions for midwives to specialise in units or teams devoted to women who require crital or high-dependency care such as women with diabetes, pre-eclampsia or those who have undergone infibulation (Lewis, 1995c; McLachlan and Yeadon, 1996). The provision of such care therefore has implications for the education of midwives to extend their role in keeping with the United Kingdom Central Council for Nursing, Midwifery and Health Visiting (UKCC, 1992).

There are of course a multitude of other user groups, organised at national and local level, that also continue to influence policy development and practice by providing research and information, advocacy services and support for those they represent, e.g. The Foundation for The Study of Infant Deaths, the Stillbirth and Neonatal Death Society, the Marce Society to name but a few. The factor which seems to unite them all is the will, motivation and time to address important consumer issues. Perhaps not having to muddle along within an imperfect and unsatisfying system as many midwives do is advantageous. Consumer groups consist of members who by the nature of their detatchment from service provision, harbour no qualms about whether to 'whistle blow', risk causing trouble or career progression by stating their viewpoint clearly and persistently.

There has always been the critisism that such groups however are not representative of the whole, and that the opinions and values researched and expressed by them reflect a mainly middle class, largely affluent strata of society, for example where home birth, water birth, and the increasing trend towards alternative therapies are concerned. Whilst this viewpoint has some validity, care must be taken not to deny the needs of that specific sample of the population, who although relatively privileged still have care needs which must be recognised. Changes in attitude towards considering the consumer viewpoint, seeking to improve communications and asking a client what she wishes for her pregnancy is applicable to all and would not have come about without such consumer pressure.

In assessing the place of user groups in relation to empowering childbearers, the Association of Radical Midwives should not be forgotten. Although not a user group as such, this National movement originated in 1976 to provide support for student midwives. Espousing a similar philosophy to other groups in seeking respect, autonomy and choice for women, the Association can also be considered influential in shaping policy development through its series of debates, discussions and publications most notably the 'Vision' a blueprint for the maternity services (Association of Radical Midwives, 1986; Sandall, 1995).

Part of the Association of Radical Midwives' philosophy is that with greater recognition of midwifery practice and autonomy of midwives, women too will benefit. Midwives would automatically seek to regard women as partners and disregard the hitherto unequal balance of power between the professional and the client.

INFLUENCES ON POLICY DEVELOPMENT FROM 1995

The most recent and influential report upon policy development in relation to the maternity services is that of the Expert Maternity Group *Changing Childbirth* (DoH, 1993). The group was established in response to the publication of the House of Commons Select Committee report on the maternity services, with a remit to review current NHS maternity care services and to make recommendations for change.

Whilst accounting for the views of expert panel members drawn from professional, voluntary and consumer groups, the report states that the wider issues related to childbearing such as nutrition, socio-economic factors, family planning, smoking and drug abuse were beyond their remit (DoH, 1993). As Sandall (1995) highlights, these issues greatly influence women's health, pregnancy outcome in relation to poverty and peri-natal mortality rates, and to disregard them also disregards the fact that approximately one-third of children are born into families on means-tested benefit. Rothwell (1996) suspects that there were larger political decisions involved in not examining these areas including resource implications.

However, those issues which the report does address as part of its remit are nonetheless important and relevant to all childbearing women. *Changing Childbirth* seeks to address those issues related to choice, continuity and control namely those listed in Box 4.1.

BOX 4.1	*Issues important to empowering women through maternity services*

- The woman must be the focus of maternity care, feel in control of what is happening to her and be able to make decisions about her care based on her needs, having discussed matters fully with the professionals involved.
- The maternity services must be readily and easily accessible to all. They should be sensitive to the needs of the local population and based primarily in the community.
- Women should be involved in the monitoring and planning of maternity services to ensure that they are responsive to the needs of a changing society.
- Care should be effective and resources used efficiently.

(Adapted from *The Challenge of Changing Childbirth*. ENB 1995)

With these issues in mind, ten indicators of success were suggested as guidelines to purchasers and providers of care. These indicators encompass the principles listed in Box 4.2.

BOX 4.2	*Nine indicators of success in providing maternity care within 5 years of implementation*

1. All women should be able to carry their own maternity notes.
2. All women should know one named midwife who will coordinate their midwifery care.
3. 30% of women admitted should do so under the lead management of the midwife.
4. Midwives should have direct access to some beds in all maternity units.
5. The total number of antenatal visits required in normal pregnancy should be reviewed.
6. Paramedic services should be available to support the midwife in instances where emergency transfer to hospital is deemed necessary.
7. There should be ease of access to information to all women regarding services available.
8. The midwife should be the lead professional for 30% of women.
9. 75% of women should know the person caring for them at delivery.
   (DoH, 1993).

Changing Childbirth has shadows of the *The Vision* (Association of Radical Midwives, 1986) within it, especially in relation to the implementation of midwifery-led care, group practices and the emphasis upon choice, communication and control. For the first time the notion of client centredness and empowerment of the consumer has emerged as a guiding principle for practice. The motivation for these initiatives to provide total woman-centred care would seem to be heavily influenced by the need to make efficient use of resources and providing a cheaper service. The risk of litigation which is ever increasing in the field, may also have served a large part of the impetus to provide choice, continuity and control than we would like to admit. It would seem almost that the recommendations of *Changing Childbirth* have the potential to enhance the part women play in their care, but to do so incidentally rather then directly. Initially there seems to be more to empower the midwife than her client within the *Changing Childbirth* report, but throughout comments are made upon the willingness of midwives to improve the service offered to women and it would seem that the spirit of the report is aligned to the spirit of midwifery. The inference is that in empowering midwives, those they care for are also empowered (Page, 1995). We have been provided with an ideal opportunity to revamp the service, an opportunity taken on board by every Trust, region and district in England who commenced their 5-year strategy for development in 1994/1995.

Having examined, albeit briefly, the background to policy development, the role of user groups in informing new policy and the current influence upon policy development, it may now be pertinent to examine in more depth some of the issues offered as solutions to the notion of health promotion in the maternity services through the empowerment of its clients. Those issues chosen for examination are the concept of choice, the use of communication skills, education and the appropriate use of technology.

USE OF COMMUNICATION SKILLS

A consistent thread throughout the recommendations of the Expert Maternity Group (DoH, 1993) is the emphasis which is placed upon the midwife/client relationship. Studies have highlighted the importance of this relationship and its potential to influence the quality of care, the outcome of labour and the woman's memories of childbirth for years afterwards (Flint, 1993). The most recent Confidential Enquiry into Sudden Deaths in Infancy recommends communication skills training for all professionals, citing poor communication between professional and client as a contributing factor to the avoidable infant deaths in its final report (DoH, 1993). The current author personally feels that good communication between the two is the gateway to a solid foundation of understanding and a true sense of rapport. This foundation can then be used to plan care together offering real choices, seeking informed consent and as continuing trust develops, increasing satisfaction for all.

This type of working partnership undoubtedly requires the use of good communication skills, something which midwives generally have been critsised for in the past. Kirkham (1989) described the manner in which midwives give information in labour. The outcome of this study related to the ways women tactically glean information from midwives using a variety of methods such as self-denigration, eavesdropping and humour. Kirkham also observed a number of midwifery tactics used to avoid answering questions such as changing the subject, ignoring the question or providing blanket reassurance. Hunt and Symmonds (1995) described an emergent theme from an ethnographic study of labour ward practice related to midwives devaluing the opinions, previous knowledge and experiences of the women they cared for. This attitude was explained as the midwives' means of maintaining control. Oakley (1980) also observed that women's own knowledge of what was happening to their bodies was largely disregarded by the experts, especially in relation to the dating of pregnancy and the description of symptoms which were largely ignored.

Women may inadvertently collude with this behaviour as a direct result of the disempowering effects of the childbearing experience and this was demonstrated by Bluff and Holloway (1994), who observed 11 women during their contact with the maternity services. The women observed trusted the midwives' expertise, even when they did not fully understand the basis for the care they were given. A currently ongoing and small study of the manner in which midwives seek to develop relationships and open communication pathways with their clients indicates that if the clients seem uninterested in themselves and are not inclined to develop a relationship with the midwife, then this has a demotivating effect upon the midwife's desire to keep trying. There is a feeling emerging that from the midwive's perspective many of their clients do not make a effort to communicate with them (McLoughlin, 1997). Notably these women come from areas of high unemployment, with large numbers recieving income support and for whom English is not their first language. Such a pattern of communication then becomes cyclical and no matter how much we espouse the notions of clients' centredness and a desire to empower women in accepting responsibility for their own care, this will not be achievable. One way perhaps of breaking this cycle is to increase the amount and level of communications skills training within midwifery and nursing programmes of education.

ISSUES OF INFORMATION AND CHOICE

Much has been spoken of the need to respect the autonomy and rights of the mother in order to empower her during the childbirth experience. It is recognised that midwives and obstetricians also have a responsibility to the unborn. Conflicts may arise when, in the name of informed choice and woman-centred care maternal wishes have a negative effect upon the health or the very existence of the child. This may be evident in the desire of a woman to continue the use of nicotine during pregnancy, or to undertake selective fetal reduction in the case of multiple pregnancy. Additionally, what becomes of those women whom we seek to empower and who choose not to let us do so? Such women are labelled as being 'difficult' or 'persistent non-attenders with 'social problems' and the wrong sort of attitude. Caring professionals may reserve the right to approach women and offer to assist those they can. However, it would seem to be the ultimate example of empowerment for a woman to request the use of the service as and when she feel she needs it rather than only when the professionals determine that she should. The difficulty lies in the fact that non-conformist behaviour disrupts the system and individualised care by its very definition does away with the concept of a standard 'normal' type of woman. Childbearing is unique in that by providing care for the mother, care is also provided for the unborn child and however much a woman wishes to exert her right to opt out of care this provides us with ethical difficulties when considering the infant although in the UK the fetus has no status in law (Dimond, 1993).

In some instances, fetal rights and empowerment have taken precedent over those of the mother. In the USA a woman may face criminal charges regarding health behaviours considered to be neglectful of the developing fetus (MacReady, 1996) and cases have been reported in the UK where women faced undue pressure to have Caesarian sections despite expressing a strong desire not to (Dimond, 1993; Kenny, 1996), and despite the fact that the absolute right to decide on treatment rests with the mother. Similar pressures have also been brought to bear upon women in relation to the uptake of screening tests. Evidence exists that women may be offered procedures such as amniocentesis on the understanding that they would opt for termination of pregnancy should the fetus be diagnosed as having an abnormality (Stacey, 1988).

Part of the solution is to provide enough information to empower the woman to make an informed choice about her care, and to enable her to select from a range of services. This may be concerned with discussing the place of birth, analgesia or screening for example. This timely information exchange relies upon the relationship between the information giver and the woman, incorporating the need for good communication between both. It is also reliant upon ease of access to such information. This raises issues concerned with service provision and its uptake, and is particularly relevant to those groups who traditionally under-use the maternity services, for example adolescent mothers, women from lower socio-economic groups, or women for whom English is not their first language. Within the confines of these groups, those who may attend may be unable to make full use of the services due to the disempowering effect of their situation, and because the service was originally established for a client group which was more closely aligned to the social norm. As Rothwell (1996) discusses, the *Changing Childbirth* document, in its initial acknowledgement that social issues were not within its remit, dismisses the needs of women from vulnerable groups. She suggests that midwifery is thus firmly placed within the medical domain and ignores the complex social issues and climate within which the majority of midwives work. Until such issues are directly addressed the concept of empowerment through informed choice appears to be something of a platitude.

Additionally, by using information, education and choice as a means to empower maternity service users, an assumption is made that all areas provide the same standard and range of services. Attempting to provide choice in this way has great financial costs implications for service providers (Roberts, 1996) and emotional costs for midwives and women seeking a service which a hospital or community trust may not make available (Dimond, 1995).

Even in the context of a full, flexible range of alternatives available, the professionals providing the information are required to have suitably up-to-date information and skills. This includes all professionals involved, not just midwives but obstetricians and GPs too. Again this is not easily achievable and wide discrepancies have been highlighted in the quality of information, bias in its delivery and whether it is consistently reinforced by all team members. This may best be illustrated in the arena of pre-natal testing where some procedures may not be wholly reliable, or there is insufficient time and professional skill to impart accurate, pertinent information (Kuba, 1995; Rosser, 1996).

We should not assume that only professionals have an influence upon a woman's knowledge base; there is an element of social support for most women from whom they obtain knowledge and who may influence their decisions. This has been referred to as 'social support' and has been defined by Thoits (1986) as consisting of two main components: expressive and instrumental support. Expressive support encompasses concepts such as sympathy, empathy, understanding and acting as confidante, whilst instrumental support takes the form of information giving, supplying advice and material aid (Thoits, 1986). Koniak-Griffin (1993) identified that social support of an informal and formal nature are of importance in successfully attaining the transition to motherhood and in developing confidence and buffering stress. Such support was also identified by Norbeck (1981) as being spontaneous and forthcoming from family and friends who undoubtedly would bring with them their own network of advice and information. Such information may include beliefs regarding regulating nutrition during pregnancy, spacing of pregnancies, umbilical cord care, medication and help to be given during pregnancy (Mead and Newton, 1967). This network of information being referred to by MacIntyre (1982) commenting that women had potential access to 'a considerable body of information and advice about pregnancy and childbearing from friends and relatives, specialist advice literature and women's magazines, television programmes and the NHS or NCT preparation classes.'

A study examining mothers' views about information and advice in pregnancy and childbirth conducted by Jacoby in 1988 examined a random sample of 1508 women. Of these, 628 were having their first baby and they most frequently mentioned books as their source of information about childbirth. Over half said they had attended antenatal preparation classes and over three-quarters had discussed the birth with their partners. A total of 60% had had discussions with their mother, another pregnant woman or a friend. What was most apparrant was that discussions with health professionals were less frequent (43%). Groups less likely to discuss childbirth with their mothers or friends and who were most likely to receive less information from health professionals were single women or those from minority ethnic groups (Jacoby, 1988). Interestingly, it is again the least empowered groups who seem to be further disadvantaged. In terms of empowering women and assisting them to make informed choices about their care, pregnancy itself seems to have a beneficial effect. The experience of childbirth would appear to convey knowledge upon women on a par with that of professionals; this was most readily demonstrated in a small sample of women who more readily challenged care given in subsequent pregnancies (Cornwell, 1995). This finding supports earlier work by Parsons and Perkins (1980) and O'Brien and Smith (1981), who both identified a similar group of women who do not attend for antenatal care. Parsons and Perkins (1980) called this group the 'competent childbearers' – they did not attend for care because they had had a baby before successfully and did not feel it was necessary. This finding reflects upon the point made earlier about empowerment and how users of the service may utilise the service when it pleases them to, rather than at the behest of the professionals involved.

It would seem then that women obtain information both on a formal and informal basis and that informal sources are readily available and used. There is little evidence regarding the exact nature of information exchanged informally and whether it serves to empower women. However there is a plethora of evidence expressing women's dissatisfaction with the information they receive from formal health care sources. This related particularly to postnatal care where conflicting professional advice about breastfeeding and baby care has caused confusion amongst mothers, and to antenatal care where the impersonal manner, minimal amount and poor quality of information imparted has left women feeling doubtful about its usefulness rather than equipping them to make informed decisions (Garcia, 1982; Reid and Garcia, 1989).

INITIATIVES FOR CHANGE

The evidence presented so far illustrates that the concept of empowerment with maternity service provision is complex and there would seem to be many pitfalls along the way. Whilst there are many areas of the maternity service which are justifiably open to criticism, there are many initiatives being undertaken at national and local level to attempt to address and improve the situation.

Amongst one of the first notable schemes was the 'Know Your Midwife Scheme' piloted in the 1980s (Flint, 1993). This scheme introduced the concept of team midwifery, continuant and consumer-orientated care. Midwives and mothers expressed greater levels of satisfaction with the 'Know Your Midwife' scheme and it would seem to be the forerunner for developments of team-based and case-load practice since that time.

Changing Childbirth has continued with the theme of continuity of care, emphasising that maternity service provision should be community orientated and that midwives work in small teams to facilitate this. Many areas are developing team or group midwifery practices but not without difficulties. The Royal College of Midwives (1996) has identified problems in making such schemes workable. These relate to the unstructured and long working hours accompanied by increased stress and burdens of responsibility for midwives who also face a flatter career structure with fewer opportunities for promotion.

Pilot schemes face funding difficulties either through a lack of new monies to resource new projects, or through the withdrawal of funding at the last moment by reticent purchasing authorities (Royal College of Midwives, 1996).

There are many successful examples of initiatives undertaken to bring the promise of *Changing Childbirth* to life. Such examples are documented in the midwifery press and include those initiatives funded originally by the *Changing Childbirth* implementation team (Jackson, 1995). In June 1994, 14 projects were awarded funds to support the initiatives of *Changing Childbirth*. They were country wide and were selected on the basis that they would serve as sources of information useful to others within the service. Evaluation methods were incorporated into each project which covered the areas listed in Box 4.3 (ENB, 1995):

BOX 4.3	*Areas covered in the projects arising from Changing Childbirth initiatives*

1. Developing a maternity bus in Bradford to provide mobile maternity services
2. Providing parenthood education for local schools in Horton
3. Improving access to information and choice in specialist areas such as non-English speaking women
4. Women with complicated pregnancy
5. Supporting GPs who wished to be involved in home deliveries.

Many of these initiatives are service led. There only seemed to be one in Greater London which indicated that it came directly from consumer groups, that being the Greater London Association of Community Health Councils' initiative to support lay members of the Maternity Services Liaison Committee.

Within the midwifery press, information appears about successful projects outlining how they were set up and evaluated. Such evaluation generally appears to incorporate health outcome measures as well as expressed levels of satisfaction. Much focus is placed upon establishing schemes and the effects of change upon the working practices of the midwives involved and there does seem to be an air of wanting to share experiences and learn how to improve the service (Hauxwell and Tanner, 1994; ENB, 1995; Lewis, 1995 a & d; Walker J, 1996; Royal College of Midwives, 1996). There is slightly less information about the effects of change upon the clients involved and how they manage change in relation to new demands made of them. It has been acknowledged that to empower women we need to educate them to take responsibility for their own decisions (Schott, 1994); this is something which the current author forsees as a major cultural change in the client role.

Various means of assisting this change have been undertaken, most notably in the form of leaflets providing information for mothers and midwives alike, e.g. the Midwives Information and Resource Service (MIDIRS) Midwifery Digest 'informed choice' leaflets, or 'how to get the best from the maternity services' leaflets. Additionally the trend for women to carry their own case notes and actively participate in care planning potentially makes them more autonomous. However, such initiatives also rely upon communication and literacy skills and for those who are disadvantaged in either respect, the onus is again laid at the midwife's door to seek suitable assistance. There is some doubt as to the effectiveness of birth plans and case notes as tools for empowerment. Concern arises when expectations remain unfulfilled as a result of unforseen emergency events, a lack of available choices or non-adherence to the planned care (Too, 1996a, 1996b; Moore and Hopper, 1995; Waters, 1996).

Independent midwifery practice represents the ideal opportunity to provide all the elements of good communication, choice and continuity but independent midwives are few and far between. Thus there is unequal access to this service, both for women who cannot afford to use the service and for midwives who would wish to practice in this way but for whom the indemnity insurance costs remain prohibitive.

The problem remains in attempting to address this vast complexity of issues (not all of which have been addressed here), of finding a model of health promotion which facilitates women in retaining control of decisions about their lifestyle and care during pregnancy. This latter aspect the current author has found hard to address. Whilst acknowledging her role as an empowerer, educator and health promoter, she like many other midwives is unsure as to how to best 'promote health'.

It would seem that the areas discussed in relation to empowering women focus upon informed choice, decision-making skills, and utilising the relationship between the client and the midwife. Any chosen model of health promotion would also need to incorporate aspects related to change management and, education whilst acknowledging lay concepts and knowledge of pregnancy. Does such a model exist?

Health promotion is commonly regarded as the prevention of ill health and disease and the increase of a sense of well-being (Kemm and Close, 1995). The two former, ill health and disease are not always directly applicable to midwifery, which is for the majority of women a normal life-changing event. If one accepts the intrinsic normality of pregnancy, then a medical model of health promotion may not be appropriate.

Some of the other approaches to health promotion as described by Ewles and Simnet (1992) are on a simplistic level more applicable, e.g. the educational, holistic, client centred or behavioural approaches, and are within the scope of daily midwifery practice.

Changing Childbirth as a policy document would seem to have adopted a multiplicity of approaches, incorporating recommendations for societal and client centred change. Concerns still remain regarding women and families who are unable to take on board health education information, or who are contented as they are without wishing to change. This is particularly relevant in relation to nicotine, alcohol and recreational drug use or the use of contraception.

In the ideal situation women would seek pre-conceptual care, with the opportunity to discuss lifestyle, options for delivery, care planning and screening long before a pregnancy is embarked upon. This would require major input into the provision of pre-conceptual services and another cultural change in raising the profile of health promotion with regard to maternity service provision. We do not live in an ideal world and the pressures of surviving within it on a daily basis suggest to me that health promotion activity is not viewed as a priority by midwives or by the women they care for. As health promoters, midwives need to be reawakened to their responsibilities, and that they need sound education to assist them in promoting health, supporting women and in challenging them appropriately when neccessary. Midwives may currently be fearful of disrupting the relationship between themselves and their client when giving health promotion advice. Colleagues have spoken to me of the 'tightrope' that is walked when discussing issues such a smoking behaviour, breastfeeding or adolescent pregnancy. They are anxious to give appropriate support without alienating a woman who needs continued maternity service care for months ahead (McLoughlin, 1997).

CONCLUSION

The messages we receive are that choice, continuity and control will sufficiently revolutionise current midwifery practice and create a happier, healthier child-bearing population (DoH, 1993).

This is not enough. We have to recognise the value and worth of each individual and yes, provide the magical three 'C's but not because the latest government policy has told us to in an effort to streamline the service and increase cost efficiency, nor because it is pleasing to our professional ears to be told that the midwife should be the lead professional for at least 70% of clients. To successfully empower women takes a great deal of skill and expertise. It also demands a shift in the balance of power in the midwife – client relationship. To fully implement the recommendations of *Changing Childbirth*, we need to encourage women to utilise the maternity services in a new and innovative way. We must also re-educate ourselves to view women differently, to really value their individuality, culture, opinions and personhood. These principles are documented in many unit policies and philosophies of care, and spoken of in many job interview scenarios. Empowerment is about converting words into action and really believing in ourselves and each other. As Kroll (1996) states 'midwives can provide the efficient and personalised service that is central to the new National Health Service reforms'. She advocates that midwives become part of the means of assessing and responding to community needs in relation to pregnancy care. Midwives should then adapt care to suit the assessed needs of an ever-changing population rather than provide care based upon the secure but complacent basis of custom and practice. When the client is at the centre of our motivation then we begin to truly empower her.

REFERENCES

Abbott, P. & Wallace, C. (1990) *The Sociology of the Caring Professions*. Ch. 2 pp. 18–20 London: Falmer.

Association of Radical Midwives. (1986) *The Vision – proposals for the Future of the Maternity Services*. Ormskirk: Association of Radical Midwives.

Bluff, R. & Care Holloway, I. (1994) 'They know best': women's perceptions of midwifery during labour and childbirth. *Midwifery*, 10: 157–164.

Churchill, H. (1995) The conflict between lay and professional views of labour. *Nursing Times*, 91(42): 32–33.

Cornwell, J. (1995) Hard earned lives: experience of doctors and health services.

In *Health and Disease: A Reader*. eds Davey, B., Gray, A. & Seale, C. pp. 115–118 London: Open University.

Department of Health and Social Security (DHSS). (1970) *Domiciliary Midwifery and Maternity Bed Needs: Report of the Sub-Committee*, Peel Report. Standing Maternity Advisory Committee, London: HMSO.

Department of Health (DoH) (1993) *Changing Childbirth: Part One and Two*, Report of the Expert Maternity Group. London: HMSO.

Department of Health (DoH) (1995) *Confidential Enquiry into Stillbirths and Deaths in Infancy* (CESDI) 3rd Annual

Report. 1 Jan–31 Dec, 1994. London: HMSO.

Dimond, B. (1993) Rights for whom? *Modern Midwife*, 3(6): 18–19.

Dimond, B. (1995) Trusting midwives. *Health Professional Digest*, 9: 4–6.

Donnisson, J. (1977) *Midwives and Medical Men: a History of Interprofessional Rivalries and Women's Rights*. London: Heinemann.

Durward, L. & Evans, R. (1990) Pressure groups and the maternity services. In *The Politics of Maternity Care*. Garcia, J., Kirpatrick, R. & Richards, M. eds Ch 14 pp 256–273. Oxford: Clarendon.

English National Board (ENB) (1995) 'The Challenge of Changing Childbirth'. A Midwifery Educational Resource Pack. London: ENB.

Ewles, K. & Simnet, A. (1992) *Promoting Health: A Practical Guide*. London: Scutari.

Flint, C. (1993) *Midwifery Teams and Caseloads*. London: Butterworth Heinemann.

Garcia, J. (1982) Women's views of antenatal care. In *Effectiveness and Satisfaction with Antenatal Care*, eds Enkin, M. & Chalmers, I. London: Heinemann.

Hauxwell, B. & Tanner, S. (1994) Developing an integrated midwifery service. *British Journal of Midwifery*, 2(1): 33–36.

Houldsworth, A. (1988) *Out of The Doll's House*. London: BBC.

Hunt, S. & Symmonds, A. (1995) *The Social Meaning of Midwifery*. Ch. 5, pp. 92–95. London: MacMillan.

Jackson, K. (1995) Changing childbirth. The work of the implementation team. In: English National Board, *The Challenge of Changing Childbirth*: a Midwifery Education Resource Pack, 4(6): pp 53–60 London: ENB.

Jacoby, A. (1988) Mothers views about information and advice in pregnancy and childbirth findings from a national study. *Midwifery*, 4: 103–110.

Kemm, J. & Close, A. (1995) *Health Promotion Theory and Practice*. Chs 1&2. London: Macmillan.

Kenny, C. (1996) Against her judgement. *Nursing Times*, 92(41): 16–17.

Kirkham, M. (1989) Midwives and information giving during labour. In *Midwives Research and Childbirth*, eds Robinson, S. & Thomson, A. Vol 1 pp 176–188. London: Chapman & Hall.

Kitzinger, J. (1990) Strategies of the Early Childbirth Movement: A Case Study of The National Childbirth Trust. In *The Politics of Maternity Care*, eds Garcia, J., Kirkpatrick & R., Richards, M. Ch. 5, Oxford: Clarendon.

Koniak-Griffin, D. (1993) Maternal Role Attainment. *IMAGE Journal of Nursing Scholarship*, 25(3): 257–261.

Kroll, D. (1996) Working for women: assessing needs, planning care. In *Midwifery Care for the Future Meeting the Challenge*. ed. Kroll, D. pp. 1–22. London: Ballière Tindall.

Kuba, L.M. (1995) The prenatal testing roller coaster: one mother's story. *Journal of Perinatal Education*, 4(4): 19–22.

Leap, N. & Hunter, B. (1993) *The Midwife's Tale: An Oral History From Handy Woman to Professional Midwife*. Ch. 1, pp. 1–18. London: Scarlet.

Lewis, P. (1995a) Developing a group practice approach to care. *MIDIRS Midwifery Digest*, 5(1): 104–108.

Lewis, P. (1995b) Refining the model-group practice midwifery. *MIDIRS Midwifery Digest*, 5(2): 219–223.

Lewis, P. (1995c) Group practice-moving the vision on. *MIDIRS Midwifery Digest*, 5(3): 353–356.

Lewis, P. (1995d) Group practice midwifery – a time for reflection. *MIDIRS Midwifery Digest*, 5(4): 475–478.

MacIntyre, S. (1982) Communications between pregnant women and their medical and midwifery birth attendants. *Midwives Chronicle*, November. 387–394.

MacKay, L. (1990) Nursing: just another job? In *The Sociology of The Caring Professions*, eds Abbott, P. & Wallace, C. pp. 20–20. Hampshire: Falmer.

McLachlan, B.K. & Yeadon, D. (1996) Care of the critically ill woman. *MIDIRS Midwifery Digest*, 6(4): 449–450.

McLoughlin, A. (1997) Unpublished MSc Thesis. Ongoing study. Manchester Metropolitan University.

MacReady, N. (1996) Fetal homicide charge for drinking while pregnant. *British Medical Journal*, 313(7058): 645 (Extracts).

Mead, M. & Newton, N. (1967) Cultural patterning of perinatal behaviour. In *Childbearing: Its Social and Psychological Aspects* eds Richardson, S.A. & Gittmacher, A.F. pp. 1–22. Baltimore: Williams & Williams.

Ministry of Health (1959) *Report on the Maternity Services Committee*, Cranbrook Report. London: HMSO.

Moore, M. & Hopper, U. (1995) Do birth plans empower women? Evaluation of a hospital birth plan. *Birth*, 22(1): 29–35.

Newburn, M. & Hutton, E. (1996) Women and midwives: turning the tide. In *Midwifery Care for The Future. Meeting the Challenge.* ed. Kroll, D. pp. 209–231. London: Ballière Tindall.

Norbeck, J. (1981) Social support; a model for clinical research and application. *Advances in Nursing Science*, **3**(4): 43–49.

Oakley, A. (1980) *Women Confined*, pp. 293–300. Oxford: Martin Robertson.

O'Brien, M. & Smith, C. (1981) Women's views and expectations of antenatal care. *Practitioner*, **225**: 123–126.

Page, L. (1995) A vision for the future. In English National Board, *The Challenge of Changing Childbirth*, 7–16. London: ENB.

Parsons, W. & Perkins, E. (1980) Why Don't Women Attend for Antenatal Care? *Leverhulme Health Educational Production.* Occasional Paper No 23, University of Nottingham.

Reid, M. & Garcia, J. (1989) Women's views of effective care during pregnancy and childbirth. In *Effective Care in Pregnancy and Childbirth*, eds Chalmers, I., Enkin, C.M. & Kierse, M.J.N.C. Vol 1, pp. 131–142 Oxford: Oxford University Press.

Roberts, J. (1996) Changing childbirth – choices and costs. *MIDIRS Midwifery Digest*, **6**(3): 261–263.

Rosser, J. (1996) Towards informed decisions about prenatal testing: a review. *MIDIRS Midwifery Digest*, **6**(2): 162–163.

Rothman, B.K. (1996) Women, providers and control. *Journal of Obstetric, Gynaecologic and Neonatal Nursing*, **25**(3): 253–256.

Rothwell, H. (1996) Changing childbirth – changing nothing. *Midwives*, **109**(1306): 291–294.

Royal College of Midwives. (1996) *Woman Centered Care Supplement*. No 3, October.

Sandall, J. (1995) Choice, Continuity and Control: Changing Midwifery, Towards a Sociological Perspective. *Midwifery*, **11**: 201–209.

Schott, J. (1994) The importance of encouraging women to think for themselves. *British Journal of Midwifery*, **2**(1): 3–4.

Silverton, L. (1995) Professional empowerment. In *Changing Childbirth: An Educational Resource Pack for Midwives.* No 2. London: ENB.

Social Services Committee (1980) *Perinatal and Neonatal Mortality.* Second Report. London: HMSO.

Stacey, M. (1988) *The Sociology of Health and Healing.* London: Unwin Hyman.

Tew, M. (1990) *Safer Childbirth? A Critical History of Maternity Care.* Ch. 1, pp. 1–37 London: Chapman and Hall.

Thoits, P. (1986) Social support as coping assistance. *Journal of Consulting and Clinical Psychology*, **54**(4): 416–423.

Tong, R. (1989) *Feminist Thought.* Chs 1&2. London: Unwin Hyman.

Too, S. (1996a) Do birthplans empower women? A study of their views. *Nursing Standard*, **10**(31): 33–37.

Too, S. (1996b) Do birth plans empower women? A study of midwives' views. *Nursing Standard*, **10**(32): 44–48.

United Kingdom Central Council for Nursing, Midwifery and Health Visiting (UKCC) (1992) *The Scope of Professional Practice.* London: UKCC.

United Kingdom Central Council for Nursing, Midwifery and Health Visiting (UKCC) (1993) *Midwives Rules.* London: UKCC.

United Kingdom Central Council for Nursing, Midwifery and Health Visiting (UKCC) (1994) *The Midwife's Code of Practice.* London: UKCC.

Walker, I. (1996) Personal Communication Action on Pre-Eclampsia Study Day.

Walker, J. (1996) Interim Evaluation of a Midwifery Development Unit. *Midwives*, **109**(1305): 266–270.

Waters, J. (1996) High hopes. *Nursing Times*, **92**(42): 16–17, Reprinted in MIDIRS *Midwifery Digest*, **7**(1): 1997. pp 16–17.

FURTHER READING

Audit Commission (1997) *First Class Delivery: Improving Maternity Services in England and Wales.* London: Audit Commission.

Buckley, E.R. (1997) *Delivering Quality in Midwifery.* London: Ballière Tindall.

Department of Health (DoH) (1998) *Midwifery: Delivering Our Future*. Report by Standing Nursing and Midwifery Advisory Committee. London: HMSO.

English National Board (ENB) (1995) *The Challenge of Changing Childbirth: A Midwifery Educational Resource Pack*. London: ENB.

Teenage pregnancy

Karen Dignan

INTRODUCTION

Teenage pregnancy should be the concern of every health professional whose sphere of practice it touches. The concerns are not just limited to the health and welfare of the teenager and the subsequent baby, but there are concerns in relation to a wider agenda which incorporates social, psychological and educational considerations. It is the intention in this chapter to explore the reasons why there is still a consistent level of unintended pregnancies in the teen years and to offer a way forward through a multiprofessional approach in a dynamic and positive way. The author sees the development of a health empowerment model which will integrate all the interested agencies as the foundational block on which to build the type of multiservice that will be specifically designed in order to meet the needs of sexually aware and sexually active teenagers.

It is very alarming, but Britain must face up to the fact that it has the highest rate of teenage in western Europe (Andrews, 1997). There has been a decrease in the 16–19-years age group during the 1990s but unfortunately the under 16-year-olds have not mirrored the same trend (Office for National Statistics, 1996). This is a worrying situation when one considers that there is free availability of contraception from a number of sources which are accessible to these young people and easier access to abortion since the passing of the Abortion Act in 1974. It must be realised that teenage pregnancy is perhaps only a facet of the whole issue of teenagers and sexual activity. The earlier in terms of years that a person embarks upon sexual activity the greater their risk of sexual health problems. This statement applies to both young women and men. On the wider plane of sexual health there is an increase risk of sexually transmitted infections, such as genital warts (Dignan and Turnheim 1996), cervical cancer (Dignan, 1993; Kerr, 1995), human immunodeficiency virus (HIV) and acquired immuno deficiency syndrome (AIDS) (Cook, 1995). It is not only the physical health of these young people that suffer but there are also adverse educational, social and economic outcomes associated with teenage pregnancies (Wellings et al, 1996; Kiernan, 1995). So whose responsibility is it to educate these young adults about matters of a sexual nature? Is it the parents'; the schools' or is it the health professionals' responsibility? The author doubts if there is one easy single answer, but suggests that the way forward is to adopt a tripartite approach, with each approach feeding into the young person in the form of education, service provision, and support and counselling.

Teenage pregnancy may be a traumatic experience at whichever end of the teenage spectrum it occurs, however it has greater physical, social and psychological consequences when it happens to the under 16-year-olds. In the World Health Report (WHO, 1995) it stated that, maternal mortality rates for those girls aged between 15–19 years of age were double the rates at 20–24 years of age. An alarming and unacceptable statistic is that for those countries where it is culturally acceptable for the young girls to become mothers at an early age, some becoming mothers as young as 13 years of age, then the mortality rate is five times higher (WHO, 1995). In China, the average age for women becoming first time mothers is 23 years old and the benefits of delayed motherhood is demonstrated in their lower mortality statistics.

It is because of the worrying morbidity and mortality figures that concerns about the holistic effects upon the health of these teenagers that the Royal College of Obstetricians and Gynaecologists (1991) and the Government in their *Health of the Nation* document (DoH, 1992b) expressed concerns. The government has set as one of the targets in the document that by the year 2000 there should be a 50% reduction in conceptions in the under 16s. The *Health of the Nation* document highlighted sexual health as one of the key areas where most benefit would be achieved in terms of delaying sexual activity in the young, reducing the number of teenage conceptions and promoting safer sexual practices. This aspect was further highlighted on *Our Healthier Nation* Consultation Paper (DoH, 1998). It is strikingly clear that it is too serious a problem for the individual agency to tackle, but one which requires a firm public policy and multi-agency approach if a positive strategy to this serious situation is to be achieved and effective. The avenue to pursue would be one of community participation and intercollaboration between the relevant health professional, educational and government representatives.

FACTORS TO BE CONSIDERED

The problems associated with teenage pregnancy are many and may be grouped into spheres which interlink. The inter-relating spheres, can be categorised into the physical, educational, social and psychological aspects all of which may have an effect upon the holistic health of the young adolescent. The extent to which these factors may affect the young girl will vary depending on her age, that is whether she is under or over 16 years of age when conception occurs. The girl who is under 16 years old will have very different needs than those of a girl who is 17 years of age. This is because the associated factors differ according to which end of the teenage spectrum the girl is at.

INTER-RELATED SPHERES

Physical considerations

Pregnant teenagers are at risk from medical and obstetric problems such as pregnancy-induced hypertension (Creatsas, 1995), a low birth weight infant (Doyle, 1992), or a pre-term delivery, all of which have a detrimental effect upon the fetus that she is carrying. The physical complications that the young teenager may suffer often has a detrimental effect upon the ultimate outcome in terms of mortality and morbidity.

Social considerations

There is now recognition of the role that society plays in relation to health and this is very evident when looking at the social factors which may have an influence upon teenage pregnancy rates. Teenage pregnancy rates are higher in areas where there is social deprivation (Smith, 1993). This again underlines the class differences in terms of the health arena. Poor housing, poverty and lack of social skills are all considerations to be borne in mind as contributing factors that will have a damaging effect not only upon the pregnant teenager but also the subsequent infant.

Educational considerations

The girl who is under 16 years old by law has to attend mainstream education, and this in itself may present difficulties. The school may request that the girl, once pregnancy is confirmed and evident, leaves and attends a special school for pregnant teenagers where peer support and special educational needs are met. This can be a most valuable service for several reasons. It provides a peer-support network for the girl and helps her to realise that she is not alone, it educates her in aspects of baby care skills as well as providing main educational curricula subjects and provides access to a midwife with whom a continuous and trusting relationship may be formed (DoH, 1992a). These are all positive considerations from the health professionals' and the educationalists' viewpoint. However, the young girl may view it entirely differently. She may not wish to be parted from her already established peer network, the move may be viewed as differentiating her from her peers and therefore emphasising the negative aspect of her situation. She may see it as further highlighting the differences between her and an older teenager who is pregnant.

Psychological considerations

The psychological considerations for a pregnant teenagers are considerable as there is a great deal of readjustment taking place. The girl may feel that she is shunted through her adolescent years into adulthood because of the pregnancy and quite understandably may feel that she has missed out on the adolescent phase of her life (Hudson and Ineichen, 1995). The adolescent years are particularly important for the development of self-esteem and self-awareness and in which body image plays an important part. The physical body changes that occur during pregnancy, such as enlarged breasts with visible veins and the growing abdominal size accompanied by the increase in weight may be viewed in a negative light. This is particularly true within Western society, where the ideal image seems to be one of slenderness. There is also the role change from being a free and single young girl to being a mother, responsible for her baby's well-being and care, the enormity of which may not be fully appreciated.

The physical, social, educational and psychological factors mentioned above are only a small part of the whole picture in relation to teenage pregnancy. It is important that all factors which affect the teenager are dealt with appropriately and these factors will differ from one person to another. This is where the tripartite approach may begin, with the education system, the health service and hopefully the support of the parents – or is it? The tripartite approach may be more evident in some areas of the country than in others. The special educational facility may not be available in some parts of the country but the service of a home tutor will be organised to provide private tuition to the girl in her own home but at a considerable financial cost to the educational system. This situation may sound very good educationally with the provision of one-to-one teaching. However, this situation can be isolating and depressing for the girl and may confirm the fact that she is viewed as being different. It can also entrench the idea that she is the only girl to become pregnant at this age and therefore she is often reluctant and fails to attend antenatal and parentcraft classes, and is denied access to the services that she will find most valuable in the days ahead. The relationship with the midwives is one that should start as soon as possible in order for the special relationship to be formed and for the trust of the girl to be gained. The teachers employed in teaching these girls often have contact with the maternity services and therefore collaboration between the two professions is fostered. The total support of the parents for the girl is crucial and should be cultivated by the teachers, midwives and the girl herself. It is rare in this day and age that a girl in this situation is made an outcast of her family due to the more liberal view of sex outside of marriage and the continuation of bringing up of the baby outside wedlock. The working together of all the concerned parties will achieve a more positive outcome for both the teenage mother and her baby.

There may be the legal position to consider if the girl is under the legal age of consent for sexual intercourse. In the eyes of the Law, the male responsible for the pregnancy has committed an offence for which he can be prosecuted; however this situation does not often materialise due to reluctance on the part of the girl to pursue this option.

The financial situation is obviously an important one when dealing with a minor. Financially the girl under the age of 16 is not entitled to State benefits as she is still a minor under parental responsibility and benefits can only be claimed for by the girl's parents or guardian. The financial cost of acquiring the necessary equipment, such as a pram, nursery equipment and clothes for the baby can be astronomical, even if good quality second-hand equipment is acquired. The ongoing costs continue for a good many years.

The older teenager is in many ways in a better position. The older girl may have a steady relationship in which marriage or cohabitation may be an option embarked upon. She may also be in paid employment, which depending on how long that employment has been in existence may mean that she is entitled to maternity leave with the option of returning to paid employment after the baby's birth. By Law she is able to claim state benefits on her own behalf and the male is not deemed to have committed an offence unless conception was achieved after a rape offence took place.

Why then do teenage girls still become pregnant when there is freely and readily available contraception? Again this is not an easy question to answer because there are so many reasons cited as to why untimely conceptions still occur. In our Western society, girls as young as 9 years of age are menstruating due to a generally improved nutritional state. Physically these young girls are able to menstruate, but ovulation may not materialise for some time after. Emotionally and psychologically they are far from ready to understand the implications of the messages that their bodies are sending out to them. In today's society, religion plays less of an important and influential role, which could be seen to lead to a decline in moral standards (Cook, 1995). This may be an influencing factor in the increase and early sexual activity embarked upon by the physically able young girls. The lack of full understanding of the maturing process which is taking place in these young people's bodies and their lack of knowledge about contraception and how to access the service no doubt play a very influential part in teenage sexual activity.

There are several other explanations offered as to why young girls become pregnant and sadly many are due to ignorance or the result of peer/boyfriend pressure. The schoolyard talk about sexual activity and how often girls have indulged in sexual intercourse without becoming pregnant, only serves to fuel the innocent girl's imagination and the fear that she is missing out on this wonderful experience. The girl then succumbs to sexual intercourse with the disappointing thought of: Was that it? The misnomer that you cannot conceive the first time is often when the most innocent of girls do.

Low self-esteem and low self-worth is often a reason for teenage girls to become mothers. This is perhaps one of the saddest reasons given. The girl may have little educational achievements, making employment less of a likelihood; this can then lead her into the cycle of little future prospects, which results in low self-esteem and low self-worth. Motherhood is seen as the answer to this because she will have a baby to love, and who she feels will love her and she will also have achieved the status of mother, making her, in her eyes, socially acceptable.

Konje et al (1992) conducted a retrospective study in Hull of 1548 pregnant teenagers under the age of 16. The purpose of the study was to discover the reasons why these young girls became pregnant and the most common reasons given are included in Box 5.1:

BOX 5.1	*Reasons for teenager's becoming pregnant*

1. Non-use of contraception
2. Overcrowded accommodation
3. Unstable home life
4. Lack of satisfaction at school
5. Their own mothers were teenagers when they first conceived.

This study further supports the need for a tripartite approach to the problems of teenage motherhood from the parents, the education system and the health care professionals. It is only through this approach that the cycle may be broken.

Whatever the reasons given as to why these young girls become pregnant with increasing regularity, there can be no doubt that the full implications of their actions are not considered or understood. These young girls do not envisage that they may actually become pregnant even if they are aware of the risk involved in not using contraception. They have little comprehension of what obstacles may lie ahead. These may range from obstetric complications to social and psychological difficulties in acceptance and adaptation to this often stressful situation.

COMPLICATIONS OF TEENAGE MOTHERHOOD

Adolescence is a time of transition from child to adult and it is not without its own stresses. To embark upon a pregnancy at this time, which in the majority of instances is unplanned, only further compounds the stresses endured by these young people. Often these young girls feel unable to confide in either their family or friends about the situation they find themselves in, which results in their being too advanced in the pregnancy for a termination should that be an option open to them. The girl will then continue with the pregnancy unsupported by family, friends or the health professional until the advanced stages of the pregnancy. The situation may continue until labour commences and the girl presents at the delivery suite or delivers the baby at home without the expert help of the midwife. This situation causes great distress for all concerned but particularly for the girl's parents, who have been totally unaware and therefore totally unprepared for their new role as grandparents. In this situation, the girl has had very little or no antenatal care and therefore no contact with the midwife, who is the prime care giver. The young girl will be totally unprepared for the stresses of labour, the degree of severity of pain that she may experience and the enormous responsibility that a new baby brings to her life.

In the case of the young woman who does present for antenatal care, this is often late and erratic. Parent education classes are not well attended by this young group of women, which results in their going into labour with little knowledge and preparation for what lies ahead in terms of labour options but also in the puerperium with respect to parenting skills. One of the most dangerous complications of pregnancy is pregnancy-induced hypertension, which is increased in frequency and severity in the young pregnant adolescent (Creatsas, 1995), which if antenatal care has not been attended for and the condition diagnosed, serious consequences may arise. Labour may be entered into in an anaemic state, with a pre-term or low birth weight baby or with all these complications. The mode of delivery might be expected to be by surgical intervention, however this is not the case according to Creatsas et al (1991) and vaginal delivery is the most achieved outcome. It must be remembered that all too often the babies of these young mothers are compromised through low birth weight or growth retardation, which makes the baby smaller than normal and therefore a vaginal delivery is often possible.

The psychological adaptation which is required by the young woman is tremendous. She has to come to terms with her change in role as she is no longer a single young woman with no responsibilities and often has the sole responsibility for providing the every need of this new baby. Coupled with this, as if adaptation to motherhood in the teen years is not enough to cope with, she also has the stage of adolescence to transit through. She has to adopt the role of mother very quickly with all too often little or no preparation. She will have been shunted through the transitionary phase of adolescence to womanhood with great speed which will not have allowed her time for adaptation or change. The true stark reality of motherhood is not as typically portrayed by the media, which the picture is often of a serene mother with a cherub looking contented baby. This in many cases is far from the truth with many of these young girls experiencing little support, financial deprivation and social isolation. These factors impinge upon her chances of providing a good stable environment in which to bring a baby up in. The stresses often felt by this young woman are transmitted to the baby which in turn responds by being a difficult baby to handle, which in turn increases the stresses felt by the young woman and so the cycle continues. The early weeks after delivery of the baby has been termed as the honeymoon period (Julian, 1983), but once the honeymoon period is over and support that was given withdrawn, then the realities of motherhood set in and the true realisation of the enormous responsibilities it brings. It is doubtful whether there is a mother out there who when asked will readily admit that the reality and responsibilities of being a mother cannot be fully appreciated until that status is achieved. Having to provide physical and emotional care in order to sustain and allow that very dependent human being to grow is an enormous responsibility. That is only one aspect to motherhood. It is coupled with the financial, social and educational responsibilities that are required in order to form this tiny human being into a member of society. All these aspects together are needed in order to provide the necessary skills for that baby to grow into an adult.

FUTURE DEVELOPMENTS

Teenage pregnancy has been brought to the fore in order to heighten people's awareness of the problems faced by the far reaching implications that this has upon the physical, emotional, psychological, social and educational spheres of a young girl's life. It is such a huge area of concern that it is not just the responsibility of one sector of professionals, it is a multifarious problem which requires a multiprofessional approach. So how can a multiprofessional approach be achieved in order to reduce the number of conceptions in the teen years but also improve the services for those who do unintentionally conceive? It is not possible, even with all involved parties concerned pulling together, to bring about the desired outcomes in a quick and dramatic style. It is a slow but forward process which may be viewed as a cause and effect situation. Perhaps the starting block is with those teenagers who are at this moment in time already pregnant. There is no doubt that the majority of pregnant teenagers either do not attend for antenatal care or if they do it is sporadic, so this chapter will now examine this service and perhaps refashion it so that it is an attractive option to these young people.

ANTENATAL CARE

The earlier these young pregnant teenagers attend for antenatal care the better the outcome in terms of reduced antenatal complications, improved neonatal outcome (Scally, 1993) and increased support from the health professional team. There is now an increasing number of units providing special antenatal clinics and parent education classes for this special group of women with positive outcomes. Antenatal clinics, where this special group of young women receive their antenatal care from the same team of midwives and other relevant health professionals, whether that be in a hospital setting, a general practitioners (GPs) surgery or on a one-to-one in the home, has proven to be of significant benefit (Dickson et al, 1997).

One very important aspect of antenatal care is the provision of parent education and this is perhaps a vital component of care in relation to these young people. Attendance at parent education classes by these young women has in the past been very poor, and this has been attributed to the low self-esteem felt by these young women (Michie, Marteau and Kidd, 1992). They have often felt stigmatised by the older women at these parent education classes who they feel may display judgmental attitudes towards them. This may also be the reason why attendance at antenatal clinics is so poor. However, changes in the way antenatal care and parent education classes are now delivered in a significant number of maternity units should be instrumental in increasing the attendance figures at both of these important services. Many maternity units are offering a special package of care for these young women, which includes providing special antenatal classes which are attended only by this client group and in which parent education is also included. Routine antenatal care is provided and any special needs are met on an individual basis.

The same team of midwives are responsible for providing this care and ensuring that referral to other professionals, such as the health visitor or the social worker is carried out. It is easier to provide the package of antenatal care and parent education as a full session for many reasons, such as because it requires less financial outlay for the young women, longer time as a group to form relationships and trust and it is often easier for the midwives to provide care in this comprehensive way. This special client group will have often very different fears and anxieties not only relating to the pregnancy, labour and the care of the baby after birth but also social and educational worries. It is because of these different identified needs that the way forward has not been from the top-down approach as described by Flick (1991), where professionals design a programme of education and have control over the content and delivery but with a bottom-up approach, where professionals and the clients plan and implement the programme of education that is designed to meet the needs of this young client group. This is the approach that has been adopted when trying to address the needs of the pregnant adolescent. The midwives work with the teenagers to provide a planned programme of education that they themselves have identified as being what they require. This is a new strategy that has been adopted in several institutions as a way of trying to address the problems associated with this minority, although increasing group. It is hoped by this collaboration the young women will feel empowered and therefore more positive about their situation. The boyfriends of the these young women, if they are still in contact with them are welcome to attend in order to offer support to their girlfriend and also to be educated themselves in relevant and important aspects relating to childbirth. If the male partner is not in contact, then whoever the pregnant teenager wishes to accompany her and be her support person are also encouraged to do so. If this support person is the client's mother, then this is often beneficial for her also. It serves the purpose of re-educating her in changes that have occurred in the whole area of childbirth and also it may help her to come to terms with the situation and her new changing role of grand-mother.

Education should be an interwoven thread throughout the whole strategy which is designed to promote and improve the health and care of this special client group. Education of the young in matters of sexual health should be of interest to every agent involved in the maturation process of these adolescents. The changes in social structure and moral views on matters of a sexual nature perhaps should alert the powers that be to the fact that the young do have a voice and an opinion on such important matters. The way forward is not to ignore their voices, but to work in harmony with them to provide information that is both accurate and sensitive to their needs. It is also important that people in positions of power and authority set the parameters for good behaviour, and this includes parents, teachers and health professionals. It is also important that respected people who are in positions where they are able to influence change are involved in the process. The organisation which springs to mind is the government ministers, because they are able to effect change and make policy decisions.

There are those who do not subscribe to the concept of educating the young in matters of a sexual nature for fear of robbing them of their childhood, which may in turn lead them to make adult decisions for which they are not ready. However, the National Union of Teachers in a recent pamphlet stated that:

> 'There exists a common myth that providing sex education for children will damage their innocence. All children have some sexual knowledge and children will learn about and hear about sex outside of the classroom. However, the danger is that much of the information they receive is misinterpreted and imprecise. This will happen whether or not schools have a policy and actively implement sex education.'

The influence that schools have as an institution plays a major role in shaping the health and lifestyle behaviours of the future generations. There is strong evidence, which should not be ignored, that states that providing sex and contraceptive education within the school environment does not lead to an increase in sexual activity or unplanned pregnancy (Peerman et al, 1996; Oakley, et al, 1995; Kirby, et al 1994; Frost and Forrest, 1995; Stout and Rivara, 1989) but does lead to empowering these young people to make responsible decisions. Careful thought and discussion with the relevant parties should be undertaken in order to provide this aspect of education at the most timely stage of not only the educational curricula but also the age of the young people. The optimum time would be before these young people began sexual activity of any kind and in that way sexual habits would not have developed. This is the time when they would be more receptive to this specialised educational programme, and no change in their behaviour would be required.

It is important to consider who is best able to deliver this specialist knowledge on sexual health matters. Is it the school teachers, the health professionals or is it neither of these and should it be tackled by the parents? It would appear that on the whole, parents are not the best able or equipped to discuss such sensitive and personal matters with their children because often they themselves are ignorant in such matters and also they frequently report feelings of embarrassment about such personal and sensitive matters. It is therefore left for the school teachers or the health professionals. It is also debatable whether or not the school teachers are themselves best able to provide this type of education for several reasons. The teachers are in a position of authority and therefore perhaps not seen as very approachable should a sensitive issue arise. They are also products of the organisation, which again in the young people's eyes gives them power, but they may not have the required skills to communicate to these young people on such intimate issues. That leaves the health professionals and perhaps these are the best equipped group to deliver this kind of information with the communication skills and knowledge required. The role of the school nurse has developed greatly over recent years but still perhaps the school nurse is not the most specialised professional to be involved in this aspect of education. The school nurse is still seen as part of the educational establishment and therefore perhaps not as approachable because of their status as a known figure. Midwives, family planning nurses and health visitors who have the knowledge and a special interest this topic area are probably the best able group to provide this service. A considerable advantage is that these health professionals are seen by these young people as being outsiders and therefore more approachable because of their impartiality and lack of personal knowledge about them as individuals. A pooling together by these health professionals of knowledge and resources in order to provide good quality sex education can be a powerful driving force in the forward strategy aimed at reducing teenage conceptions and increasing teenagers' knowledge in sexual health matters.

There have been positive strides made since 1992 when the EC Commission and the European Council in collaboration with the World Health Organization (WHO) launched a new project: the European Network of Health Promoting Schools. The aim of his project was to develop a network of schools committed to health promotion in as many European countries as possible while trying to link these national efforts in terms of close international cooperation. This innovative concept aims to put health firmly within the school curriculum and also to promote attitude and behavioural changes towards healthy practices. The WHO endorses a health promotion programme which involves other health-directed institutions, such as hospitals in endorsing primary health promotion and disease prevention.

Health related activities have been around the school curricula for some time now, however, the fairly new mainstream curricula is a recent development and one in which sex education is still not an actively seen thread. Because of the growing concerns regarding teenagers' sexual activity, there has been a review of the school curriculum in respect of how the issue of sexual health is addressed. Perhaps because schools are the institutions where adolescents meet on a regular basis with the purpose of increasing knowledge in various fields, it seems right and fitting that this institution should be a cornerstone for future development in sex education. It must however be recognised that schools are not without their limitations, such as limited time and teachers with the appropriate skills to deal with such a sensitive issue. Sex education in schools requires not only an increase in knowledge about such topics as contraception, sexuality and pregnancy but also requires a change in behaviour and attitude which is far more difficult to achieve and to measure. This situation is compounded by the age of these young people in whom adolescence and hormonal changes brings its own set of physical, psychological and emotional changes and adaptations.

The Education Bill with its recent amendments has created a degree of vacillation with regard to the future integration of sex education. Prior to the amendments under the terms of the 1986 Education Act (no. 2) responsibility for sex education rested with each school's governing body. Educational legislation introduced into England and Wales during the late 1980s had two main factors. It established central control of the curriculum but also devolved responsibility for management of individual schools. There was now opportunity at national level to take responsibility for establishing sex education within the educational curriculum. The department of education supported this theme allbeit a contentious one because it was caught up in traditionalist vs progressive arguments. There was also conflict between the schools and the parents. There is growing evidence that sexually active teenagers, unplanned pregnancies and early sexual activity needs to be tackled by a multiplicity of agencies in order to formulate an effective programme of sex education. Sex education is now a compulsory part of the curriculum in secondary schools, however parents do have the right to withdraw their child from these sessions on religious grounds.

In 1992, the Government recommended that sex education should be an integral part of the school curriculum. Whether the recommendation is taken up by the individual schools is largely dependent on the school governors and the parents and the teachers involved.

Europe still lags behind in carrying out substantial research studies on the effectiveness of sex education as compared with the USA. As far back as WHO (1976) and Lewin (1986), observations were made that most countries in the WHO European regions do implement to varying degrees sex education in schools, however, where the difficulty lies is in the fact that the resources in both time and money are not available to conduct a proper evaluation of the service provided. The USA is much better equipped at evaluating their programmes and this is an outcome of years of conflict that has been endured between the proponents and opponents of sex education.

The theory that including sex education in the school curriculum will only serve to encourage the young and often immature to indulge in practices that they are not totally ready for or feel at ease with yet, has not been proven (Stout and Rivara 1989, Eisen et al 1990). Earlier studies by McKillip et al (1984) and Braspenning et al (1987) observed an increase in young people's intention to use contraception after attending sex education lessons. This then demonstrates that sex education can be effective in reducing unplanned and untimely pregnancies by providing information and promoting effective and acceptable methods of contraception. Teenagers who had received sex education were much more likely to use effective contraception than those who had not. The argument put forward by opponents of sex education in schools is that it will encourage the young to participate in sexual activities appears to be unfounded.

The evidence put forward suggests that pregnancy rates and abortion rates are reduced, there is a delay in the timing of sexual onset and definitely an increase in the positive use of reliable and effective methods of contraception. There does appear to be overwhelming evidence to support the fact that sex education does empower these young people and has a positive effect upon knowledge, attitude and contraceptive use (Kirby et al 1994), which ultimately will lead to a decrease in conceptions, and therefore teenage pregnancies.

How can we empower these young individuals to enable them to take more control and have choices in their lives? This is not so easy to address but an attempt will be made to find a way through this tangled web of information, resources, policies, laws and interested parties. The two choice words here are 'enable' and 'control' and one leads on to the other, that is enabling somebody allows them to have control. Raymond Jack in his book *Empowerment in Community Care* (p11) states that: 'enablement is about developing a person's capabilities and this is a professional skill; and empowerment is about the struggle for power and control which is essentially a political activity.' Now as already stated earlier, to address the problem of teenage pregnancy requires a multi-agency approach which includes political investments.

THE EMPOWERMENT APPROACH

When one looks at how to enable these young teenagers to become empowered in order to take control and have a choice in their situation then the situation becomes a very complex one. There does however appear to be four factors which are fundamental to facilitating self-empowerment as listed in Box 5.2.

BOX 5.2	Basic elements affecting self-empowerment
	1. The environment, which can act as either a facilitator or a barrier to control 2. Skills possessed by the individual which enable them to overcome environmental barriers 3. Individual beliefs about the degree of control they have 4. Emotional traits, such as feelings of self-worth.

Wallerstein (1992) sees empowerment as an ecological construct that applies to interactive change on multiple levels: the individual, the organisation and the community. This view sits nicely with the empowerment of teenagers in issues around sexual health, because if headway is going to be made in this field, then the teenagers, the school, health services and the family as the community component must all interlink to help produce effective change.

The empowerment model seeks to increase the individual's ability to choose and to influence their environment (Kemm and Close, 1995) Its aim is to equip individuals with the skills and information that will give them power to take control of their own health. How better to develop these young people's sense of ownership and partnership in their own health but to enable them to become empowered. One of the essential ingredients of the empowerment approach is value clarification, that is helping people be clear about what they really want. By enabling adolescents to value themselves and to have information upon which to make informed choices, empowerment can be achieved.

Self-empowerment is a healthy state but in order to achieve that optimum state of health, other factors also play an instrumental role but may be viewed as coming under the umbrella of self-empowerment. These other spokes to the self-empowerment umbrella are self-worth, self-esteem and body image. These factors are aspects which are raised with great regularity in relation to the issue of teenagers and sexuality. Tones and Tilford (1995) suggest that a person who is self-empowered has high self-esteem. The concept that an individual who has a high level of self-esteem and therefore is self-empowered is less likely to succumb to peer pressure to conform. This is a very important consideration in relation to teenagers. Teenagers form a social group which has its own set of rules and codes of dress. Take a wander around any shopping precinct on a Saturday afternoon and note the behaviour and dress of the teenagers. You will not be surprised to see that many of them are dressed alike. Many have conformed to the same dress and behaviour code. Taking this conformity a step further it is then easy to see how conforming to other codes of behaviour, that is sexual conformity, is succumbed to through peer pressure. It is seen by Tones and Tilford that in order to break this conformity cycle, one has to first work on improving the teenagers' self-esteem, which then leads to enabling them to become self-empowered and therefore less likely to conform to peer pressure with regard to sexual activity.

Perhaps the most workable approach to adopt in order to empower these young people is through an educational approach. The educational approach of Ewles and Simnett (1995) supplies the knowledge and as far as is possible ensures knowledge and understanding of health issues on which informed decisions can be made. This approach fits nicely with the whole issue of teenagers and their health requirements, because it values the educational process in providing the information, it respects the teenagers as individuals and when after being given the necessary information allows them to make the choices for themselves. The process of enabling and empowering is the fundamental thread which weaves throughout the educational model as it facilitates development of beliefs and values and from which self-concept grows.

RECOMMENDATIONS

Adolescence is a time of great change and adaptation in life and one in which there are great risks attached, particularly in relation to health behaviour activities. Bringing about changes in young adult lives calls for not just information advice and counselling but needs to be attacked from a health promotion standpoint and one which will take into account the social and psychological adaptations required at the difficult stage of maturity.

Teenage pregnancy has been brought to the fore in order to alert, particularly health professionals, to the problems and dangers of this situation. The devastating consequences are not confined just to the girls' health but takes in the wider arena which impinges upon health; the social, psychological and educational spheres. The concerns are not restricted to one area but do require a concerted effort by all disciplines involved in order to ensure a reduction in teenage pregnancy in the future which will meet the *Health of the Nation* (DoH, 1992b) target to reduce the conception rate to the under 16s by the year 2000.

Let us begin first by looking at the school education system to see how that may be improved in order to be an effective agent in bringing about a reduction in teenage pregnancies. It is sad to think that the area of sexual health is still seen, although to a lesser extent, as a taboo topic. It can be seen from the literature available that including sexual health in the school curriculum does not encourage teenagers to be more sexually active but serves to ensure better safe sexual practice (Hurrelman, Leppin and Nordlohne, 1995). This is where lessons from our colleagues in the other European countries can be learnt because sex education is a more prominent theme within their curriculum and because of this it is not seen by the teenagers as a topic to be giggled at and shied away from. Perhaps the time to begin planting the seeds of safe sexual practices is not in senior schools but to take it a step further back and introduce the topic in primary schools. Some no doubt would disagree, however waiting until the teen years may indeed be too late for some who may have already experimented. It is also important that this area of education includes both sexes and not just the young girls. Encouraging both sexes of this young group to be educated and work together in this field should prove to be productive not just in terms of educational information in relation to the subject area but also hopefully they will learn to respect each other as responsible mature adults.

The health professionals involved play a very significant part in teenage sexual health matters. The teenager who finds herself pregnant should have easy access to a midwife at an early stage in order to minimise the health risks attached to early childbearing and also in order to build up a trusting relationship with a team of midwives that she will see throughout her pregnancy. The development of special antenatal and parent education classes for this special client group is a must and one where the health visitors and social workers are also closely involved. It might be said that it is like closing the stable door when the horse has bolted in the provision of these tailored services for this special client group. However, this is perhaps where there is a case for working in reverse. This it would seem goes against the present day philosophy of health care provision, which is to strive forward and not backwards. Nevertheless, this is not the retrograde step that it may first appear. Before we as health professionals can effect change in the reduction of teenage conceptions, it is important to understand the youth culture and their needs. It is vital that the teenagers who are already pregnant or have become mothers are educated in the field of sexual health and this includes contraception in order to prevent another pregnancy. The teenager who has the relevant information is more empowered to use that information in order to avoid another unintended pregnancy. It must be remembered that pregnancy is only one facet of sexual health and the avoidance of sexually transmitted infections, which includes HIV and AIDS, through the education of safe sexual practices is also an important aspect.

The health professional's involvement in school education within the field of sexual health can have a significant impact, in terms of being an independent and non-authoritative person in whom the teenagers can confide in. It is for this reason along with their special knowledge and skills in the field of sexual health that they are the prime providers of the special education. Midwives and health visitors who are in contact with teenage mothers may invite them along as part of the educational programme to paint a true picture of motherhood. This is not to say that motherhood is a negative status because it is not. Motherhood can be the most rewarding and fulfilling experience of a woman's life, however untimely motherhood is not as rosy as it may appear to be.

The provision of a contraceptive service that is specially designed to cater for the needs of this young client group must be value for money. Providing clinics not in the health service setting but perhaps in youth centres, cinemas or bowling alleys may prove to be more fruitful in terms of attendance and adoption of safe practices. All aspects of sexual health which include cervical smears, breast examination and testicular examination for young men should be an integral part of the service. This type of service is not only managed by health professionals but needs the support of ancillary staff and this is again where the tripartite approach of education, the health professionals and the parents could interlink.

CONCLUSION

A difficult realisation for any parent is the fact that their child has grown up into an adult and the state of womanhood or manhood has been achieved. This denial may be a factor in their reluctance to discuss matters of sexuality and contraception with their offspring. It must also be recognised that many of these teenagers were themselves products of their parents' teenage conceptions, and so the cycle is continued. It is now perhaps time to break that cycle in order to bring about effective change in this field of sexual health. This is where the tripartite approach can be used not only to feed into the teenagers but also where the health professionals and the educationalists can feed into the parents. Educating the parents in matters of a sexual nature will help to break down the barriers of ignorance with their children and the inclusion of social and communication skills are also important factors. The ability to communicate with their teenager on an adult level where respect for their knowledge and viewpoint is given will go a long way in breaking barriers of ignorance and hopefully will be instrumental in building bridges in their relationship.

The UK is supposedly a well-developed country, especially in the field of health and education. People from neighbouring countries are envious of our prestigious achievements within these two areas but do we always deserve such admiration? We can and must learn from those countries that have been more successful in reducing the teenage conception rates and adopt the appropriate strategies into our society's culture. The formalisation of a planned approach to sexual health implemented within the school curricula and the openness of all the appropriate parties to discuss the issue would be a big step forward and one that has been successful in other countries. It is imperative that action is taken sooner rather than later in order to meet the *Health of the Nation's* target set to reduce the number of teenage conceptions by the year 2000.

Evidence is provided to support the fact that a multiprofessional approach with an educational theme is the way forward. The support and involvement of parents is essential if the tripartite approach is to be achieved and effective. Education gives knowledge and the aim is that these young adults will be empowered to use that knowledge in relation to sexual health. It is hoped that young women will be empowered to say no to the persuasion of sexual intercourse by a persistent young man. On the other hand, one would hope that he would respect her as an individual and respond to her wishes. When a sexual relationship is formed, then the ultimate goal would hopefully have been achieved and that is that they are both empowered to draw on the knowledge that they have in the sexual health field and be empowered to utilise the services provided in order to adopt safe sexual practice. This would be the epitome of health promotion through an empowerment approach and the rewards would be healthier teenagers whether sexually active or not, and a reduction in the teenage conception rates.

REFERENCES

Andrews, G. (1997) Contraceptive advice: helping women to make an informed choice. *Practice Nurse,* 14(3): 185–190.

Cook, V. (1995) An inner urban funded maternity care programme: maternity projects: teenage pregnancies. *Midwives,* March: 76–79.

Creatsas, G. (1995) Sequelae of premature sexual life. *Journal of The Royal Society of Medicine,* 88: 369–370.

Creatsas, G., Goumalatsos, N. & Deligeoroglow, E. (1991) Teenage pregnancy comparison with two groups of older pregnant women. *Journal of Adolescent Health Care,* 12: 77–81.

Department of Health (1992a) *Changing Childbirth.* Report by the Expert Maternity Services. London: HMSO.

Department of Health (DoH) (1992b) The *Health of the Nation. A strategy for health in England.* London: HMSO.

Department of Health (1998) *Our Healthier Nation.* Consultation Paper. February 1998: J 20/628/1IP. London: HMSO.

Dickson, R., Fullerton, D. Eastwood, A. Sheldon, T. & Sharp, F. (1997) Preventing and reducing the adverse effects of unintended teenage pregnancies. *Effective Health Care,* 1–12.

Dignan, K. (1993) Testing times. *Nursing Times,* 89(44): 28–30.

Dignan, K. & Turnheim, R. (1996) Genital herpes. *Professional Nurse,* 11(12): 801–802.

Doyle, W. (1992) Preconceptional care – who needs it? *Modern Midwife,* January/February, 18–22.

Eisen, M., Zellman, G.L. & McAlister, A.L. (1990) Evaluating the impact of a theory-based sexuality and contraceptive education program. *Family Planning Perspect,* 22: 261–271.

Ewles, L. & Simnett, I. (1995) *Promoting Health: A Practical Guide.* 3rd, edn. London: Scutari.

Flick, L.H. (1991) A Critique of Community-based Teritary Prevention with the Adolescent Parent and Child. Cited in Burke, P. & Lister, W. (1994) Adolescent mothers' perceptions of social support and the impact of parenting on their lives. *Paediatric Nursing,* 20 (6): 593–98.

Frost, J.J. & Forrest, J.D. (1995) Understanding the impact of effective teenage pregnancy prevention programs. *Family Planning Perspect,* 27: 188–195.

Hudson, F. & Ineichen, B. (1995) *Taking it Lying Down.* London: Macmillan.

Hurrelman, K., Leppin, A. & Nordlohne, E. (1995) Promoting health in schools: the German example. *Health Promotion International* 10(2): 121–131.

Jack, R. (1995) *Empowerment in Community Care.* London: Chapman & Hall.

Julian, K. (1983) A comparison of perceived and demonstrated maternal role competence of adolescent mothers. *Journal of Sex Education Therapy,* 11: 38–45.

Kemm, J. & Close, A. (1995) *Health Promotion: Theory and Practice.* Basingstoke: Macmillan.

Kerr, J. (1995) Cervical cancer: Improving the service. *Nursing Standard,* 9(18): 26–29.

Kiernan, K. (1995) Transition to Parenthood: Young Mothers, Young Fathers – Associated Factors and Later Life Experiences. Welfare State Programme Discussion Paper 113. London Family Planning Association, cited in *Effective Health Care,* Preventing and Reducing the Adverse Effects of Unintended Teenage Pregnancies.

Kirby, D.B., Short, L., Collins, J. et al. (1994) School based programs to reduce sexual risk behaviours: a review of effectiveness. *Public Health Reports,* 109: 339–360.

Konje, J.C., Palmer, A., Watson, A. et al. (1992) Early teenage pregnancies in Hull. *British Journal of Obstetrics and Gynaecology,* 99: 969–973.

Lewin, B. (1986) *Sex and Family Planning: How We Teach the Young.* World Health Organization Regional Office for Europe.

Michie, S., Marteau, T.M. & Kidd, J. (1992) An evaluation of an intervention to increase antenatal class attendance. *Journal of Reproductive and Infant Psychology,* 10: 183–185.

Office for National Statistics (1996) *Birth Statistics FM1* no. 23. London: HMSO.

Oakley, A., Fullerton, D. & Holland, J. et al.

(1995) Sexual health education intervention for young people: a methodological review. *British Medical Journal*, **310**: 158–162.

Peerman, G., Oakley, A., Oliver, S. & Thomas, J. (1996) *Review of Effectiveness of Sexual Health Promotion Interventions for Young People*. London: Social Science Research Unit, University of London.

Royal College of Obstetricians and Gynaecologists (1991) *Report of the RCOG Working Party on Unplanned Pregnancy*. London: Royal College of Obstetricians and Gynaecologists.

Scally, G. (1993) Pregnancies – The challenge of prevention. *Midwives Chronicle and Nursing Notes*, July, 232–239.

Smith, T. (1993) Influence of socioeconomic factors on attaining targets for reducing teenage pregnancies. *British Medical Journal*, **306**: 1232–1235.

Stout, J.W. & Rivara, F.P. (1989) Schools and sex education: does it work? *Paediatrics*, **83**: 375–379.

Tones, K. & Tilford, S. (1995) *Health Education, Effectiveness, Efficiency and Equity*. 2nd edn. London: Chapman & Hall.

Wallerstein, N. (1992) Powerlessness, empowerment and health: implication for health promotion programs. *American Journal of Health Promotion*, 6(3): 193–205.

Wellings, K., Wadsworth, J., Johnson, A. et al (1996) *Teenage Sexuality, Fertility and Life Chances*. A Report for the Department of Health Using data from the National Survey of Sexual Attitudes and Lifestyles. London School of Hygiene & Tropical Medicine, cited in *Effective Health Care*, Preventing and Reducing the Adverse Effects of Unintended Teenage Pregnancies, February 1997

World Health Report (1995) Annual Report. Cited in McGragor, A. (1995) Preventing teenage pregnancy. *Lancet*, **345**: May 27.

FURTHER READING

Hudson, F. & Ineichen, B. (1991) *Taking it Lying Down*. London: Macmillan.

Phoenix, A. (1991) *Young Mothers*. Cambridge: Polity Press

Ewles, L. & Simnett, I. *Promoting Health: A Practical Guide 3/E* (1998) London: Baillière Tindall.

6 Promoting child and family health through empowerment

Sue Hooton

KEY ISSUES

- The present approaches to health promotion appear to do little to address persisting child health inequalities
- Co-ordinated multiprofessional and multi-agency health promotion team working is essential if child health targets are to be achieved
- There is a great deal of evidence available to identify the most vulnerable groups of children in society
- Children need to be empowered to take more responsibility for their own health
- Children understand a great deal more about health than we often acknowledge
- Professional knowledge about childrens' health knowledge and behaviour is limited
- Children may be more receptive to health education messages than their parents
- Children's existing health knowledge may be more accurate than their parents'
- Children have the right to be empowered in matters that affect their own health status but require adult support to directly effect that right

'The way a society treats its children reflects not only its qualities of compassion and protective caring, but also its sense of justice, its commitment to the future and its urge to enhance the human condition for coming generations.'

(Perez de Cuellar, United Nations Secretary General, 1990)

INTRODUCTION

This chapter aims to explore current approaches to child health promotion. It focuses on health promotion for primary school children, as this group appears to be particularly neglected within the growing range of health promotion literature. The work is felt to be of importance to any professionals who work with young children as it intends to identify and explore the significant challenges presented to those directly involved in promoting the health of young children. It is proposed that within this chapter, professional understanding of child health matters will be enhanced and a clearer understanding of the factors that influence children's rights to health will emerge.

CHILDREN IN SOCIETY

What rights do children have in society?

Social attitudes towards children are changing as children's rights are becoming more clearly established within Western society. In past years, children were afforded few rights and the dominant view and expectation was that adults should act on behalf of children to better protect them. More recent and enlightened attitudes focus on the paramount importance of the 'best interests' principle within child welfare with a resulting move towards acknowledging that children have distinct rights, opinions and choices as individuals.

This shift towards conceptualising children's rights has largely resulted from the influential work of the United Nations (UN) Convention (1959–1991) and in consequence through legislation such as the Children Act (1989). Flekkoy (1991, p214) suggests that the UN Convention represents a turning point in the way that children's rights have been promoted internationally and the consequent change in attitude towards the values societies are attributing to children and the rights of children who are viewed as individuals in their own right rather than the 'property' of their parents. However she acknowledges that there is still much to do in the pursuit of promoting the concept of children's rights and the empowerment of children.

The basic principles underpinning the UN Convention Rights of the Child are listed in Box 6.1.

BOX 6.1	*Basic Principles Underpinning the UN Convention Rights of the Child*
	■ Right of Non-discrimination
	■ Right that others should act in 'the best interests' of the child
	■ Right to life, survival and development
	■ Right that children's views should be sought and respected

These principles apply to a range of formal attitudes towards and civil rights for children such as rights within the family unit, rights to basic health and welfare and cultural respect, along with rights to education and protection (Lansdown, 1995, p536). This changing scene presents distinct challenges to adults who provide care for children to review current practices to ensure that children's rights are understood and upheld by more fully involving children in matters that affect them, from an age when they are able to understand issues and make decisions for themselves.

Do children have the right to a healthy life?

The UN Convention (1989) proposes that children are entitled to 'the highest attainable standard of health care' and that all member states should ensure that health care is provided to all children, with emphasis being placed on preventative health (Wilson, 1995, p98). As such, it would appear that the attainment of optimum health would be a fundamental right of all children, along with the individual child's right to be involved in health matters. However, the degree to which children are afforded this right would appear to vary greatly.

The complexities of involving children in health care decisions should not be underestimated as there are many legal, ethical and professional dilemmas to be considered. Rose (1997) discusses the ambiguities involved in defining 'childrens best interests' and Neighbour (1992) argues that there are situations were paternalism is justified as not all children will wish to, or be able to make such decisions. However, it could be argued that failing to attempt to involve children in health care decisions results in a situation where children only experience an 'indirect right' to be involved in health care matters, thereby perpetuating the status quo. Flekkoy (1991) maintains that this situation is not new, as historically, children's rights have more usually been indirect in nature as they have long been subsumed in the rights of adults to act on behalf of children. In this way children have been in danger from not necessarily being excluded, but rather from being ignored when it comes to having direct rights. Therefore the UN Convention presents guidance and consequential challenges to health professionals who implicitly must work towards involving children more directly in care decisions and health issues as a matter of right.

How healthy are children today?

Few could disagree that child health in the UK has improved over the years. Many more children are surviving infancy and childhood and moving into adulthood, and children today are taller and healthier than in past generations. The House of Commons Health Select Committee (1997, px) reported that childhood mortality rates have been falling steadily in the Western world and that the 'most marked long-term decrease in mortality has been among younger children in the 1–4 year age group'. However, despite the falling mortality rate, it is well acknowledged that many children will not achieve optimum health (as an automatic right) and that child health inequalities are an indisputable and unacceptable feature of our society (Bradshaw, 1990; Oppenheim, 1993; DoH, 1998).

The growing understanding of the nature and pattern of child health inequalities begs scrutiny of the relationship between the notion of equal rights to health attainment for all children, against the failure to achieve child health for so many vulnerable children within an affluent society. The prevalence of child health inequalities would indicate that there is much scope for improvement in the current approaches to child health promotion.

CHILD HEALTH IN THE COMMUNITY

Trends in child health

Traditionally, infant mortality has been a key measure of child health, however as infant mortality rates are at an all time low in developed countries, morbidity

BOX 6.2	*Trends in the UK from 1971–1991*

- For both sexes, stillbirth and infant mortality rates have halved in number
- Babies born weighing under 2500 g in 1991 accounted for 59% of neonatal deaths
- During the 1980s the rates of all multiple births increased
- There was a large fall in neonatal deaths associated with sudden infant death syndrome (SIDS)
- Childhood respiratory conditions account for nearly one-half of all general practitioner (GP) consultations
- Hospital admissions due to childhood cancers increased four-fold, whilst mortality rates fell by about half

(Reproduced from *In the Health of Our Children*, Botting, B. and Crawley, R., 1996, 61 with kind permission from HMSO.)

levels and the effects of disability on children are attracting increasing interest (Office of Population Census and Surveys (OPCS), 1996).

Box 6.2 includes selected key points from the 1996 OPCS 'Overview in Trends and Patterns in Childhood Mortality and Morbidity,' which are indicative of some of the current child health trends.

It is clear that major developments in neonatal care and management are resulting in many more infants surviving premature birth, and that successes in neonatal care are resulting in an associated increase in the numbers of children with permanent disabilities and associated complex nursing needs. This trend presents a significant challenge to those involved in antenatal care to reduce the incidence of and risks associated with premature births.

Who are the vulnerable children?

Childhood accidents

The 1996 OPCS results revealed that at all ages in childhood there was an identifiable gradient of risk of increased mortality with increasing social disadvantage which is most marked at ages 1–4 years. Much evidence already exists to identify the vulnerable children in society along with growing evidence that child health inequalities continue to persist between social groupings (OPCS, 1996). The OPCS report also showed clearly that childhood injury and poisoning continued to be the major cause for hospital referral of young children. The *Health of the Nation* initiative (DoH, 1992) concentrated upon reducing the number of childhood accidents and much of this work is carried forward into the current health strategy *Our Healthier Nation* (DoH, 1998). In support of setting new national targets to reduce childhood accidents, the Department of Health (DoH) states that: 'Accidents are the greatest single threat to life for children and young people' and that the 1996 Health Survey for England estimated that the annual childhood accident rate for children aged 2–15 years was 31 for every 100 boys and 22 for every 100 girls. Two major factors were identified in connection with trends in childhood accidents: (1) that the unacceptably high number of childhood accidents appears to be linked with social deprivation and (2) that the social 'gap' is widening (Roberts and Power, 1996).

According to the National Health Service Executive (NHSE) (1996, p33) the most vulnerable groups of children are likely to be those living within travelling families, from ethnic minority families, with disabilities, who live in lone parent families or who live in deprived areas (both inner city and rural areas). For some children the transient nature of family life may lead to social exclusion, through for example, having no permanent address, not being registered with a GP or not having continuous contact with education or child health services.

Childhood accident rates show distinct socio-economic class differences. The DoH (1998, p65) provide evidence that 'children from poorer backgrounds are five times more likely to die as a result of an accident than children from better off families'. There is also strong evidence of the social variations in childhood death due to fire, with children living in Bed & Breakfast accommodation and children from homeless families being identified as being particularly vulnerable to burns, scalds, falls and swallowing poisonous substances (Conway, 1988; Wilson, 1995). Wilson (1995) further describes the relationship between poor housing and common chest conditions such as childhood asthma, pneumonia and recurrent upper respiratory chest infections, which are the commonest causes of childhood illness and of resulting school inattendance. Road traffic accidents are also a feature of premature death or serious injury for children who live and play in deprived areas, where there is often an associated lack of gardens and poor public facilities such as safe play areas. It is obvious then that certain, identifiable children are particularly at risk.

What is the impact of low income upon parenting?

Clearly the degree of absolute poverty to be seen within society has improved over the years. However, even in today's affluent society, the adverse effects of poverty upon children's health remain a cause for concern among health professionals. Oppenheim (1993) states that just under one-quarter of children living in the UK are living in relative poverty as families with children form a disproportionate part of the poorest section of society. This continues to be particularly so for lone parent families and families of people who are unemployed or earn low wages (Benzeval, Judge and Whitehead 1996, p72).

Blackburn (1991) suggests that there are three distinct but interacting processes that impact on the health of low income families, that are physiological, psychological and behavioural in nature. As income provides the fundamental prerequisites for health, a lack of income often results in families being exposed to poor housing and poor diet. The psychological effects of parenting on a limited budget and feelings of inadequacy for parents who are unable to provide for their children is known to affect parental health resulting in stress and depression with an associated inability to provide adequate parenting skills. Blackburn further suggests that the cumulative effects of poverty upon parenting may lead to the uptake of health-damaging behaviours such as smoking and increased alcohol intake as coping mechanisms. This clear evidence of the nature and pattern of health inequalities and the influence upon family functioning offers essential data not to be ignored by those involved in child health activity. This review of child health issues reveals that child health inequalities are well acknowledged and well researched. However, the degree to which the subsequent growth in child health promotion activity addresses inequalities in child health is not so well documented.

Do health promotion models acknowledge child health inequalities?

Much health promotion work is undertaken within the community by professionals and community groups working directly with children. Generally, health promotion activity is changing from that which was previously medically dominated to activities which acknowledge the wider health experience. This redefinition of the parameters of health reflects a shift from narrow definitions of health as described in terms of illness/freedom from illness to definitions which recognise the effects of psycho-social influences upon health and health attainment.

This shift has resulted in the growth of health education models which focus upon notions of 'lifestyle'. Although this approach encompasses psycho-social theories it has been criticised for falling short in its approach as historically, it has assumed individual control over health and health attainment. In this respect, professionals have been accused of becoming involved in 'persuasive' health education activities whereby individuals would be expected to change their lifestyles according to the latest health education messages. Nutbeam (1984, p117) and others realised the limitations of health education lifestyle models and criticised this approach as being too narrow in focus in that the models failed to change established health behaviour, as they failed to address the wider context in which individuals' health behaviour is shaped. Further criticisms accuse the concept of 'lifestylism' as being overly class related, leading to sterotypical notions of health behaviours resulting in a move towards a 'professional control culture'.

The concept of lifestyle, however, continues to be acknowledged as an important feature central to health promotion and features as a fundamental concept within the majority of the emerging health promotion models along with the recognition of wider health determinants.

In compiling a health strategy to extend into the 21st century, *Our Healthier Nation* (DoH, 1998) acknowledges the role that social, economic and environmental factors play in health attainment and aims to avoid 'extremes of individual victim blaming on the one hand and nanny state social engineering on the other'. The 'contract for health' that underpins the new health strategy is based upon principles of partnership between the Government, local communities and individuals in the pursuit of healthy living. Clearly, health promotion has come to be regarded as a complex, multi-faceted activity which embraces health psychology as well as socio-economic and political dimensions of health and health policy.

Does child health promotion work?

The NHSE (1996) document *Child Health in the Community* outlines the three major aspects of health activity for pre-school children as programmes of immunisation, child health surveillance and health promotion services. Perhaps the most influential guidance for child health professionals who predominantly work with young children and their families in health promotion has been the Hall Report (1989; 1996).

Until recently, community health work with children has emphasised the health surveillance approach, involving much child health screening and measurement activity designed to monitor developmental progress. Such activities, being outcome focused and relatively easy to measure, have been received favourably by the commissioners of health services. However, Hall (1996) has suggested that it is time to recognise the failings of such a narrow approach. He more recently states that preventive health services for children should extend beyond the narrow remit of child health surveillance with its focus on detection of abnormalities, to include efforts to prevent illness and promote good health. He recommends that the term 'child health promotion' is a more helpful general term in describing the scope of activity that needs to be undertaken. The definition of health promotion offered in the Hall Report is 'any planned and informed intervention which is designed to improve physical or mental health or prevent disease, disability or premature death' with activities being described as: (1) primary promotion aimed at reducing the incidence of disease, (2) secondary promotion aimed at reducing the prevalence of disease and (3) tertiary promotion aimed at reducing disabilities and promoting the adjustment to disease (Hall, 1996, p9).

Historically, much child health promotion work has been aimed at parents in the guise of 'persuasive' models of health education. Such approaches attempted to persuade parents to change their lifestyle to enhance the health of their children. In retrospect, health professionals have been criticised as conspiring to develop a 'blame culture' through the use of persuasive health education with families who were often in no position to effect change in their lifestyles to enhance the health of their children.

More recent approaches are based on models of health promotion which aim to *empower* families in health attainment and as such these models implicitly require collaborative approaches based on professional partnership with children and their families. Such a shift exemplifies the more sophisticated understanding of the nature of health and the rights of individuals within health matters. It also further highlights the complexities involved in ensuring that children's rights within health provision are understood and upheld. Further information around the roles and responsibilities of the varying professionals are discussed later in this chapter under 'Healthy Alliances'.

EMPOWERING CHILDREN DIRECTLY

What do children have to say about health matters?

If professional understanding about the ways in which children can be empowered to take more responsibility for their own health is to develop, it would appear logical to work directly with children and explore their health perceptions and ambitions. The following activities provide examples of how this can be attempted.

Using draw and write techniques

An exercise was undertaken to establish the health perceptions of a group of primary school children aged 6–7 years. An increasingly popular technique known as 'draw and write' was used in order to provide a medium which reflected the younger children's cognitive and practical abilities, whilst focusing on their perceptions of health and ill health. Pridmore and Bendelow (1995, p473) describe the benefits to be gained from such methodologies in obtaining sophisticated data which is grounded in children's own ideas, beliefs and metaphors. They give a detailed account of the ethical and humanistic issues of using such techniques. They assert from their study that 'using children's drawings, in conjunction with writing or dialogue can provide a powerful method of exploring the beliefs of young children which may inform health behaviours and influence health status'.

The classroom-based activity undertaken by the author was informal, participative and fun to be involved in. Although it was a very small-scale exercise, it was informative in demonstrating the following associations: (See Figs 6.1 & 6.2)

A healthy person was someone who was young, dressed in sporting attire and actively engaged in sporting activity: swimming, skipping, boxing and motor car racing. There were lots of outdoor activities drawn and a strong presence of sunshine, grass and trees.

An unhealthy person was characterised as an elderly person, with a beard and moustache and largely portrayed as small and bent, and in need of a walking stick. The majority of unhealthy people portrayed were older men. These individuals did not enjoy the same outdoor pleasures of sunshine, grass, and birds as the healthy people did. Several children also drew small, extremely

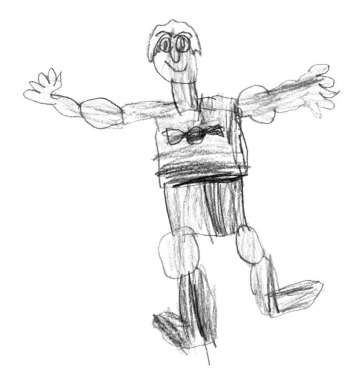

Figure 6.1A Child's drawing of a healthy person

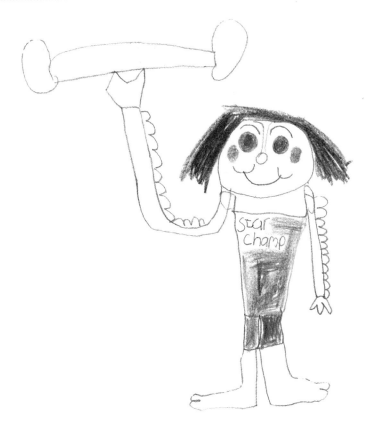

Figure 6.1B Child's drawing of a healthy person

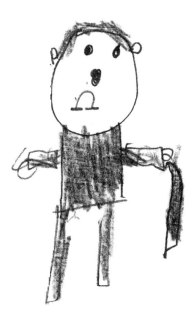

Figure 6.2A Child's drawing of an unhealthy person

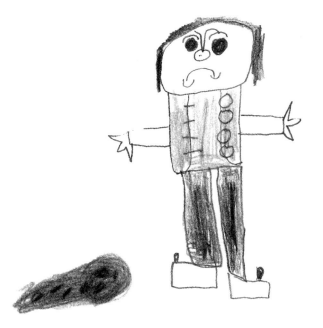

Figure 6.2B Child's drawings of an unhealthy person

detailed, circular (pizza like) pools at the side of the unhealthy people, which were later explained to be 'sick, of course'. In this way the children could symbolise their own experiences of being unwell.

A second exercise was undertaken with older children, which aimed to examine more complex health issues such as general understandings about health and in particular healthy lifestyles.

Talking with children about health

The following statements were made by children during discussions in a group of older primary school children aged between 10 and 11 years. The children (mostly young girls) were articulate and comfortable in discussing health matters. The following extracts were from conversations about the ways in which the children felt that their lives could be healthier:

'My parents could buy me less sweets. They buy me sweets as treats, especially if they are working late or going out'.

'We could exercise more as a family by doing more walking and cycling. Now my Mum wants to buy an exercise bike but we already have bikes, its just that Mum and Dad say they don't have the time to use theirs'.

'I think that we have a healthy diet. We talk about food a lot and try to eat five pieces of fruit each day, but we don't eat too many vegetables because we all like different things and it drives my Mum mad'.

'My lunch box could be healthier, I have sandwiches, crisps and a chocolate bar every day. Although when we get to school me and my friends all share out our food, that way, even the kids with strict parents get some chocolate and crisps which they aren't allowed at home'.

'My parents won't ask visitors not to smoke in our house and I think that they should because that's not good for me'.

Throughout the conversations, the children identified many major health determinants without prompting. They could relate the basic components of a healthy diet, nationally recommended exercise guidelines, and they knew about the risks of passive and active smoking upon health. They also demonstrated a keen sense of justice towards their rights to healthy living in that they complained about parental *laissez-faire* attitudes towards health issues and discussed how they shared out 'treat' foods at school, thereby bypassing parental controls over lunches.

Although few concrete claims could be made from the two studies described above, they have been useful in providing insight into the world of children and the origins of their health perceptions which, if more thoroughly researched could provide the foundations for future health promotion activity.

How do children learn about health?

Bagnall and Dilloway (1996) explain some of the complexities that lie within child health promotion and state the need to understand children's influences, interests and language if formative health promotion opportunities are not to be missed. Part of this understanding must acknowledge the varying sources of children's health knowledge.

The way in which children's learning is shaped by role modelling and conforming to social norms is well documented, indicating that much health behaviour will be shaped at an early age through behaviours observed within the family.

However, influences from outside of the family will also be influential as children are exposed to the wider world outside of the immediate family. The children who were involved in the above conversations stated that they learnt quite a lot about healthy living from input at school and at organisations such as Scout and Brownie groups.

It has been reported that children as young as 6 years old have distinct ideas about the causes of health and ill health, perceptions which might prove useful as a foundation for developing new concepts and paradigms upon which new child health promotion models might be founded. It is surely time to recognise that the next generation of health promotion models should be child focused and grounded in the reality of children's experiences and needs as opposed to those that are transferred from the adult health experience. Talking to children to elicit understanding about health attitudes and health behaviours requires the professional to enter the world of children and to use media that are familiar and attractive to the child. When working with children in his studies, Eiser (1991) used Playmobil toys, descriptive stories and photographs – methods which reflected the developmental abilities of the children. Eiser also found that as well as acknowledging maturational processes, understanding is very much determined by children's personal experiences, factors which emphasise the very individual nature of the ways in which children perceive health and make the whole exercise very complex and time consuming. Perhaps this explains why within the raft of health promotion literature, there is very little information about younger children's perceptions of health.

However, there is more literature relating to children's understanding about ill health and illness. Children under 7 years old are known to believe in illness as a form of punishment or as something that is 'caught' from others. A child between the ages of 7 and 11 years old understands the principles of contagion more thoroughly and older children are able to explain illness using increasingly complex biological terms as they have more knowledge about scientific processes (Bibace and Walsh, 1981; Eiser, 1991).

Clearly, getting to understand individual children's perceptions of health and illness is a time-consuming and complex activity requiring much knowledge about child development. Eiser (1991, p342) suggests that it is also essential to explore professional knowledge and attitudes towards children's perceptions of health if health professionals are to understand the ways in which children's health perceptions are shaped and change over time.

Whose responsibility is child health?

Health promotion activity involves making fundamental decisions regarding health responsibilities, definitions of which will determine the nature of the resources allocated and activities to be undertaken.

Consider each of the following statements:
- Parents should be responsible for their children's health
- Professionals should be responsible for children's health
- Society should be responsible for children's health

Which do you agree with most strongly and why?

Each statement has received much professional attention in recent years and in fact each could be argued convincingly from different ends of the social and political spectrum. There is growing recognition that there is a collective responsibility for child health (DoH, 1998) which implies a need for policy makers, professionals, parents and children themselves to acknowledge their responsibilities and to work collaboratively to promote children's health.

Can children be considered responsible for their own health?

From the author/children conversations documented earlier, it became obvious that the children understood very complex issues about the ways that parental health behaviours and beliefs compromised their own chances for health and conflicted with their own growing health knowledge. The children also understood and were accepting of the practical difficulties involved in providing a totally healthy home environment quoting examples of cost, time, effort and motivation involved.

Overall, these conversations demonstrated that the children in the interview group were interested in health matters and had an impressive range of health knowledge, but were largely under the control and influence of their parents. Studying groups of older children, Nutbeam et al (1993) found that the contemporary teaching and health education approaches dramatically improved young people's smoking-related knowledge but did not in fact reduce the incidence of smoking behaviour in young people. This important study identified the need to pay further attention to attitudinal change through life skills teaching, to help young people resist the social pressures to smoke. Today, there is significantly more health promotion and health education literature aimed at improving children's health, however, despite such major investment in health education resources, the relationship between children's health knowledge and ensuing health behaviour remains largely unknown.

As our understanding of health promotion theories and principles becomes increasingly sophisticated, it would appear that in relation to child health promotion, it is time to move the focus from *WHAT* to target to *WHO* and *HOW* to target. In order to take this work forward, it would appear logical to surmise that children will only achieve their rights to health and to be involved in health decisions, if adults make time and effort to understand the experiences, aspirations and pressures of childhood. This must be a prerequisite to any developing health promotion work and a fundamental issue in the way forward in empowering children to optimise their knowledge and health opportunities in support of improving their health-enhancing behaviours. The identification of such issues may help inform individuals in entering partnerships with children and their families and demonstrate how, despite sound professional intentions, children do and will continue to fall into the 'indirect care/indirect rights' trap.

Can partnership models hinder children's rights?

The concept of 'partnership' is fundamental to many contemporary child and family health promotion models and is generally felt to be a positive concept. The ideology underlying partnership is influenced by family systems theory and incorporates basic principles of equality and shared decision making between individuals and the health professionals involved in their health care. Doherty and Campbell (1990, p22) state that it is of course important for professionals to work within the framework of the family, as this is where social and health-related behaviours are learnt as children are exposed to family health beliefs and related health behaviours which they will be likely to replicate. Few child health professionals would dispute the benefits derived from family-focused care, however for many children, the reality of 'family partnership' often means professionals working directly with parents who advocate for their children. However, it is difficult to surmise exactly what form working in partnership with children might take, especially when considering working with young children and it is not difficult to understand the reasons why many initiatives that might be described as incorporating progressive 'partnership' models may in fact exclude children, in favour of regarding parents as the natural and rightful partners.

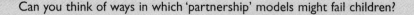

Can you think of ways in which 'partnership' models might fail children?

The notion of partnerships within health care is a popular inclusion within current health directives, however they often fail to give a description of what constitutes a 'partner'. Not surprisingly, the partnership concept rarely appears directly to involve young children as within society generally, children are not usually regarded as equals alongside adults. This situation is unlikely to change until children's rights are truly established, perpetuating the state of exclusion in what might be described as an 'adult conspiracy' to protect (control) children's affairs.

Second, the frameworks of many health promotion models/strategies include adult goals and aspirations and are based upon adult experiences of health and illness. There are few models of health promotion which incorporate child centred goals and perceptions of health. If children are to be included as true partners in health matters then there is a need to develop models of health promotion and ensuing health promotion strategies that reflect and are informed by the world of children. This inevitably involves fully utilising and developing child-centred theories of health and illness, involving children directly in this developmental work.

Questions have been asked as to whether there can ever be an equal relationship between professionals and their patients. Ross and Phipps (1986) identified the power struggle inherent within health education activity, which was found to result in patient resentment and non-compliance. McIntosh (1992) describes the dissatisfaction and parental concern regarding the intrusive and patronising attitudes of professionals which resulted in poor attendance at a children's clinic. Mayall and Foster (1989, p35) found many differences between the childrearing aspirations and expectations of health visitors when compared against those of mothers, another study which showed a consequent reduction in clinic attendances. This study found that health visitors' knowledge focused upon theories of child psychology, leading to a 'problem-based approach' to their work, largely ignoring the socio-cultural dimensions of childrearing practice which was the parents' reality. This leads to consideration of the premise for entering such partnerships and the often obligatory nature of partnership within health care.

Consequently, it can be concluded that 'real' partnership is difficult to attain, requiring mutual obligations to be negotiated and clearly stated before any health contracting process is entered into.

The case therefore has been presented for children to be regarded as partners in health care and health care decision making. Clearly, a major philosophical shift is required by adults responsible for the care of children to create opportunities which acknowledge the abilities and respect the rights of children to be directly involved in their own health decisions. This shift challenges health professionals to work innovatively and directly with children and to see them as being central to health promotion work rather than using parents or other adults as mediators.

To avoid such difficulties, professionals may be seen to fall into the 'family care' trap whereby health matters relating to children are discussed with parents in a spirit of 'partnership', failing to acknowledge the particular experiences of the child.

How might children be more directly involved in their health decisions?

It is proposed that it is timely to consider new concepts to underpin and direct models for child health promotion, which start with consideration of the fundamental relationship between individuals. Fradd (1994) states that 'caring for an individual involves respect for their personal integrity and autonomy; having a "genuine regard" and that caring is an essential prerequisite for empowerment'. Therefore, if developing health promotion frameworks are to empower children, it is necessary that they respect the unconditional rights of children within health matters.

Strategic frameworks which develop should include interdisciplinary and interagency cooperation as a fundamental principle and consider the most effective ways in which children's views should be actively sought and implemented. Professionals who work in close contact with children will be more likely to understand the dynamism of child development and the impact that social, emotional and physical maturation has upon the individual's level of understanding and abilities in decision making according to differing levels of ability. Professionals also need to be aware of the changing nature of childhood if health promotion is to be effective.

As children grow up in a technological society, children are becoming more computer literature and more interested in learning through technological media. The potential use of information technology in health promotion activity should be thoroughly explored, taking leads from what children already find enjoyable and stimulating. Creative use of media such as TV, magazines and the music industry may offer potential avenues for health promotion by using presentations which are successful and attractive to children.

Children do not have a political voice. Therefore, in relation to health policy, much activity and many resources may be centred around the implementation of health policies which are not of interest to children and therefore likely to fail. It is suggested therefore that the establishment and more full involvement of user groups might help inform policy and guide its implementation.

HEALTH ALLIANCES

Working together to achieve the national targets for child health attainment

The White Paper The Health of the Nation (DoH, 1992) presented a health strategy for England towards the year 2000 and beyond. Much of this work is being carried forward through the proposed health strategy outlined in Our Healthier Nation (DoH, 1998). The focus of The Health of the Nation initiative was to 'provide a clear focus on current health issues, highlight the need for multi-agency cooperation in improving preventative care, whilst recognising the unique role of health professionals in educating the general public in health matters' (Williams 1994, p353). The Health of the Nation targets specified for children's health are outlined in Box 6.3. This health promotion work will be ongoing and increased emphasis has been placed upon the need to further reduce childhood accidents by 20% by the year 2010 (DoH, 1998).

BOX 6.3	*Targets for Children's health in* **The Health of the Nation**

- To reduce the prevalence of smoking among 11–15-year-olds by at least 33% by the year 1994. This was not achieved in 1994 and has become a major area of health promotion activity since
- To reduce the number of conceptions among under 16s by at least 50% by the year 2000
- To reduce the number of accidental deaths among children aged under 15 by at least 33% by the year 2005

Many of the other health targets appear to be predominantly adult focused, however closer attention reveals that they are entirely relevant to the health of schoolchildren. Bagnall and Dilloway (1996, p21) suggest that concerns around the key targets identified for cardiovascular disease, lung cancer, sexual health and human immunodeficiency virus (HIV), accidents and mental health are in reality issues relevant to the health of every child. The NHSE (1996, p46) outlined the topics related to *The Health of the Nation* targets to be included in school-based health promotion as:

- Sex education and preparation for parenthood
- The dangers from smoking, alcohol, drug and substance misuse
- Accident prevention
- Environmental protection (risk of sun exposure etc.)
- Nutrition
- Oral health
- The general inclusion of positive health behaviour including both physical and psychological health.

A further document entitled *The Health of the Young Nation* (Moores, 1995) was compiled following a series of 'professional discussions' around the ways in which *The Health of the Nation* targets related to young people. Introducing this initiative, Moores (1995) stated that nurses, midwives and health visitors are in a pivotal position to improve the health of young people and emphasised the particular contribution to be made from school nurses working alongside children and young people to promote healthy lifestyles. The document includes key factors, which were identified by health professionals as being particularly influential in promoting the health of young people.

Which factors do you think were identified by health professionals as being most influential for the successful achievement of National targets for children's health?

The major factors identified are listed in Box 6.4.

BOX 6.4	*Key factor to promoting the health of young people*

1. Need for health services to be available and accessible
   - Confidential services
   - Local services in centres frequented by young people
   - Out-of-hours services

2. Health professionals who were knowledgeable about the issues and young people's behaviours
   - Need for professional understanding of the national health imperatives
   - Need for local knowledge
   - Accurate and accessible local health profiles
   - Collaborative working between local agencies (police, commerce, health and social services)

3. Effective service organisation
   - Need for professional autonomy
   - Shift from 'routine' health tasks
   - Ease of referral across service boundaries

Working collaboratively

Traditionally, child health promotion has been viewed as a community activity, undertaken by the primary health care team. Particular emphasis has been placed upon the role of health visitors who provide health care for the under 5s and school nurses working with older children, working in collaboration with GPs, who are directly responsible for child and family health. The revised 1993 GP contract emphasises the role of general practice in health promotion and the importance of multidisciplinary delivery of services. *Our Healthier Nation* (DoH, 1998) describes the ways in which professional groups can work together and form alliances to improve child health. One example provided is 'the healthy schools initiative' which is designed to raise awareness of children, teachers and local communities to the opportunities that exist in promoting the health of children at school. In setting out examples of how future health contracts might work, government responsibilities are made explicit along with actions required by schools and the commitments to be made by parents and pupils. In this way, all concerned parties sign up to a commitment to work together and acknowledge shared responsibilities.

The role of the school nurse is also identified as being important in ensuring that schools keep a clear focus on health and the new health strategy presents distinct challenges to school nurses to work creatively and collaboratively in the pursuit of child health. Bagnall and Dilloway (1996, p18) consider the scope for developing the role of the school nurse and fully explore the ways in which the present school health service meets child health needs. They discuss the valuable contribution that school nurses can make in 'opportunistic health promotion' and conclude in favour of a shift from routine health surveillance in favour of more direct health promotion activity. However, they suggest that historically, there has been a lack of understanding between school nurses and primary health care teams. Unfortunately their research revealed that GPs as commissioners of health services, appeared to know little about school nursing activity or the scope for developing the role of the school nurse in relation to child health promotion.

Much of the progress achieved in reaching the goals and targets set out in *The Health of the Nation* (DoH, 1992) is dependent upon the establishment of health alliances where professionals and groups work together in the pursuit of a common aim. In relation to reducing accidental deaths in childhood, the NHSE (1996, p56) provides examples of health authorities participating in multi-agency health alliances which serve to identify accident risk in localities and stimulate educational and environmental measures to reduce such risks. Such alliances often involve a wide range of agencies for examples in road accident prevention, increasingly health professionals, teachers, police, social workers, local authorities, societies such as ROSPA and residents are working together in a spirit of joint collaboration. The Health Education Authority (HEA) is also actively involved in primary health promotion, supporting different health alliances bringing groups together to work towards preventing teenage pregnancy, promoting adolescent health, and providing a national young person's health network (NHSE, 1996, p57).

The potential for working together with voluntary agencies and children's charity organisations within child health promotion has yet to be realised. Many of these organisations have considerable expertise in working with children and families outside of the formality of the health services. Perhaps the groups who have been most significantly involved are Action for Sick Children, The Child Poverty Action Group and the National Children's Bureau. More specialist groups such as MENCAP, Barnado's and many others have engaged in relentless publishing and lobbying to determine improved services for children by directly and indirectly influencing children's issues on the socio-political health agenda.

How might professionals work together to empower children?

It is suggested that there is much potential to develop health promotion approaches which more directly empower children and one area where there has been considerable progress is that of the self-management of childhood asthma. Asthma is perhaps the most common chronic condition of childhood with almost 25% of children in the UK likely to suffer from asthma at some stage and the amount of children being diagnosed each year is increasing (Carruthers, 1993, p41). Altogether, allergic-type conditions such as hay fever, rhinitis and other respiratory conditions account for over one-half of children's consultations with GPs (OPCS, 1996). It is not surprising therefore that the management of childhood asthma has received a great deal of professional attention.

Carruthers emphasises the importance of professionals being prepared to work together and to forego professional boundaries if asthma health promotion work is to be successful. Increasingly, school nurses, doctors, practice nurses and health visitors are working together with teachers and pupils to formulate policies to help children manage their own asthma. Strategies include positive action such as providing asthma education for teachers and pupils, and providing written information and guidelines for asthma management; all of these strategies provide support for children to manage their asthma effectively and maintain their independence during school hours.

Effective management of childhood asthma depends upon professional understanding of the psycho-social needs of the child as well as more practical matters such as avoidance of trigger factors and good inhaler technique. Clearly, success will depend upon informing and empowering the family in their abilities and their attitudes towards managing their child's asthma, but ultimately, true success will come from empowering the child directly. Children with asthma are often exposed to parental fears and anxieties about their condition and in many cases may find themselves in a role which is supportive of and protective towards their parents. They will also experience many occasions when parents will not be with them to guide or advise them about their asthma and must therefore be confident and independent in their self-management abilities. The aim of self-management programmes is to enable the child to come to terms with and more effectively cope with their asthma, requiring plans which reflect the everyday realities and challenges of the child's world. When due consideration is given to the above factors, self-management asthma plans have been found to be successful in ensuring compliance with treatment even with very young children (Ramsay, 1994).

Children will also be empowered through receiving accurate information about their condition and treatment/management options and there are now many books, leaflets, games and even clubs such as those run by the National Asthma Campaign to make learning fun and offer opportunities to learn from other children and families in the same situation.

Community children's nurse

Much asthma management work is undertaken by community children's nurses, who work collaboratively with other members of the primary health care team. Thornes (1994) described the gaps in service provision encountered by families with children discharged from hospital services and the role of the community children's nurse serves to fill this gap by providing continuity of care with primary and secondary services whilst advising, teaching and supporting children and their families in their own home. The health promotion role of the community children's nurse works effectively in preventing children with chronic conditions such as diabetes and asthma from repeated hospital admissions, decreases time lost from school and optimises 'normal' childhood activity. The community children's nurse understands the developmental needs of children and the impact of child development and maturation upon health status and receptiveness of health promotion. In this way, an infrastructure is developed which empowers even very young children to gain competence in their self-management aims. It is acknowledged however that not all children will want to take on the responsibilities and obligations involved in self-management programmes and their right to negotiate their involvement and to opt in and out of partnership arrangements must be respected.

STRATEGIES AND EVALUATION

Developing strategies to involve children and young people

Commissioning of child health services is increasingly being driven by the public health agenda (DoH, 1992; 1997) with commissioning decisions being based upon the health needs analysis of localities. However, there is a need to review the ways in which children are represented within the commissioning process and the nature of child health data being collected. It has been suggested that many 'needy' children may find themselves marginalised outside of the more usual data collection categories, such as children from minority ethnic families and travelling families who might not readily access health services. There is also growing concern about groups of children who care for adults, children who may not wish to be identified for fear of the repercussions of discovery.

Within the present emerging national health strategy, the advent of the establishment of primary care groups within localities, presents opportunities for input from user groups who advocate for children who find themselves in difficult situations. The DoH (1997) suggest that primary care groups will be built upon appropriate partnerships and will have responsibility for planning and developing services as well as contracting to and implementing local health improvement programmes. It is intended that the health improvement programmes will be central to future health provision and will focus upon individuals who are socially excluded, thereby improving health through tackling health inequalities. If child health issues are to be addressed in a radical way, then children surely must be involved in health improvement programmes, contributing their experience and expertise to inform child health issues.

How can children and young people influence service provision?

The need to involve children as service users in all aspects of health care is receiving much professional support. It is clear that future services will be increasingly needs led and a crucial point for consideration by all involved must be how to involve children and young people in commissioning activity. It is through such activities that individuals can exercise their rights to be involved in health provision and be more involved in the decision-making process. However, the ways in which children can become involved in meaningful activities rather than being involved as 'token gestures' remain to be explored. Particular attention needs to be given to the challenges presented by involving children who have mental health or learning difficulties, or children from ethnic minority groups, groups of children who are most likely to be under-represented in any consumer activity yet may be regular service users. In preparing guidelines for commissioners and providers of children's services, Hogg (1996) suggests that 'standards developed with children, young people and their families are often the best indicators of quality' and provides useful audit checklists to help this process.

How might children become more involved with decision making within the health services they use?

Although progress is slow, there is growing documentary evidence of children being involved in the ways listed in Box 6.5.

BOX 6.5	*Ways to involve children in decision making regarding health service provision*

- Inviting children to be members of quality groups within services
- Completing school projects designed to elicit children's opinions and experiences
- Involving children in building plans for new departments/services etc.
- Seeking the opinions of children at the point of service use
- Talking directly to children rather than through their parents
- The use of TV and other media, e.g. the Internet to elicit children's views
- Informing children of their rights to be involved at every stage of contact
- Establishment of child advocacy groups
- Involving children in professional conferencing activity
- Arranging for children to talk with ministers/policy makers

In the past, it was more likely that children would be involved in evaluating services that they had used, rather than directing future service delivery. Unfortunately, even within this process, many parents have been asked to evaluate services on behalf of their children as few tools have been available for use with the younger age groups.

CONCLUSION

Many health directives relating to child health have indicated the need for partnership models to develop and the need for interagency working to make for effective change within children's health services. As long ago as 1976, The Court Report *Fit for the Future* called for closer coordination of services concerned with the health and welfare of children. The vision of integrated child health services emerged and has been a constant theme in much subsequent child health literature (Audit Commission, 1993; Hall, 1996; NHSE, 1996; DoH, 1998). However robust the intentions of such health policy, Bagnall and Dilloway (1996, p4) suggest that there is little evidence of strategic vision in the provision of health care and health promotion for school-age children and call for concentrated and combined efforts to develop strategies to effect change.

The agenda for interagency working is emerging through the developing infrastructure of the 'New NHS' through the development of primary care groups and health improvement programmes. The case for involving children directly in health care issues has been presented and some of the considerable challenges have been explored. It is up to informed and enlightened individuals working for and with children to make sure that this opportunity is not missed. The above initiatives are already happening, although progress is patchy. Perhaps the ideal starting point is to invite children and young people to meet and suggest their own ideas – it might be that child-focused solutions are out there waiting to be uncovered!

REFERENCES

Audit Commision (1993) *Children First: a study of hospital services.* London: HMSO

Bagnall, P. & Dilloway, M. (1996) '*In a Different Light*'. *School Nurses and their Role in Meeting the Needs of School Age Children.* London: HMSO.

Benzeval, M., Judge, K. & Whitehead, M. (1996) *Tackling Inequalities in Health.* London: King's Fund.

Bibace, R. & Walsh, M. (1981) *Children's Conceptions of Health, Illness and Bodily Functions.* San Francisco: Jossey Bass.

Blackburn, C. (1991) *Poverty and Health: Working with Families.* Milton Keynes: Open University.

Botting, B. & Crawley, R. (1996) *In the Health of Our Children (OPCS)* London: HMSO.

Bradshaw, J. (1990) *Child Poverty & Deprivation in the UK* London: National Children's Bureau.

Carruthers, P. (1993) Asthma at School. *Community Outlook*, August, pp. 41–43

Children Act (1989) London: HMSO.

Conway, J. (1988) *Prescription for Poor Health: the Crisis for Homeless Families.* London: Shelter.

Court Committee (1976) *Fit for the Future.* Report of the Court Committee on Child Health Services. London: HMSO.

Department of Health (DoH) (1992) *The Health of the Nation.* London: HMSO.

Department of Health (DoH) (1997) *The New NHS. Modern, Dependable.* London: HMSO.

Department of Health (DoH) (1998) *Our Healthier Nation.* London: HMSO.

Doherty, J. & Campbell, L. (1990) *Families and Health.* London: Sage.

Eiser, C. (1991) It's OK Having Asthma – Young Children's Beliefs about Illness. *Professional Nurse*, March, 342–345.

Flekkoy, M. (1991) *A Voice for Children.* London: UNICEF.

Fradd, E. (1994) Power to the People. *Paediatric Nursing*, 6(3): 11–14.

Hall, D. (1989) *Health for All Children.* Oxford: Oxford University Press

Hall, D. (1996) *Health for All Children.* 3rd edn. Oxford: Oxford University Press.

Health Select Committee (1997) *The Specific Health Needs of Children and Young People*, House of Commons 2nd Report London: HMSO.

Hogg, C. (1996) *Health Services for Children & Young People.* London: Action for Sick Children.

Lansdown, G. (1995) In eds. Carter, B. & Dearnmun, A. *Child Health Care Nursing.* Oxford: Blackwell.

McIntosh, J. (1992) The perception and use of child health clinics in a sample of working class families. *Childcare, Health & Development*, 18(3): 133–150.

Mayall, B. & Foster, M. (1989) *Child Health Care: living with children, working with children.* Oxford: Heinemann

Moores, Y. (1995) *The Health of the Young Nation.* London: HMSO.

National Health Service Executive (NHSE) (1996) *Child Health in the Community: A Guide to Good Practice.* London: HMSO.

Neighbour, R. (1992) Paternalism or autonomy. *The Practitioner*, 236: 860–864.

Nutbeam, D. (1984) Health education in the National Health Service; the differing perceptions of community health physicians and health education officers. *Health Education Journal*, 43.

Nutbeam, D. et al (1993) Evaluation of two school smoking education programmes under normal classroom conditions. *British Medical Journal* 306: 102–107.

Office of Population Census and Surveys (OPCS) (1996) *The Health of our Children.* London: HMSO.

Oppenheim, C. (1993) *Poverty: The Facts.* London: Child Poverty Action Group.

Perez de Cuellar, J. (1990) In *A Voice for Children.* Flekkoy, M. (1991; 215) London: UNICEF.

Prescott-Clarke, P. & Primatesta, P. (1996) *Health Survey for England 1996; findings.* A survey carried out on behalf of the Department of Health, 1998 (series HS, 1 (6)). London: HMSO.

Pridmore, P. & Bendelow, G. (1995) Images of health: exploring beliefs of children using the draw and write technique. *Health Education Journal*, **54**: 473–488.

Ramsay, J. (1994) The psychology of childhood asthma. *Paediatric Nursing*, **6**(8): 17–21.

Roberts, I. & Power, C. (1996) Does the decline in child injury mortality vary by social class? A comparison of class specific mortality in 1981 and 1991. *British Medical Journal*, **313**: 784–786.

Rose, P. (1997) Best interests versus autonomy: a model for advocacy in child health care. *Journal of Child Health Care*, **1**(2): 74–77.

Ross, J. & Phipps, E. (1986) Physician:patient power struggles:their role in non-patient compliance. *Family Medicine*, **18**: 99–101.

Thornes, R. (1994) *Bridging the Gaps:Caring for Children in the Health Service*. London: Action for Sick Children.

Williams, S. (1994) In *Child Health: A Reader*, eds Gott, M. & Maloney, B. Oxford: Radcliffe.

Wilson, M. (1995) In *Child Health Care Nursing*. eds Carter, B. & Dermun, A. Oxford: Blackwell.

7 Youth health promotion in the community

Grainne Graham

KEY ISSUES

- Historical/legislative context
- Concentration on 'problem' issues
- Parent partnerships
- Educational alliances
- Less empowering methods
- More empowering methods
- Peer education
- Outreach and detached approaches
- Healthy settings
- Specialist services

INTRODUCTION

The health of young people is very much in vogue at the moment. It is prioritised by government and is constantly in the media. However, much of this attention is directed at dealing with problems. 'Twelve-year-old girl gives birth', blast the tabloid headlines, whilst the government pledges 'war on drugs'. Society appears to be concerned, not so much with promoting the health of young people, as preventing them from indulging in certain behaviours which society circumscribes. In reality, these behaviours are perceived by many young people either as an accepted part of their life, or more worrying for many adults, as enjoyable, life-enhancing activities, whose risks do not outweigh the benefits. This is not to say that there are no important health issues for young people, nor that the behaviour of young people does not pose a serious risk to their own and others' health. The real problem though is that whilst health promotion is targeted at negative behaviour change approaches which seek to stop young people from smoking, drinking, taking illegal drugs and having sex, we are not enabling them to be empowered to make their own health choices. Instead, we are telling them that the only healthy choice is to 'say no'. Not only that but we, the adults, are setting the agenda. We are focusing on issues that cause us as adults problems, rather than looking at the issues which young people themselves raise. Although many professionals working with young people are aware that this is the case, they are stuck with a social and political agenda which makes empowering work on young people's health very difficult. This chapter will explore this contention by first of all setting the context of young people's health in the late 1990s. It will go on to explore the ways in which prevailing attitudes and strategies in this area are disempowering to young people and it will identify what the real issues are for young people. It will then look at ways in which the different agencies can work together in a more empowering way. Finally it will identify strategies which are negative, less empowering and less successful and contrast these with more positive, empowering strategies. Throughout the chapter, reference will be made to health promotion and health education. Within this chapter, health education will refer specifically and only to educational activities, whilst health promotion will refer to the range of broader activities including policies, legislation and environmental initiatives.

CONTEXT

Successive governments have prioritised the health of young people. This has usually been through legalisation relating to education and health. There have also been developments in social services and the international arena which have had an impact on young people's health. This section examines these initiatives and then goes on to explore professional developments in relation to young people's health throughout the 1980s and 1990s.

Educational context

In the 1980s there was a commitment to building sex education into the taught curriculum of schools (DES, 1987) and a high profile media campaign against drug misuse was aimed at young people. Many people working with young people, especially teachers and youth workers took on board the need to undertake health education with young people, particularly around the issues of sexual health, human immunodeficiency virus (HIV)/acquired immunodeficiency syndrome (AIDS), illegal drugs, smoking and alcohol. In schools, health education focusing on these issues was taught as part of personal, social and health education lessons. Whilst in youth service settings more informal, health education was taking place. With the advent of the National Curriculum in the 1980s, health education in schools was somewhat marginalised, as health education was not included as a core subject. It was however classed as a cross-curricular area, that is a subject which could be covered as part of other subjects, for instance science, English and religion, and schools were encouraged to address health education issues through other subjects (National Curriculum Council, 1989). In order to help schools with this, guidance was issued by the National Curriculum Council, detailing which issues should be covered at which ages, with suggestions of which national curriculum areas they could be fitted into (National Curriculum Council, 1990). This guidance, whilst not mandatory, was potentially important for young people's health. It suggested a framework of health education in schools which was comprised of nine components. These included the traditional 'problem' areas of drugs and sex, but the framework was wider, more encompassing, it included family life education, environmental issues and psychological aspects of health education. The content of each component was also progressive as it emphasised the importance of attitude and values clarification and skills building, rather than merely concentrating on the acquisition of knowledge. The drawback was the lack of statutory requirements, which meant many schools, especially in the secondary sector were unwilling or unable to implement a programme of planned and progressive health education such as the curriculum guidance had encouraged. Development of health promotion initiatives in youth service settings was also impeded by a similar lack of statutory obligation. Then in the late 1980s, with the appointment of local education authority drugs and health education coordinators and the expansion of health promotion departments, a degree of impetus, coordination and cohesion began to emerge. In both the formal and informal educational settings therefore health education was growing and developing through the 1980s and 1990s. However, much was still left to the interest and commitment of individual professionals initiating projects which were often ad hoc and short term.

Health service context

The Department of Health has prioritised young people's health in both of the national health strategies produced in the last decade. The first such strategy was *The Health of the Nation* (DoH, 1992). It set five priority areas for the nation's health:

1. Accidents
2. Coronary heart disease
3. Sexual health
4. Cancers
5. Mental health.

Within these areas targets were set which related specifically to young people. These were:

■ To reduce the prevalence of cigarette smoking among 11–15-year-olds
■ To reduce deaths caused by accidents among the under 15s
■ To reduce pregnancies for girls under 16 years old

Other targets were set in the key areas which related to changing the behaviour of the general population and many of those targets could also be applied to young people, for example in increasing exercise, improving dietary habits, reducing the incidence of skin cancer, and reducing sexually transmitted diseases. The potential for health-promoting work with young people inherent in *The Health of the Nation* was realised by many professionals working on young people's health. It gave some sense of purpose and order to their work. This was further developed when the Government launched a new *Health of the Nation* initiative, aimed specifically at young people: *The Health of the Young Nation*. This was not however a coherent programme of work on promoting young people's health. It merely highlighted the importance of young people's health and encouraged health professionals and others working with young people's to use the existing targets within *The Health of the Nation* to promote young people's health. The problem with this approach was the limitations inherent in *The Health of the Nation*, namely its concentration on change of lifestyle. Whilst both *The Health of the Nation* and *The Health of the Young Nation* did acknowledge the issue of youth health promotion and they did provide a framework within which to promote young people's health, they both failed to provide an holistic, empowering approach to young people's health. Instead they continued to contextualise young people's health in terms of problem issues.

It was because of the problems inherent in *The Health of the Nation* that many people involved in young people's health looked forward to the new national health strategy which was promised in 1997 by the Labour government soon after they were elected. The draft strategy was published in January 1998 as a discussion document entitled *Our Healthier Nation* (DoH, 1998). Many were pleased to see a clear acceptance of the societal and economic influences on health, and a pledge to reducing inequalities in health. However, the document is long on narrative but short on practical commitment. It reduces the many targets for health found in *The Health of the Nation*, but has possibly made the mistake of throwing the baby out with the bathwater. Although the new strategy's main targets are four of the five health areas identified in *The Health of the Nation*, it excludes the fifth area – sexual health – the one which possibly has the greatest impact on young people. The Government has said that sexual health is still a priority issue and that it has been excluded merely because a separate strategy on sexual health will be produced. However, this diminishes the impact of having one overarching health strategy which identifies the key issues that should be addressed nationally. There is the possibility that an individual sexual health strategy will have a lot less force than the national health strategy and may well be sidelined in favour of the areas which are highlighted in the national strategy.

The positive aspect of *Our Healthier Nation* is that in addition to the key health areas, it identifies three key settings, one of which is healthy schools. The strategy clearly puts the emphasis of young people's health on the holistic healthy school concept. However, there is little concrete information on the way it sees the healthy school idea developing in practice and although money for healthy schools was promised in the document, this has already been handed out to eight areas, with no promise of any more money for the many other areas that are developing, or wish to develop healthy school initiatives.

The final document is still to be produced and only time will tell whether it will have an empowering effect upon young people's health. The signs would seem to be that the health service is changing radically, but as yet there is no evidence of that creating a more enlightened or empowering ethos.

Social services context

Whilst the Departments of Health and Education were seeing young people's health from a rather narrow perspective, a more interesting and more empowering attitude to young people was being adopted at the Department of Social Security through The Children Act, which was passed in 1989 (HMSO, 1989). The Children Act is primarily aimed at the responsibilities of Social Service Departments (SSDs), in regard to individual children deemed to be in 'need'. However, it had general implications for health promotion and young people, through the ethos and the implications of the Act. At the heart of the Act is the need to act in the best interests of children and as such it is based on the premise of parental responsibility, rather than parental rights. The Act has been described as a charter for children, whose overriding purpose is to promote and protect children's welfare (DoH, 1993). The Act states that children have the right to be kept informed about what is happening to them. They also have the right to participate in any decisions which are made about their future. The Act talks about the need for young people to achieve or maintain a reasonable standard of health or development and the importance of not impairing the health or development of young people. The Children Act also highlights the need for interagency cooperation in the planning and provision of services which affect young people. The Act placed responsibilities on SSDs, health and local education authorities to cooperate to consider overall development needs, including physical, social, intellectual, emotional and behavioural ones. The need for health practitioners to work together with local authorities, for instance in identifying needs was also recognised. The Children Act is important in considering empowerment and young people's health, because it stipulates that children's wishes, feelings and best interests should be taken into account in any decisions which affect their health and development. In so doing it sees that the heart of young people's issues is not the problems that young people create, but their rights which need to be respected and protected.

International context

The empowering approach to young people found in the Children Act reflected international developments in relation to young people's rights. The Convention on the Rights of the Child was adopted by the United Nations in November 1990 (UNICEF, 1995). It is a document which seeks to enshrine in international law the rights of young people under 18 years old all over the world. By 1995, 176 of the world's 191 countries had ratified the convention. It contains 54 articles pertaining to young people's rights and responsibilities. In the Convention, the notion of young people's rights as expressed in the Children Act is seen in a much broader context and developed much further. As a consequence, the implications for young people's health are more obvious and much greater. The articles relate to the areas listed in Box 7.1.

These general principles have clear bearings on the rights of young people to health. In particular, development and participation rights can be seen as

BOX 7.1	*Areas covered by the Articles of The Convention on the Rights of the Child*

- *Survival rights* – this refers to their most basic needs and includes access to health care
- *Development rights* – to enable children to develop to their fullest potential
- *Protection rights* – to guard them against all forms of abuse and exploitation
- *Participation rights* – to enable children to have free expression and take an active role in decisions which affect them.

(UNICEF, 1995)

ensuring that children and young people have the right to information, education and services which will enable them to grow and develop healthily and make healthy decisions. Of the 54 articles there are several which have specific bearing on health and young people as detailed in Box 7.2.

| BOX 7.2 | *Articles of The Convention on the Rights of the Child specifically relating to young people* |

Article 3 – This states that the best interests of the child should be the primary consideration of any decisions, actions or legislation which affect the child

Article 12 – This states that a child who is capable of forming its own views has the right to express those views and they should be given due weight in any decisions affecting the child

Article 17 – This recognises a child's right of access to appropriate information, especially that which promotes her/his social, spiritual, moral, physical or mental health and well-being

Article 23 – This states that children with disabilities have the right to a full and decent life. Signatory states should promote the exchange of appropriate information in relation to disabled children and preventative health care

Article 24 – This states the right of the child to health and health services. In particular signatory states should: '... develop preventive health care, guidance for parents, and family planning education and services'.

(UNICEF, 1995)

The Convention therefore by acknowledging the rights of young people to involvement in decisions affecting their health and to information, education and services which promote and protect their health, can be interpreted as an endorsement of health promotion for children and young people. It should be possible to use the Convention to argue for the provision of progressive, planned and empowered health promotion initiatives.

Professional context

Despite the lack of real government commitment to meaningful health promotion work with young people, a range of key professionals, including teachers, youth workers and health professionals continued to implement health education initiatives throughout the 1980s. What became increasingly apparent, particularly to health promotion specialists, was the need to move away from ad hoc, one-off, issue-based health education and to adopt not just a more planned and progressive approach, but a holistic and empowering one, based on young people's needs, rather than society's concerns. The concept of health-promoting settings was gaining ground in Europe and out of this was born the idea of 'health-promoting' schools, whereby not only would young people be educated about personal health, but they would be educated in an environment which reflected the ideas and ideals which they were being encouraged to adopt. *The Health of the Nation* whilst being primarily concerned with encouraging individual lifestyle change, did acknowledge the importance of the healthy settings concept, including the health-promoting school. In fact, *The Health of the Nation* pledged support to a European Network of Health-Promoting Schools. With the advent of *Our Healthier Nation*, a much firmer commitment has been made to health-promoting schools by the Government. As a result, more and more practitioners working with young people on health are adopting broader approaches, developing healthy setting initiatives and in general working towards a more empowering practice. Unfortunately the legacy of *The Health of the Nation* and its individualistic approach, coupled with the lack of statutory educational requirements, mean that many other practitioners are still locked into a narrow, information giving approach. Whilst *Our Healthier Nation* should have a positive effect, the limitation inherent in its approach may mean that it will be a long time before professional practice becomes more empowering.

COMMUNITY DEVELOPMENT

As stated in the introduction, much health promotion work undertaken with young people, tends to be problem focused and as such is not empowering in nature. This section will explore these issues more deeply in relation to community development/participation as a means of ensuring a more empowering approach. The main issues which much of youth health promotion has focused on is sex and drugs education. Generally the purpose of the education has been to stop young people from becoming involved in either of these two activities. However, evidence suggests that many young people are using both legal and illegal drugs (HEA, 1992; Parker et al, 1995) and that many are becoming sexually active at younger ages (Johnson et al, 1994). As a result, health education has often set up a conflict situation, with the professionals trying to stop young people doing what they enjoy. This in itself causes a problem for enabling the empowerment of young people through health promotion. Another problem this causes is that it sees young people's lives in isolated compartments, whereby they choose to indulge in these separate health-compromising activities. In reality, young people smoke and have unsafe sex for a whole range of inter-connected reasons. For health promotion with young people to be effective and empowering, it must be holistic by seeing at the heart of the issues not problems which young people create but the young people themselves.

At the centre of health promotion for young people is the need for positive self-esteem (Lloyd, 1994). If young people have a good sense of self-esteem they can make decisions which are healthy for them. Health promotion should therefore be approached in a way which, while providing the necessary knowledge, enhances young people's sense of self-esteem by building up essential skills. Unfortunately the concentration on problem issues and behaviours and some of the methods used to tackle these issues, actually diminishes young people's self-esteem and in so doing depowers them. Many approaches have taken a victim-blaming approach by seeing drug misuse, poor diet etc. as being choices which individuals make freely. These approaches assume that informing young people of the consequences of these behaviours will stop them from practising them. In fact, behaviour is affected by a whole range of factors and some of the most important factors are beyond a young person's control, for example socio-economic circumstances and family background. Evidence suggests that children from families from lower socio-economic backgrounds will have a high chance of developing poor health-related behaviours, because they are in a low income situation and because their parents already practise health-compromising behaviours (Klerman, 1993). Similarly evidence shows that young people from low income and socially deprived backgrounds are more likely to become teenage parents than people from more affluent backgrounds (Smith, 1993; Babb, 1993). For these reasons, education alone has been shown to be an ineffective way of affecting young people's health behaviour in relation to illegal drugs (Royal College of Psychiatrists, 1987) and alcohol (May, 1991). Given this, it is both inappropriate and disempowering to merely tell young people about the risks of such behaviours and expect them to either not start or change them. Once it has been established that the context in which young people make health choices is important, it is possible to see that it is not information that young people need to dissuade them from certain activities, but the skills to:

- assess the information accurately
- recognise risk situations
- explore their own feelings, values and attitudes
- make informed decisions.

Information does need to be given in providing effective health promotion for young people, but it also needs to encourage the development of the above skills. It should not be solely focused on affecting problem-related behaviour – such approaches to drug and alcohol education have failed in the past (Coggans et al, 1991; May, 1991). It could be argued that the reason they have failed is that they have not been empowering to young people because they have not addressed the wider factors affecting health and they have not allowed young people the freedom to determine the outcomes they want.

To be truly empowering, health promotion for young people should be based on the Rogerian principle of student-centred learning (Rogers, 1983) and the Frierian principle of praxis (Friere, 1972). Both approaches are built upon the notion of community participation, in that the learner is truly at the centre of the process. This is achieved through the learner:

- defining their own needs
- directing the course of their own learning
- being actively involved in the learning process
- reflecting on what they have learnt and the learning process.

In relation to youth health promotion, this entails young people being actively involved in defining their own health needs, developing the strategies to address those needs and directing how those strategies are implemented. This notion of student-centred learning has far-reaching implications for youth health promotion, as indeed it does for all education. No longer is the young person merely the recipient of information, nor are they just participants in the learning process – they are in control of their own education. The power is therefore taken away from the adult, be it a teacher, a youth worker, or even a parent and placed squarely with the young person. Such an approach is radical and likely to arouse opposition in those it takes power away from, for example the health and education professionals. However, only by accepting the principle of consulting and involving young people in meaningful ways will youth health promotion overcome the difficulties of being problem based and victim blaming, and therefore alienating young people. Too often in the past young people's views were ignored. No-one knew what young people wanted because no-one asked. Unfortunately this is still true for much of health promotion. *The Health of the Nation* targets which relate to young people (DoH, 1992) were not arrived at by consultation with young people, but by the Government in consultation with adults. Targets have therefore been set which affect young people but about which they have had no say. This is also true for most of the health education young people receive in school. It is devised and implemented by teachers and where there is consultation, it is usually on the topics of drugs and sex education because they are considered contentious, and even then the consultation is only with parents and governors. The truth of the matter is that despite the fact that the Children Act enshrined the principle of consultation with young people in British law, young people are seldom, if ever, consulted about the health care, or the health education they receive, or about what their health needs might be.

This is not to say that the issues which society highlights in relation to young people's health are not important. There is evidence to back up the concerns of many professionals and parents as the information in Box 7.3 illustrates.

BOX 7.3	*Statistics of drug and alcohol use, and pregnancy rates in the UK*

- The UK has the highest teenage pregnancy rate in Europe and the second highest rate in the developed world, second only to the USA (HEA, 1997a)
- The use of illegal drugs is widespread among young people, with recent studies showing over a third of all 15–16-year-olds use some sort of illegal drug (Turtle, Jones & Hickman, 1997)
- In England, 30% of 15-year-old girls and 29% of 15-year-old boys smoke cigarettes regularly (Office of National Statistics, 1997)
- 11% of 13-year-olds drink alcohol regularly (HEA, 1992).

These statistics make it plain to see that these are important health promotion issues for young people. It would be an interesting dilemma however, if young people were consulted about their needs in relation to health promotion and they said they did not feel sex and drugs were important issues to address. In reality, there has been little consultation in the UK on the health issues young people think are important. In the USA, there has been research into adolescents' health concerns (Millstein, 1993). These studies have shown that adolescents acknowledge a wide range of health concerns, but only a few were consistently ranked highly. These were:

- school issues
- acne
- mental health.

- dental health
- interpersonal relationships

If UK adolescents have a similar perception of health concerns, the priorities for youth health promotion will need to change somewhat. Until young people are consulted about what they want from health promotion and they start to be actively involved in the subsequent strategies, empowering and therefore effective health promotion work will not be possible. However, it remains to be seen whether schools, youth clubs and society at large will accept the need to truly empower young people. It is likely that they will feel threatened by such an approach, seeing it merely as depowering to themselves. There are some examples of good practice though, where steps are being taken in the right direction, at least in so far as young people are being more involved, for example:

1. The health-promoting school concept has the involvement of young people central to its ethos. The concept is also one which could be adapted to other settings for young people, for instance youth clubs.
2. Young people have been consulted on their needs in relation to sexual health services (HEA, 1996) and there are examples up and down the country of service provision modelled on the expressed views of young people (Aggleton, 1996). The section on strategies explores other examples of good practice.

HEALTHY ALLIANCES

This section will explore the different settings for health promotion work with young people and the opportunities for healthy alliance work within these settings. For health service workers, the community health care setting provides opportunities for health promotion work with young people. General practitioners (GPs), practice nurses, community drugs and alcohol workers and family planning nurses have clear roles in youth health promotion. They may have patients/clients who are young people and they can give health promotion information and advice to them. Unfortunately there are limitations implicit in these settings. The formal nature of the GP surgery can make young people feel depowered as they lack experience in social skills and they feel unsure that confidentiality will be maintained. As a consequence, young people do not like to attend their general practice for health information or general family planning clinics for sexual health services (West et al, 1995; HEA, 1996). Community drugs and alcohol teams usually provide a more informal environment and so might be more conducive to health promotion work with young people. However many are orientated to the needs of dependent users who are usually adults. This leaves little time for the workers to develop work with young people and may serve to give these services an image which puts young people off using them.

For these reasons, there is probably greater scope for health promotion work with young people in settings outside the health service. By the very fact that they are outside the health service, these settings provide opportunities for healthy alliances as health professionals can work in partnership with people from other settings, with the common goal of promoting young people's health. These settings are:

- homes
- youth clubs
- schools
- universities and colleges.

By looking in depth at these settings and the people who have a health promotion role within them, we will be able to see both the opportunities and difficulties for healthy alliance work in these settings.

Homes

One of the primary and probably the most influential settings for health promotion with young people is the home. Parents and other family members often have a far greater impact on young people's behaviours than any outside agency or professional, as it is suggested that patterns of behaviours and attitudes which influence health are well established by the time a child is 5 years old (DES, 1986). This does not mean that outside professionals do not have a valid role in promoting the health of young people, but rather it provides an opportunity for professionals to work with parents on promoting the health of their children. Such an alliance is necessary because the information that parents impart to their children is usually from an adult perspective, not one which is negotiated with the child (Brannen and Storey, 1996). In addition, many parents feel ill-equipped to undertake certain aspects of health education, for example sex education, and would welcome help and support from schools (Young, 1991, HEA, 1995) and possibly health professionals. The health promotion role of parents is an area where there has been relatively little work on a planned basis, however there is growing interest in health professionals working with parents to facilitate their health promotion role (Young, 1991). This can encompass:

- information sessions for parents on health issues which affect young people
- in-depth work with groups of parents over a period of time to build up their skills in health promotion.

Unfortunately, most of the work so far has tended focus on the first method and was limited once again to drugs and sex education. However, more in-depth work on a broader range of health issues could be adopted and it is likely that initiatives of this nature will be developed over the coming years. An important issue will be how the work of these alliances with parents are developed. There is the possibility that the professionals will dictate which issues are addressed and in which ways. If they are to be truly empowering though, the alliances need to be rooted in community participation and development. This means they need to be developed jointly with parents/carers and based on their expressed views, in consultation with young people. There are however many young people who are not cared for by their parents, but are cared for in local authority homes. There are also those who have parents who are unwilling or unable to take on the role of health promoter for their child. For these young people, settings outside the home, and professionals from those settings, may well be the best people to take on the main health promotion role. Even where parents are interested and involved in the health education of their child, they often want their own work to be supported and developed by professionals in the other settings where their children spend their time. Chiefly these are educational settings.

Schools

The setting where young people spend most of their time outside the home is school. It is here that there is possibly the greatest potential for health promotion and also the greatest limitations. Its potential lies in the sheer amount of time young people spend there and in the educational purpose. Where better for 'education' about health to be carried out than in an educational establishment? The difficulty is that there is little statutory requirement for schools to undertake health education. Despite this most schools, both primary and secondary, do provide some health education, although the quantity and quality is very diverse.

It is in primary schools that perhaps the greatest amount of health education takes place. The nature of primary education, with one teacher being responsible for all the education of a class for a whole year, lends itself to the holistic nature of health education, where different themes can be developed across different subjects in a congruent manner. There are also many elements of the national curriculum at primary level which deal with health-related issues. In particular, primary science is concerned with growth and development (Brown, 1996), which brings in many physical, emotional and social health issues. The problems are that many primary schools do not recognise the work they do as health education, whilst others do not recognise the opportunity to introduce health-related themes and so do not develop them. It is because of this that healthy alliances are necessary, to enhance teachers' understanding and abilities in relation to health education and to involve other relevant health professionals in programmes of health-related work.

In contrast to primary schools there is little in the national curriculum for secondary schools which necessitates health education. However, its classification as a cross-curricular subject means there are opportunities to develop health-related themes in many subjects (Brown, 1996), but these are left very much at the discretion of schools and individual teachers (Jamison, 1993). Most secondary schools do provide health education for their pupils, but usually as an isolated subject, in the form of personal and social (health) education (PSHE). It is here that issues important to young people's health can be considered, but again it is up to individual schools to do as much or as little health-related work as they wish. Although some schools do take health education seriously and have planned programmes within PSHE, for many others the discretion they are allowed results in a concentration on information about sex and drugs education, with little emphasis on emotions, skills or wider health issues.

The reality therefore, is that most secondary and many primary schools are unable or unwilling to provide comprehensive programmes of holistic health education within their existing resources. One of the crucial problems has already been alluded to; lack of statutory provision. There are however other limitations, principally:

1. The national curriculum is so demanding that it leaves insufficient time for health education.
2. Teachers did not train to become health promoters and so many do not have the skills or possibly the interest to carry out health promotion.
3. Other professionals, for example school nurses, are not trained as teachers and may be wary of taking on what they see as the teacher's role by becoming involved in classroom-based education around health.
4. Many of the issues relating to young people's health involve personal reflections and feelings and the lack of confidentiality which the classroom affords may not be an appropriate place to consider these issues.
5. Health promotion and young people revolves around not just knowledge, but attitudes and skills. This means that didactic teaching styles are not appropriate. Interactive techniques involving discussions, small group work and role play are necessary. However, this is often not possible either because class sizes are too large or teachers are not skilled in these techniques.

In order to minimise these limitations and to provide more rounded health promotion to young people, healthy alliances with outside health professionals are important. There is a range of professionals who work with schools on health issues and in so doing are creating healthy alliances. School nurses are the professionals who perhaps spring to mind most readily. This is not surprising as they can play a vital role in complementing the health education work of teachers in schools; the role of school nurses tends to vary greatly though. In some areas it goes little further than routine health checks, whilst in other areas they have a more extensive role. This can include working in partnership with the school and other health service staff, for example health promotion specialists, to support and train teachers in health education (Simpson and Went, 1994). There has certainly been interest in recent years in developing school nurses' health promotion roles along more extensive and innovative lines (Bagnall, 1991; Reid, 1991; Few et al, 1996; Bailey, 1994). This could involve school nurses in the following ways:

- Participating in the planning and delivery of health education in the classroom
- Providing health advice to pupils and staff
- Working in partnership with staff and parents on health-related school policies etc.
- Running drop-in health clinics within the school to provide specialist help, advice and information on a range of health issues for young people
- Providing similar drop-in health services outside of school hours, in nearby health centres, youth clubs etc.

The advice and support nurses give, both to individual pupils and to staff in school can be on general health issues and on more specific issues, e.g. sexual health, diet and exercise, smoking cessation etc. Often the extent of the school nurse's role reflects the amount of resources available for the service; little money means fewer nurses and therefore a more limited role. The amount of funding for the service in turn reflects the commitment of the local trust or health authority to the service. Obviously the more extensive role of the school nurse provides the most scope for enabling healthy alliances which can facilitate the empowerment of young people. School nurses are one part of the wider school health service, which as well as medical support also provides dental health support to schools. The main difficulties for all these professionals are:

1. Their own time constraints. Often there are too few school health professionals and this is usually because of limited health service resources, which results in 'soft services', i.e. those which aren't directed at acute care, having been cut back.
2. Time constraints imposed by the schools, which won't allow the health professionals the time they need to provide comprehensive inputs.
3. Communication difficulties between the health professionals and the teachers where they do not know what each other is doing.

Often it is the very fact that it is a healthy alliance which causes the problems. The health professionals and the schools belong to two different organisations with different priorities, different processes and different structures. This can lead to a misconception of roles and responsibilities which hampers the planned provision of effective health education.

Despite the problems associated with the school setting, many schools and many health and education professionals do prioritise health promotion. This is illustrated in the growing popularity of health-promoting school schemes. A recent publication listed 75 such schemes in England (HEA, 1997b). In practice these schemes are true healthy alliances with the health and education sectors working together to identify barriers and solutions to the wider health promotion role of schools. This is possibly the way forward for successful, empowering health promotion work with young people in a school setting.

Youth clubs

The other setting outside the home where there is great potential for health promotion work with young people, is in youth clubs. There is a large network of statutory and voluntary youth clubs and centres throughout Britain where young people spend their leisure time. Although the primary purpose of youth clubs is not education in the academic sense - they are certainly concerned with the broader social education of young people and for that reason State-run youth services are often part of local education authorities. The concern with social education means that there are natural links with an empowering approach to health promotion, which is concerned with health in a social and environmental context, rather than an individualistic one (Tones, 1995). The nature of the youth work setting is informal as attendance is purely voluntary and young people choose whether or not to go there. For this reason many youth workers feel that it is a better place for health education than school, as the atmosphere is more relaxed and so more conducive to discussions, debates and small group work (Graham, 1996). Throughout the 1980s and 1990s youth workers have taken on a health education role with young people. There has been little research in this area, but what there is shows that for the majority of youth workers health education is an important part of their work. Although some youth clubs have planned programmes of health education work, this is probably not the norm. For many youth workers health education happens in an ad hoc manner and is almost inseparable from their general day-to-day youth work. Issues are often discussed and debated as and when they arise rather than through a planned programme. For many youth workers this is how it should be, as it lets young people raise the issues when they want to (Graham, 1996). In that sense it is more empowering than a planned programme, which is usually based, whether knowingly or not, on the agenda of the youth worker. The difficulties with health promotion in a youth club setting are as follows:

- Many youth workers have little or no training in health education and may feel ill-equipped to deal with the issues.
- The informal nature of the setting means that in the long term, in depth work is difficult.
- Many youth centres do not have policies on health-related issues and therefore broader health promotion work is difficult.
- Community nursing staff tend not to be involved in health education in youth clubs because few have recognised roles in this setting.

These problems highlight the need for healthy alliances, where health professionals support youth workers to develop their health promotion role. Such alliances have already been developed and provide examples of good practice. Youth Clubs UK is a national youth organisation which in 1992 worked with the Health Education Authority (HEA) and local youth clubs, colleges and health promotion departments to organise a series of health fairs. These were actually workshops for people who work with young people and they looked at the skills and issues important to youth health promotion (Rogers, 1995). In terms of empowerment this alliance was interesting because it looked at holistic health issues. There were workshops on sexuality and gender, self-image, health and disability, massage and aromatherapy. It also recognised young people as a partner in the healthy alliance, involving them in the planning and development of the workshops. The healthy setting concept could certainly be appropriate to youth clubs in the same way as it is to schools. In Northern Ireland, one such scheme has already been set up (Fermanagh Herald, 1996). To enable this to happen healthy alliances would need to:

- ensure youth club staff were trained to increase their knowledge and skills in relation to health promotion
- provide advice on health-promoting policies relevant to youth clubs, for example no smoking, healthy eating and physical environment policies
- look into the feasibility of involving community nursing staff in the life of youth clubs, for example through regular health sessions or the provision of young people's health services within the club.

The health-promoting youth club might experience particular problems though, because of the informal nature of youth clubs and the financial restraints which many youth services experience. This can be overcome to some extent if:

- health professionals adapt to the informal nature of youth clubs and do not expect them to be like schools
- health authorities and local authorities work together in setting young people's health as a priority for youth services

Universities and colleges

Apart from schools and youth clubs, other educational settings can provide opportunities for health promotion with young people: colleges of further and higher education and universities. Although they are establishments for formal academic education, the scope for health education on a planned basis to groups of students is limited, because students choose what they study, so curriculum-based work is not usually possible. Instead health promotion potential lies with tutors who have pastoral responsibilities, either for individual students or for groups of students. This would be an informal role, similar to that of the youth worker's, whereby a whole range of health-related issues could be discussed and advice and information given in an ad hoc manner.

There is also scope for broader work in this setting, such as developing and implementing health policies and the provision of health-related services (O'Donnell and Gray, 1993). This would necessitate the involvement of health professionals, who have the relevant skills and experience to undertake such work. These professionals could be:

- Occupational health nurses
- Staff in student medical/health centres, i.e. doctors, nurses and counsellors
- Community nurses with a brief specially widened to include these establishments
- Health promotion specialists/health education coordinators

The policy work could involve discreet work on specific policies, e.g. no smoking, healthy eating or drugs policies. On the other hand these could be widened to a health-promoting college approach, tackling the same physical, environmental and psychological issues which the health-promoting school does. These professionals would also be involved in more general health promotion work, on a one-to-one basis with young people as clients. Many of the issues which young people will go to the occupational health nurse or the student health service about will be health promotion issues, e.g. contraception. Many others will have health promotion implications, or will provide opportunities for health promotion issues to be addressed. The issues of smoking, alcohol consumption, healthy eating and use of illegal drugs, could all be addressed in this way. In relation to empowerment, there is a potential problem though, as health professionals may be giving unsolicited advice on issues which young people have not identified as a priority.

In order to overcome the difficulties inherent in these healthy alliances and to progress the wider health-promoting role of schools, colleges, youth clubs etc., the health education co-ordinator and health promotion specialist for young people are important. The former is usually employed by the local education authority and the latter by the local health authority or trust. They have similar and complementary roles: to develop health promotion initiatives aimed at young people and to provide specialist support on health promotion to other professionals who work with young people. This can comprise of:

- initiating and developing specific long-term and short-term programmes
- training other health promoters on specific, as well as general, health promotion issues and skills
- advice on health education policy and programme development
- advice on wider health promoting initiatives, e.g. smoking and healthy eating policies
- an interface between the establishment and the outside health professional, enabling other healthy alliances to operate more smoothly.

Although the prime responsibility of these professionals might be to work with schools, they often have a wider role to work with anyone who might have a health promotion role with young people. This can include youth workers, social workers etc. Not all areas have these professionals though. It is at the discretion of the education authorities' whether they have a health education coordinator and although most health districts have a health promotion service, they do not necessarily have a health promotion specialist to work on young people's issues. Without these dedicated and specialist workers healthy alliances between health, education and social services still occur, however their frequency and efficiency can be very much limited. Even where both workers are in existence there can still be problems though, as they are employed by different organisations. This can mean that although they work broadly to the same aims they may have different priorities. A greater difficulty often arises with professional rivalry and protectionism. In these times of shortage of resources and consequent short-term contracts, job insecurity is very high. As a result both professionals can feel that the other represents a threat to their job. This can lead to a reluctance to engage in too much joint working. This can be compounded by the fact that health education coordinators usually come from educational backgrounds whilst health promotion specialists are often from health service backgrounds. Given the other difficulties which exist in relation to progressing health promotion with young people, this is in fact short sighted. It would be far more beneficial to combine resources, thereby providing a more comprehensive and better quality service and a good argument for continued funding for both professionals. It would also greatly increase their ability to engage in meaningful and empowering health promotion work.

STRATEGIES AND EVALUATION

There has been a significant amount of research which demonstrates the less effective health education strategies for involving young people. Unfortunately evidence for more effective methods of both health education and health promotion proves elusive. However, it is true to say that the less effective methods are also the least empowering, and that whilst recent new directions have not yet been proven effective, they do appear to be more empowering.

Less empowering methods

The following strategies have limited effectiveness and limited potential for young people's empowerment:

- Shock horror approaches
- Didactic methods.
- Single issue approaches

Shock horror approaches

Shock horror approaches have been proven ineffective since it was demonstrated that graphic and gruesome depiction's of the adverse effects of smoking or illegal drug use did not have any long-term effect on behaviour (Tripp and Davenport, 1988/1989). In the short-term, people were horrified and often changed their behaviour, but the images and messages were so disquieting that people sublimated their memories of them and soon reverted back to their original behaviours. Another reason that shock horror approaches proved so ineffective is the simple fact that many of them did not tell the truth and young people realised this. Even if just one part of the message is false young people often reject the whole message. Drugs education is perhaps the best example of this failure of the shock horror approach. The Heroin Screws You Up mass media campaign in the 1980s with its 'shocking images' of young people destroyed by the ravages of heroin failed to have an impact on the vast majority of young people (Whitehead, 1989). It failed because most young people did not identify with dependent heroin users and they knew from their own and their contemporaries' experiences that the drugs they were interested in – cannabis, speed etc. – had relatively little ill-effects on most users. Drugs prevention campaigns have also shown another fault of shock horror approaches, namely their counterproductive effect. It was felt that the campaign in the 1980s actually glamorised drug use and may have encouraged experimentation with drugs (Royal College of Psychiatrists, 1987), as the campaign posters became pin ups on bedroom walls. Unfortunately lessons were not learned and the experience was repeated in a later drugs prevention campaign in the early 1990s. It should be no surprise however that these shock horror methods are not effective, because they undermine the whole notion of empowerment in the following ways:

- They manipulate young people's emotions
- They preset the agenda
- They take away young people's choice to make their own decisions
- They are setting young people up to fail because they have a pre-determined behavioural outcome that is often unrealistic.

At best, shock horror approaches simplify the message so much that they distort the truth and at worst they lie to young people. By setting up such a dishonest environment, young people will not have the freedom to make up their own minds and decide what behaviour is best for them as an individual. They can never therefore be empowering.

Single issue approaches

As discussed earlier, much health education with young people has concentrated on single problem issues such as drug use and sex. This has been proven ineffective because it ignores the context in which young people make decisions. A behaviour is rarely determined by a discreet set of factors - it is more often the consequence of many interconnected factors and the environment in which it is carried out (Tones, 1995). Often the factors and the environment are beyond the young person's control because they are political, social and economic in nature. As illustrated earlier, young people's smoking, illegal drug taking and unsafe sexual behaviour is often caused by:

- lack of money
- poor job opportunities
- lack of family support.

Teaching young people techniques to quit smoking, resist peer pressure or put a condom on, is not going to change the young people's socio-economic environment, and so are likely to fail in changing behaviour. Political and social changes are necessary to provide the environment in which young people can make free choices about their health behaviour. Given that these changes are not forthcoming, an empowering approach to health promotion must:

1. accept the right of young people to make decisions which might compromise their health, because those are the ones which best suit their circumstances
2. work with young people to help them identify:
   - the factors affecting their health

- which of those factors they want to address
- how they want to address those factors.

Within this pragmatic approach to empowering health promotion, single issue approaches can have some use, if implemented in the right way. Often schools and other settings have difficulty with general concepts of health education and promotion, which are seen as too woolly and vague. Instead they want something concrete to latch onto, and this can be true of the young people too. Highlighting a specific issue can therefore be used to arouse the interest, either of the young people themselves or the schools or youth club etc. Once they are on board, young people can then identify the issues they are interested in and the ways they wish to address them.

Didactic methods

Empowering health education should afford young people the opportunity to debate health issue in such a way that they are enabled to:

- examine their own and others' attitudes to health-related issues
- form their own opinion
- make their own decisions on health-related issues.

Unfortunately much health education in the past has not made this possible because of its didactic nature. A didactic approach presents health issues as facts and gives information in a value-laden way. Clear black and white messages are given, portraying certain health behaviours as acceptable and others as unacceptable. For example, illegal drug use, smoking and underage sex are seen as wrong. The problem with this approach is not merely that it is ineffective (Dorn and South, 1985), but that it is oppressive. It tells young people that they have a choice between the right behaviour and the wrong behaviour. If they choose the wrong behaviour they are seen to have failed. Young people who come from backgrounds where illegal drug use, smoking, pre-marital sex or unhealthy eating are the norm are immediately confused, marginalised and put down by such an approach. As shown earlier, the influence of their social environment is such that they are more likely to adopt the health behaviours which are portrayed negatively. They have in effect been set up to fail. The result of this is that rather than raising their self-esteem, which is vital if they are to make free and therefore healthy choices, it actually undermines their self-esteem, depowering them even more.

More empowering methods

It is clear from the failure of the three approaches discussed earlier that effective health education which is also empowering needs to be:

1. Holistic – looking at the many factors which affect young people's health, for example healthy setting work, such as health promoting schools schemes.
2. Interactive and participative – actively involving young people in the process of health promotion. This can be through games, quizzes, role plays, small group work and discussions.

3. Young person led – young people are not merely the passive recipients of health promotion, but are at the centre of the process. They are able to express their needs and identify possible strategies for the health education/promotion work they will be involved in.

There are few practical examples of really empowering approaches to youth health promotion. Outlined below are two programmes which demonstrate how avowedly empowering methods can work in practice and some of the problems and potential associated with such work.

The 'Kids in Action' programme from Canada was a health promotion strategy for children which used a school-based community development approach (Kalnins et al, 1994). It aimed to enable empowerment through community development, using the educational ideas and methods of Paulo Friere. The Frierian approach entails the action by a community to first name the problems they face in everyday life. The community then engages in a dialogue about those problems which will lead to critical thinking, whereby the root causes of the problems and possible solutions to those problems are identified (Friere, 1972). Kids in Action worked with 9–10 year olds, in 90-minute weekly sessions over one school year. The children were involved in identifying community health problems, choosing a priority problem, designing and implementing activities to solve the problem and evaluating their experiences. A facilitator conducted the sessions, but there were few parameters established at the beginning of the programme. Activities were devised weekly in response to decisions made by the children. The first few sessions consisted of discussions on the notion of community and community health, including how children keep themselves healthy, how their decisions and the decisions of others affect their health and the impact of the environment on their health. The children then walked in small groups around the local area, pointing out things they considered good and bad, healthy and unhealthy. Back in their classroom they used this information to map out their neighbourhood. They were then asked to identify the issues of most concern to them. Through a process of voting, the class reached a consensus on the issues they thought most important. The facilitator then worked with the children to help them design and implement strategies to deal with their problem. Methods used by the programme included extended conversations, dialogue with invited community 'experts', brain-storming sessions and games. The problem the children identified was drugs and drug dealers across the street from the school. Their strategies consisted of posters, a video of sketches and a rap song describing their feelings about the issue, a petition to the city mayor and a stall at a local drugs awareness day.

At the end of the programme the children hosted an open day for parents, teachers and the local community to celebrate their achievements and show the community what they had achieved. Kalnins et al felt the programme demonstrated that children can engage in a community development process. They found that children on their own do not think of health in its broadest terms, or conceptualise it as a collective concern, but they can learn to do so. However, they also felt the programme raised several important key issues in relation to community development and young people as listed in Box 7.4.

The second practical example of empowering youth health promotion is the Adolescent Social Action Program (ASAP) in New Mexico, USA (Wallerstein and Sanchez-Merki, 1994). This was also based on the work of Paulo Friere,

BOX 7.4	*Key issues identified for involving young people in community development*

- What is the definition of community, when children come from varied geographical, social and religious backgrounds?
- There was a contradiction within the programme: whilst it was empowering it was also controlling, in that adult professionals were the active agents who preset the health agenda
- The programme was bound by the school timetable and progress was required within a pre-determined timescale
- The larger societal culture was a limitation because it does not expect nor foster empowerment

and was aimed at adolescents from high-risk, low-income, predominantly minority communities. It comprised of small groups of pupils going into a hospital for three sessions and into a gaol for one session, to interview patients and goal residents who had problems related to alcohol, drug misuse, violence, teenage pregnancy and HIV. After the interviews, but while still on site, a facilitator took the young people through a structured group dialogue. This enabled them to reflect on the lives of the people they have met, their own lives and what they could do to address problems in their own communities. They also participated in an extensive curriculum of decision making, conflict mediation, communication skills and resistance to peer pressure. After this experience, the young people were trained back at their schools to become peer educators in their schools, feeder schools and community settings. The facilitators were specially trained college students. The programme was qualitatively evaluated and it was found that students went through three stages of change. In the first stage, they developed an action orientation of caring about the problem, about each other and about their ability to act in the world. In the second stage, they began to act for individual changes, expressing an ability to help others who were close to them. In the third and final stage, they reached a level of understanding of the need for social change and the possibility of larger social actions. Wallerstein and Sanchez-Merki conclude that ASAP shows that young people involved in a Frierian programme can evolve beyond powerlessness to create a sense of empowerment enabling them to make a real difference to the world. They argue that the role of the health educator as facilitator is of crucial importance. The facilitator needs to be effective in the process of structured dialogue. They need to constantly raise questions in the group reflection sessions which highlight:

- the role of societal forces
- the limitations of individual action
- the difficulties of social action
- the role that members of a community can take in social action.

In doing this, the young people can be enabled to develop and maintain a commitment to their involvement in listening, dialogue and action. The Frierian approach also has benefits for the health educator as well as the young people. Through the process of praxis (action and reflection), the health educator can model and promote their own growth as they promote the growth of the young people they are working with.

The Kids In Action and the ASAP programmes have as their objective empowerment for social change. It is interesting that they are both examples from North America. With the UK's concentration on individual decision making and lifestyle choices, it is difficult to imagine similar programmes being implemented here. However, there are movements in the UK towards newer and more innovative approaches to youth health promotion. These explicitly acknowledge the importance of empowerment and could therefore have empowering potential. These approaches will discussed next.

Peer education

At present peer education is an extremely popular approach to health education with young people (Neesham, 1997a). It is used extensively in the USA and Canada and appears to be growing in popularity in the UK. It is based on the premise that peer influence has a large impact on young people's behaviour and that young people themselves may be in the best position to enable their peers to identify the problems which are important to them and appropriate solutions (Neesham, 1997b). Many peer education projects are rooted in the notion of community development, through the involvement of young people in their own education and in the form, content and delivery of their peers' education. This approach embodies the notions of community participation and social action intrinsic to empowerment. Furthermore, by enabling young people themselves to become health educators or facilitators, they are being given access to roles normally denied them and in that way they are being given an element of power.

In peer education programmes, a group of young people are recruited to become peer educators. These young people are then trained by adults, usually health professionals to undertake health education with another group of young people. The peer educators present positive role models, advocating healthy behaviour, whose views and actions the recipients will hopefully identify with and emulate (Milburn, 1995). The approach would certainly appear able to afford results in terms of positive effects on behaviour. Both the Postponing Sexual Involvement Programme in the USA (Howard and McCabe, 1992) and the programme reported by Mellanby et al (1995) in the UK showed success-ful results for sex education with the use of peer education. It is also being used for sex education in informal youth groups (Hamilton, 1992). It has not just been used for sex education though. A major national peer education project was undertaken by Youth Clubs UK, the HEA and the DoH, with 18 schemes being set up across the country (Vautrat, 1996). It recruited at-risk and disaffected young people as peer educators. They could choose an issue from the five *Health of the Nation* key areas, which in itself was limiting. However, the content and organisation of the training programme was very much what the peer educators wanted. The training materials developed from the programme are very much based on empowerment ideas. They incorporate a substantial degree of self-determination for peer educators and encourage them to challenge their own attitudes and values, rather than merely training them to deliver pre-set health messages (Harvey, 1995; Harvey and Smith, 1996). Results of the success of this and other similar programmes are awaited with interest, however, it is probable that meaningful results, as with most health promotion interventions, will only be available in the longer term say after 5 years. Unfortunately too few programmes are followed up for that length of time.

Although there is reason for some optimism regarding the success of peer education, it is advisable to sound a cautionary note when considering issues of empowerment as illustrated in Box 7.5.

BOX 7.5	*Cause for exercising caution in considering empowerment in peer education*

1. Peer education programmes take many very different forms. There is no one set peer education approach to follow – instead programmes have a variety of different aims, objectives and methodologies (Milburn, 1995). There is no consensus even on what the term 'peer' means. Does it refer to someone of the same age, or a few years older or younger? Are different social and cultural backgrounds taken into account?

2. There are ethical issues over whose agenda is being set – the young person's or the adults who set up the programme to deal with perceived health problems? Are the peer educators and the recipients being educated, or manipulated by adults into 'acceptable behaviour' (Milburn, 1995; Neesham, 1997b). If it is the latter option, the peer educators are actually being exploited by the adults running the programme (Neesham, 1997a).

3. Many programmes used older peer educators and the age difference may mean that the young people do not identify the educators as their peers. The scope for shared exploration of common problems and solutions would therefore be limited, as the peer educators may not be facilitators in the Frierian sense, but teachers in another guise, representing the same power imbalance. The result of this is that the young people are unable to articulate their true feelings.

4. Programmes tend to be single issue based and, as with other types of youth health promotion, they have tended to focus on sex and drugs education. This takes way from young people the power to identify their own problems, which is crucial to Frierian notions of empowerment.

5. There is a lack of good evaluation into the effectiveness or otherwise of peer education (Milburn, 1995).

In general the difficulty for peer education to be truly empowering has been described as the extent to which power, control, authority, responsibility and leadership will really be ceded to young people in peer education projects (HEA, 1993). These criticisms do not undermine peer education as a whole. The examples of existing peer education projects show a very definite potential for benefit (Neesham, 1997a). It is important however that peer education programmes:

■ are clear about their aims and objectives
■ choose peer educators who are truly from the community of young people they will be working with, in terms of age and experience
■ ensure that the peer educators are adequately trained, supported and supervised
■ wherever possible rigorously evaluate their effectiveness.

Outreach and detached approaches

Two related strategies which are potentially empowering methods of health promotion for young people are detached and outreach approaches. They have traditionally been associated with youth work, where youth workers will go onto the streets and work with those young people who do not want to access the youth clubs, but choose instead to hang out on street corners, in bus stops, on waste ground etc. (Jarvis, 1992). This way of working is usually seen as more empowering, because it is going to where young people are and negotiating an agenda with them. In fact outreach and detached workers have themselves said that the ethos of this approach is empowering (Jarvis, 1992). If young people are not interested they can simply walk away and there are no imposed rules, as there are in youth clubs, schools and at home, and no threat of sanctions can be imposed. In order to be successful it truly has to start where the young people are. Outreach usually refers to informing young people about pre-existing services and increasing their awareness of them and encouraging them to use them. Detached work usually refers to taking services or information out to where young people are and working with young people there on the streets (Driscoll, 1993).

Outreach and detached work has for several years been used as a way of taking health messages to young people (Driscoll, 1993). Workers, who are often a mix of youth workers and community nurses, go onto the streets and disseminate health-related information. This can either be information on services which are available for young people, in an attempt to reach out to young people and bring them into the service provision, or it can be merely giving educational information in an informal way, usually about safer drug use and safer sex. An example of a HIV-detached project is the Under the Stars project in Norwich, UK (Driscoll, 1993). Youth volunteers were recruited and trained to become detached HIV educators, giving advice, information, leaflets and condoms to young people on the streets in Norwich at night. The project was judged a success with 20–27 contacts being made per night. It was also felt to be empowering to the volunteers, as the training was ongoing, based on the volunteers expressed needs and facilitated to encourage feelings of equality and empowerment.

The problem with outreach and detached health programmes is that in the very fact of attaching health to the brief of the worker the agenda is shifting from being the young person's programme to that of the service provider's. Young people are not necessarily saying they want drugs and sex advice on the streets, but that is what they are being given. The whole premise of outreach work, which is to bring people into existing services, raises dilemmas as it may be telling young people who have chosen not to attend certain services that they should be attending them. At the centre of the problem could be misconceptions about what empowerment really means. One outreach worker in an interview described his work as trying to empower people to make their own choices. He felt that by giving young people the relevant factual information they were being 'empowered' (Jarvis, 1992). In reality no-one can empower someone else, and certainly not by merely giving information. It is not enough to tell young people they have a choice; they need to be supported to develop the skills which will enable them to make their own choice, whatever that might be. This does not mean that outreach and detached work cannot be empowering – they can if:

- the work is long term and the outreach/detached workers have time to build a relationship with the young people and work with them on a truly negotiated agenda
- consideration is given to why this approach has been adopted. It could be that a service has been established which is based on young people's expressed needs and outreach is merely a way of publicising the service

- the work does not start with a pre-existing agenda of sex and drugs. It can start where the young people are and work with young people on the health issues they are interested in, in ways that they find acceptable.

Healthy settings work

As discussed earlier the concept of the health-promoting school is increasing in popularity and is based on a notion of healthy alliance work. It can also embody an empowering ethos, which acknowledges the holistic nature of health and the importance of involving the pupils in a meaningful way (Lloyd, 1994, Boddington and Hull, 1996).

In health-promoting school schemes, schools are supported to promote health in an holistic way, looking beyond the classroom to provide a healthy environment for the whole school community (Scottish Health Education Group/Scottish Consultative Council on the Curriculum, 1990). Typically they would look at the full range of health issues including physical activity, diet, mental health, safety and substance misuse, including smoking. However, they also address issues related to the physical environment, for example whether the toilets are clean and tidy, and the social environment, such as relations with parents and the wider school community. They then identify practical ways in which the whole school community can tackle these issues. Examples would include: classroom-based work, school policies, improving the school meals and training for staff and governors. Most schemes advocate that young people should be involved at all stages in the process and their views and ideas, incorporated in the actions the school takes. Representatives of the different year groups, racial and religious groups etc. can work alongside members of staff, governors and parent representatives to identify the health issues important for the school and appropriate solutions. The representatives can then feed information on progress and possible strategies back to their peers for comment and consent.

The theory of the health-promoting school approach is therefore empowering, however there is a problem with ensuring that the reality matches the theory. This is because, despite agreement on the concept and ethos of a health-promoting school, there is no agreement on what the practical process should be. In practice each scheme and each school will vary in the approach taken; this means that the amount of power that pupils have in the process will vary with different schemes and different schools. Pupils may merely be informed about what is happening, with little chance to influence it, or they may be consulted on a pre-set agenda of issues which the school wishes to address. Given the power balance in the majority of schools, it is likely that many health-promoting school schemes may experience severe restrictions on the extent to which they can be truly empowering.

Despite the limitations which the approach poses in practical terms for empowerment, it is likely that it will continue to be developed, as early results from a major evaluation project are looking positive (Hamilton, 1997). The European Network of Health Promoting Schools' current evaluation project in England has recently demonstrated that pupils in health-promoting schools in comparison to pupils in matched control schools recorded better health-related behaviour and self-esteem. As discussed in the healthy alliance section, the health promoting school concept could be applied to other youth settings, for example youth clubs and care homes. However, there has been little documented work on this approach in those settings. If the current health-promoting school initiatives continue to show successful results, albeit in behavioural rather than empowerment terms, then it is possible that the concept will be developed in other youth settings. Although the apparent affect on self-esteem is encouraging, the real impact such schemes will have on young people in empowerment terms has yet to be established. It is to be hoped that the Government's current commitment to healthy schools as set out in *Our Healthier Nation*, will result in more resources being invested in this area.

Specialist services

Health promotion with young people can also be carried out through the provision of specialist services. Young people's health services are becoming commonly established, though the majority of these have a specific sexual health remit. A recent publication listed 65 young persons' sexual health services in the UK (Aggleton, 1996). However, research into sexual health services for young people, shows that what young people really want are not specialised sexual health services. Instead they want general services offering a wide range, or menu, of health-related information, advice and treatment (West et al, 1995; HEA, 1996). A service marketed as just a drugs or sexual health clinic would put young people off attending because they would not want other people, especially parents, to know they were attending a service for sexual health or drugs advice. A general health service for young people provides ample opportunities for health professionals, especially community nurses to offer an holistic service, comprising a range of health promotion interventions for young people, which could include advice and information. In practice, a service primarily aimed at providing information and advice on drugs and drug misuse would have more success in attracting customers if it were advertised as a general health service for young people, offering drugs advice amongst other things. Some community nurses would be in the position to provide both the drugs advice and the general health advice. Where it is felt necessary for a specialist drugs worker to provide the drugs advice, there is still scope for a community nurse to offer the other wider health advice. The fact that these services are usually offered in an informal, drop-in style means that they have to meet young people's needs and provide what young people want for them to be successful. As such they should be more empowering than traditional health services, which are usually based on what the service provider is willing to offer the client.

The Woodhouse Park Clinic in Manchester is an example of a successful young person's health service, which offers advice on a wide range of health issues, including sexual health (Williams, Kirkman and Elstein, 1994). It was established in 1988 and has had success in attracting young men under the age of 16 who are normally reluctant to access services. A more holistic young person's health service is Base 51 in Nottingham, UK (Read, 1993). Unlike other services, it does not operate for a few hours a week from an existing health or community venue, but is a specific young person's drop-in health centre, housed in a converted factory in the centre of Nottingham. It offers a wide range of health services and referrals and is designed to meet the needs of disadvantaged young people, including those who are homeless. It is open during the day and evening and has showers, clothes washing and crèche facilities. It also offers dance, drama and aerobics sessions. The ethos of the service is very much one of empowerment and young people were actively involved at all stages of the design of the service and the building. The Teenage Health Club in Alexandria, Scotland is another a young person's health service, which actively involved young people in running the club, deciding what health issues to consider and what changes were needed to be made to the service (Little, 1997).

There is a view that specialist services are themselves disempowering as they marginalise young people from mainstream services. The argument is that rather than setting up new services, and letting existing providers off the hook, we should be making the existing services more accessible to young people (Burke, 1995). Although this may be true in the long term, in the short term it is clear that existing services do not meet young people's needs and it may take a long time for the attitudes of health professionals and society at large to change. Until such changes do take place, if they ever do, specialist service may well be the most empowering way of providing for at least some of the health needs of young people.

CONCLUSION

There would appear to be plenty of scope for youth health promotion in the community. However, the current situation is very much a patchwork of provision, primarily because of scarce resources and the lack of statutory requirements. There is also a paucity of good evidence as to what constitutes effective interventions, at a time when calls for value for money are ever increasing. With these constraints in the general field of youth health promotion, it is perhaps no surprise that work on empowering approaches to youth health promotion have not been very well developed. There is potential though in some of the newer approaches which are more holistic and young person centred. The Government has also made a firm pledge to public health with the appointment of a minister for public health and the revised health strategy, *Our Healthier Nation*. It is still unlikely however that truly empowering approaches, which devolve substantial amounts of power and control to young people, will become the norm, unless the adults who currently hold the power, be it in government, in schools or within families, are prepared to lose some of their own power.

Within the limitations that exist, practitioners must judge for themselves how empowering their practice can be. It is important to consider that no matter who the health promoter is, or what the constraints are, effective and empowering health promotion should take the social and cultural contexts of young people into account. It should seek to validate young people's experiences, by rooting practice in the reality of their everyday lives and expressed needs. Only by working in these ways can we begin to help young people learn what they are and what they could be.

DISCUSSION QUESTIONS

- To what extent can empowering practice in youth health promotion be developed within the current health, education and social contexts?

- Is there greater potential for empowering youth health promotion in the health than the education sector?
- In what ways can community health workers become involved in more empowering practice?

REFERENCES

Aggleton, P. (1996) *Promoting Young People's Sexual Health*. London: HEA.

Babb, P. (1993) Teenage conceptions and fertility in England and Wales 1971–91. *Population Trends*, **74**: 12–17.

Bagnall, P. (1991) The way forward for school nursing. *Health Education Journal*, 50(3): 115–118.

Bailey, C. (1994) New frontiers for school nurses. *Health Education*, 2: March, 12–14.

Boddington, N. & Hull, T. (1996) *The Health Promoting School*. London: Forbes.

Brannen, J. & Storey, P. (1996) *Child Health in Social Context*. London: HEA.

Brown, T. (1996) *Opportunities for Health and Education to Work Together*. South Thames: NHS Executive.

Burke, T. (1995) A healthy approach to partnership. *Young People Now*, March, 20–21.

Coggans, N., Shewan, D., Henderson, M. & Davies, J. (1991) Could do better, an evaluation of drug education. *Druglink*, September/October, 14–16.

Department of Education and Science (DES) (1986) *Health Education from 5–16: Curriculum Matters 6*. London: HMSO.

Department for Education and Science (1987) Circular 11/87, *Sex Education in Schools*, London: Department for Education.

Department of Health (DoH) (1992) *The Health of the Nation*. London: HMSO.

Department of Health (DoH) (1993) *The Children Act Report 1992*. London: HMSO.

Department of Health (DoH) (1998) *Our Healthier Nation*, A Consultation Paper. London: HMSO.

Diamond, A. & Goddard, E. (1995) *Smoking among Secondary School Children in 1994*. London: HMSO.

Dorn, N. & South, N. (1985) Return of the topic, developments in drug education and training. *Health Education Journal*, 44(4): 208–212.

Driscoll, J. (1993) Detached, that's a sort of house innit? *Youth Clubs*, 74: December, 22–23.

Fermanagh Herald, Health Promotion Award Scheme for youth clubs launched, 21 February 1996.

Few, C., Hicken, I. & Butterworth, T. (1996) *Partnerships in Sexual Health and Sex Education*. Manchester: University of Manchester.

Friere, P. (1972) *Pedagogy of the Oppressed*. London: Penguin.

Graham, G. (1996) The Health Education Role of Youth Workers, unpublished MSc thesis, University of Manchester.

Hamilton, V. (1992) HIV/AIDS – A peer education approach. *Youth and Policy*, 36: March, 27–33.

Hamilton, K. (1997) *The Health Promoting School: a summary of the ENHPS evaluation project in England*. London: HEA.

Harvey, M. (1995) *A Framework for Peer Learning*. London: Youth Clubs UK.

Harvey, M. & Smith, G. (1996) *Yes Me! A self development programme for peer educators*. London: Youth Clubs UK.

Health Education Authority (HEA) (1992) *Tomorrow's Young Adults*. London: HEA.

Health Education Authority (HEA) (1993) *Peers in Partnership*. London: HEA.

Health Education Authority (HEA) (1995) *Parents, Schools and Sex Education*. London: HEA.

Health Education Authority (HEA) (1996) *Promoting Sexual Health Services to Young People*. London: HEA.

Health Education Authority (HEA) (1997a) *Health Update – Sexual Health*. London: HEA.

Health Education Authority (HEA) (1997b) *Health Promoting School Schemes – Contact Names and Addresses*. London: HEA.

HMSO (1989) *The Children Act*. London: HMSO.

Howard, M. & McCabe, J. (1992) An information and skills approach for younger teens. In *Preventing Adolescent Pregnancy*. eds. Miller, B., Card, J., Playoff, R. & Peterson, J. New York: Sage.

Jamison, J. (1993) Health Education in Schools: A survey of policy and implementation, *Health Education Journal*, 52(2): Summer.

Jarvis, M. (1992) HIV who knows best? *Youth Clubs,* **68**: June, 28–30.

Johnson, A.M., Wadsworth, J. & Field, J.

(1994) *Sexual Attitudes and Lifestyles*. London: Blackwell.

Kalnins, I., Hart, C., Ballantyne, P. et al. (1994) School based community development as a health promotion strategy for children. *Health Promotion International*, **9**(4): 269–279.

Klerman, L. (1993) The influence of economic factors on health related behaviours in adolescents. In *Promoting the Health of Adolescents*. eds. Millstein, S., Petersen, A.. Nightingale, E. New York: Oxford University.

Little, L. (1997) Teenage health education: a public health approach. *Nursing Standard*, **11**(49): August, 43–45.

Lloyd, J. (1994) Health promoting primary schools: a settings context. In Morton, R. & Lloyd, J. (1994) *The Health Promoting Primary School*. London: Fulton.

May, C. (1991) Research on alcohol education for young people: a critical review of the literature. *Health Education Journal*, **50**(4): 195–199.

Mellanby, A., Phelps, F., Crichton, N. & Tripp, J. (1995) School sex education: an experimental programme with educational and medical benefits. *British Medical Journal*, **311**: 414–420.

Milburn, K. (1995) A critical review of peer education, with young people, with special reference to sexual health. *Health Education Research*, **10**(4): December.

Millstein, S. (1993) A view of health from the adolescent's perspective. In Millstein, S. Petersen, A. & Nightingale, E. *Promoting the Health of Adolescents*. New York: Oxford University Press.

National Curriculum Council (1989) *The National Curriculum and Whole Curriculum Planning: Preliminary Guidance*, Circular Number 6, York: National Curriculum Council.

National Curriculum Council (1990) *Health Education, Curriculum Guidance 5*. York: National Curriculum Council.

Neesham, C. (1997a) Hey teacher leave them kids alone. *Healthlines*, July/August, 14–16.

Neesham, C. (1997b) Peer power: giving young people a voice. *Healthlines*, September, 12–14.

O'Donnell, T. & Gray, G. (1993) *The Health Promoting College*. London: HEA.

Office of National Statistics (1997) *Smoking among Secondary School Children in 1996, England*. London: Office of National Statistics

Parker, H., Measham, F., Aldridge, J. (1995) Drug futures, changing patterns of drug use among English youths. *ISDD Research Monograph 7*. London: Institute for the

study of Drug Dependence.

Read, C. (1993) Safe Haven based on West Side Story. *The Independent*, 15 June.

Reid, J. (1991) Developing the role of the school nurse in public health. *Health Education Journal*, **50**(3): 118–122.

Rogers, C. (1983) Freedom to learn for the eighties. New York: Merrill Press.

Rogers, A. (1995) *Analysis of a healthy alliance*. London: Youth Clubs UK.

Royal College of Psychiatrists (1987) *Drugscenes*. London: Royal College of Psychiatrists.

Scottish Health Education Group/Scottish Consultative Council on the Curriculum (1990) *Promoting Good Health*. Edinburgh: Scottish Health Education Group.

Simpson, A. & Went, H. (1994) West Sussex school nurses teach the teachers. *Education and Health*, **12**(2): 25–27.

Smith, T. (1993) Influence of socio-economic factors on attaining targets for reducing teenage pregnancies. *British Medical Journal*, **306**: 1232–1235.

Tones, K. (1995) Health education as empowerment. In *Health Promotion Today*, London: HEA.

Tripp, G. & Davenport, A. (1988/89) Fear advertising – it doesn't work. *Health Promotion*, Winter 17–18

Turtle, J., Jones, A. & Hickman, M. (1997) Young People and Health: the health behaviour of school–age children. London: Health Education Authority.

United Nations International Children's Fund (UNICEF) (1995) *The Convention on the Rights of the Child*. London: UK Committee for UNICEF.

Vautrat, D. (1996) Peering into a healthy future. *Healthlines*, February, 22–23.

Wallerstein, N. & Sanchez-Merki, V. (1994) Frierian praxis in health education: Research results from an adolescent prevention programme. *Health Education Research*, **9**(1): 105–118.

West J., Hudson, F., Levitas, R. & Guy, W. (1995) *Young People and Clinics: Providing for Sexual Health in Avon*. Bristol: University of Bristol.

Whitehead, M. (1989) *Swimming Upstream, Trends and Prospects in Education for Health*. London: King's Fund.

Williams, E., Kirkman, R. & Elstein, M. (1994) Profile of a young person's advice clinic in reproductive health 1988–93. *British Medical Journal*, **309**: 24 September

Young, I. (1991) Encouraging parental involvement in school. In *Youth Health Promotion*. Nutbeam, D., Haglund, B. Farley, P. & Tillgren, P. London: Forbes.

FURTHER READING

Millstein, S., Petersen, A.C. & Nightingale, E.O. (1993) *Promoting the Health of Adolescents, New directions for the twenty first century*. New York: Oxford University Press.

This book is divided into two sections. The first section contains articles on: (1) adolescents, health and society, including the effects of economic factors on young people's health; (2) cultural considerations for ethnic minority young people, (3) adolescents perceptions of their health needs and social influences on young people's health; including family, peers, school and community. The second section focuses on specific health issues. All the articles are from an American perspective, but they still contain much relevant and interesting information.

Nutbeam, D. et al (1991) *Youth Health Promotion, from theory to practice in school and community*. London: Forbes.

This book is also divided into two sections. The first contains articles on the theories underlying youth health promotion, particularly community-wide approaches. The second section looks at different international approaches to youth health promotion from Europe, the USA and Australia; the emphasis again is on community-wide programmes, but there are also articles on holistic and student-centred programmes.

Aggleton, P. (1996) *Health Promotion and Young People*. London: HEA.

An up-to-date overview of young people's health in relation to specific health issues. Looks at mortality and morbidity, risk factors and effective interventions for The Health of the Nation areas and drug use. Useful for gaining a current picture of young people's health and health behaviour, but very topic specific and little reference is made to issues of empowerment.

National Curriculum Council (1990) *Curriculum Guidance 5, Health Education*. York: National Curriculum Council.

Outlines the nine areas for school health education. Contains guidance on the issues that should be addressed within those areas for children at different ages. Concise, yet comprehensive and holistic in nature.

Scottish Health Education Group/Scottish Consultative Council on the Curriculum. (1990) *Promoting Good Health*. Edinburgh: Scottish Health Education Group.

Outlines the features of a health-promoting school and the ways in which schools can move from traditional health education towards a more health-promoting school ethos.

8 Homeless women and primary health care

Melanie Ibbitson

- Homelessness
- Health
- Women
- Primary health care
- Feminist research

INTRODUCTION

This chapter will focus on the relationship between homelessness and ill-health, focusing primarily on women. It will begin by examining the low uptake of mainstream primary health care services by homeless people and some of the obstacles confronting them when seeking access to services. The chapter will move on to discuss the current lack of research into homeless women's health as well as the importance of utilising a feminist research framework both to facilitate the empowerment of homeless women and also to expand the current body of work. Some of the arguments for and against specialist provision for homeless people will be set out later in the section, illustrated by several examples of a coordinated approach. Finally, some strategies will be suggested for health promotion which would aim to improve the health care of homeless women and men.

CONTEXT

This section will examine the nature of homelessness and its impact upon women, the link between health and homelessness, and some of the factors which may complicate the delivery of appropriate primary health care to homeless women.

Homelessness: definitions, prevalence and trends

The use of the term 'homeless' is problematic for it may be interpreted in many different ways. For some, the term applies only to those sleeping rough, who are literally 'roofless'. For others the word 'homeless' is broader, describing those people living in Bed and Breakfast or other temporary accommodation and those staying with friends, as well as those sleeping rough. The term could also be applied to people about to be released from institutional accommodation (such as prison or foster care), families forced to live apart, friends forced to live together, or tenants under notice to quit.

Watson and Austerberry (1986) attempted to reflect this spectrum of housing status by envisaging a continuum of 'home ... to ... homelessness'. Most people would agree that a home is more than a shelter from the elements. Even the most luxurious house may not feel like home if a person has no key to the front door, no right to decorate, or may be asked to leave at any moment. For most people, housing status changes throughout their lives. A young person who has enjoyed a secure home for 18 years for example may leave the parental home to study in another part of the country, and may then experience 3 years of insecure housing.

In 1994, 146 119 households (families) were accepted as homeless by local authority housing departments in England and Wales (Guardian, 1996). This term is thought to represent approximately 419 400 individuals. Although it is the official statistic, this figure is likely to only represent the tip of the iceberg. The term 'hidden homeless' is used to describe people who either do not choose to present themselves as homeless to the local authority although their current housing situation is insecure, unsafe or inappropriate, or in cases where they do present, are not accepted as eligible for rehousing. These people are not included in official statistics.

It is almost impossible to compile statistics which accurately quantify the numbers of 'hidden' homeless people, as many are squatting, staying with friends or family, tolerating domestic violence and unhealthy living conditions, or sleeping rough. Furthermore, the very nature of homelessness is such that those affected are forced to lead a transient life, often moving regularly and are therefore difficult to trace. A report from Single Homelessness in London in 1995 estimated that in London there were 45 000 single homeless people staying in squats, hostels, Bed and Breakfasts or sleeping rough, and a further 32 000 staying with friends in overcrowded conditions (Guardian, 1996). Shelter estimates the number of people unofficially homeless throughout the country as a whole to be approximately 1 200 000 (Guardian, 1993).

Whatever the discrepancy between official and unofficial homelessness statistics, it is generally agreed that the rate has risen dramatically during the last 10–15 years. In 1979, 57 000 households were accepted as homeless by local authorities in England and Wales (Platt, 1989) compared with 146 119 households in 1994 (Guardian, 1996). This reveals an *official* increase of more than 150% in just 15 years.

The largest increase in homelessness is thought to be occurring among single people with no dependants. There are no national statistics for single homelessness, although in 1990, CHAR, the pressure group for single people and housing estimated that there were 2 million single homeless people in Britain, of whom 45% were situated outside London (Shelter, 1990). Under the Housing Act 1985, local authorities only have a statutory obligation to rehouse those people who are considered to be in 'priority need'. Single homeless people are excluded from this group unless deemed 'vulnerable' because of old age, physical disability, mental handicap or illness. Other forms of vulnerability such as being lesbian or black (and thus susceptible to homophobia or racism) for example would not be taken into consideration. An estimated one in 10 young homeless people are lesbian or gay. They may be rejected by their families because of their sexuality or may be coming out of local authority care:

'Homophobia and fear work to drive thousands of people out from families or state institutions on to what can be a very hostile street environment.'

(Burns, 1996)

Women: the hidden homeless

Although men are more likely to approach the local authority for rehousing, and are thus more often recognised in official statistics, homelessness is also a problem for women. Women are thought to account for approximately one-quarter of the homeless population living in temporary accommodation (Roof, 1994). More difficult to assess however, is the level of women's potential homelessness as much of it remains concealed. Although some women do present themselves as homeless, many remain in unsatisfactory or violent relationships and unsuitable housing because they lack any alternative or escape. Although they may literally have a roof over their heads, many of these women would perhaps choose to leave if they had somewhere to go (Watson and Austerberry, 1986). This group of women can be perceived as the 'hidden homeless'. The fact that much of women's homelessness is so hidden in nature may cause women's housing needs to remain unrecognised and unmet. Although all single homeless people are discriminated against by the current legislation, which does not recognise them as officially homeless, women face additional barriers in accessing good quality, affordable housing for the following reasons, which will be discussed in turn:

1. Economic status
2. Role of women in society
3. Private sector
4. Domestic violence
5. Emergency provision

Economic status

In spite of the increasing numbers of women in the labour market and the Equal Pay Act of 1975, women's average full-time earnings still only amount to two-thirds of men's. Moreover, women are far more likely to work in low-paid, part-time and insecure jobs with the result that only one in 10 households headed by a woman can afford to take out a mortgage. Indeed, mortgage companies refused mortgages to single women until relatively recently. Low income levels often restrict women's housing options, causing them to rely heavily on local authority housing (Miller, 1990).

The 'Right to Buy' policy introduced in 1981 has encouraged local authority tenants to purchase their homes at discounted prices. One consequence of this policy is that housing has been transferred from the relatively accessible local authority rented stock to the less accessible home-ownership sector (Connelly and Crown, 1994). A large proportion of the rented properties 'left behind' in the local authority sector are in poorer condition and less desirable locations compared with those which have been bought. Tenants who are able to benefit from this policy tend to be relatively well off:

> 'people who purchase through this scheme are, in general, those who are in employment and have earnings at the top end of the income distribution of local authority tenants.'

> *(Connelly and Crown, 1994)*

Such policies which encourage home ownership indirectly exclude most single women, who generally have less purchasing power than men in the housing market. A woman's income is generally too low to repay a mortgage without recourse to a second wage.

In spite of the large numbers of women who depend on social housing however, council housing stocks have been decimated over the last 20 years. The number of houses built by local authorities between 1968 and 1990 fell from 133 145 to 13 434 per annum (Guardian, 1993), almost a ten-fold decrease.

Role of women in society

Assumptions about women's role in society as primarily wives and mothers rather than independent individuals has led to the development of housing policy geared towards the needs of the conventional nuclear family. State intervention in housing provision has invariably catered for 'family' housing needs:

> 'British housing policy and the housing market operate in favour of the traditional nuclear family household.'
> *(Watson and Austerberry, 1986)*

Single women are marginalised by current policy which does not consider them to be in 'priority need' unless they are pregnant, have children, or are vulnerable because of mental health needs or learning difficulties (Connelly, Roderick and Victor, 1990). Women are apparently considered valuable only when they have children. There seems to be a dichotomy between the 'deserving' and the 'undeserving' homeless woman where government policy is concerned. Policies which promote owner occupation above all other forms of housing inevitably work to the detriment of single women.

Private sector

Rarely able to purchase their own home and denied access to priority rehousing by the council, many single women are forced into the private sector. Although renting privately is the norm in many European countries, the private sector now accounts for only 7% of the housing market in the UK (Connelly and Crown, 1994). It is characterised by high rents, low standards of accommodation, and deposits or rent in advance. Moreover, since the Housing Act 1988, tenants have had less security as shorthold assured tenancies have become commonplace, giving landlords the option of terminating the tenancy after only 6 months. The 'fair rents' system has also been discarded, resulting in rent rises to 'market level'. Illegal eviction and harassment (sexual or otherwise) of tenants by landlords is also a major problem with 150 000 cases reported every year by the Housing Projects Advisory Service (HPAS, 1994). As private rented accommodation is in very high demand, landlords are able to be selective, hence discrimination exists against people who are homeless, claiming social security benefits, or who are black, lesbian or members of other minority groups (HPAS, 1994).

Domestic violence

Domestic violence accounts for 25% of all reported crime. Home Office figures of incidents of domestic violence began to soar at the end of the last decade, when cases escalated from 12 000 to more than 26 000 per year (Guardian, 1996). Relationship breakdown is the largest cause of homelessness among women. In 1990, approximately 50% of women placed in Bed and Breakfast accommodation by local authorities were escaping domestic violence (Ross, 1990). In spite of these figures however, there are only 270 refuges in the country, housing just 3000 women. A parliamentary report in the 1970s stated that a further 800 refuges be set up, and only last year the Police Federation and the Association of Directors of Social Services maintained that more bed spaces are urgently needed (Guardian, 1996).

Women without children, who are fleeing domestic violence or sexual abuse are not automatically in 'priority need' when they approach the local authority, as interpretation of the current legislation varies widely. Women may be required to take legal action against their violent partner before they will be accepted, or may be expected to show evidence that violence has taken place. Mental abuse is unlikely to be easily demonstrated. Some women may decide to tolerate or return to a violent situation rather than risk rejection or humiliation at the Housing Department. A CHAR report found that sexual abuse is also a significant cause of young women's homelessness. Young women leaving home as a result of sexual abuse however are not necessarily eligible for priority rehousing (CHAR, 1992).

Emergency provision

When single women *are* accepted as officially homeless, and accepted for priority rehousing, the majority of emergency hostel provision caters for homeless men. Women-only hostels for single women are scarce, and due to high demand rarely have vacancies. Many women are consequently forced into unsuitable Bed and Breakfast accommodation, where cooking and washing facilities are inadequate, and rooms are often shared (CHAR, 1991). Where emergency hostel accommodation is available, it is likely to be mixed, and thus may not provide a safe environment for a single woman:

> 'In most hostels, the rooms and dormitories are segregated by gender and kept locked to protect the girls and women from rape and sexual harassment.'
>
> *(Grant, 1997)*

Some women may opt to return to their previous living situation, however unsuitable, in preference to remaining in temporary accommodation for several months.

The situation regarding emergency provision is now likely to become even more problematic since the 1996 Housing Act came into effect. This legislation dilutes the local authority's statutory duty to secure emergency accommodation for homeless people in 'priority need'. In effect the proposals alter the definition of homelessness to rooflessness. Once provided with emergency accommodation, a homeless woman will no longer be eligible for permanent rehousing. The few hostels and women's refuges that do exist will therefore fill up very quickly and remain full (HPAS, 1994).

As has been demonstrated, single women's experience of housing contrasts with that of single men, for women are doubly disadvantaged due to both their single status and their sex. As the public and private rented sector has become gradually less accessible and available, good quality affordable housing for a single woman unable to purchase her own home seems in short supply. Current housing policy which promotes home ownership as the desired norm works against women who are not situated in a conventional family.

Homelessness and health

Homelessness is generally accepted as a serious challenge to public health. In 1990 the Department of Social Security Health and Homelessness Unit conducted a survey of single homeless people staying temporarily in Bed and Breakfast accommodation in Manchester, UK. The report concluded:

'We found their general health was worse than any comparable groups in the settled population ... if steps are not taken to meet these needs the cumulative health effects will be disastrous.'

(DSS, 1990)

Numerous studies have acknowledged a correlation between homelessness and poor health (Connelly and Crown, 1994; Department of the Environment, 1993; George, Shanks and Westlake, 1991; Pleace and Quilgars, 1996; Pickin and Ramsell, 1991; Whynes and Giggs, 1992). In 1990, Wright conducted a study in which 63 000 homeless people were interviewed in the USA. Wright (1990) found that homeless people 'suffer from most disorders at an elevated and often exceptionally elevated rate.'

Some of the most common physical problems suffered by single people who are homeless are chronic chest or breathing problems, skin complaints, pneumonia, ulcers, musculo-skeletal problems, and gastrointestinal disorders. Frequent headaches, foot problems, seizures and tuberculosis are also common.

Estimates of the prevalence of mental illness among homeless people vary widely, but studies suggest that between 40% and 50% of all homeless people may be suffering from mental illness (Fischer and Breakey, 1986; Morrisey and Levine, 1987; Scott, 1993; Vergare and Aarce, 1986). Although the results from studies are inconsistent, it is clear that the mental health of the homeless population is significantly worse than that of the domiciled population. Rates of anxiety, depression, deliberate self-harm, personality dysfunction and psychoses, (especially schizophrenia) appear to be particularly high (Scott, 1993). In Bines' study (1994), the self-reporting of 'depression, anxiety and nerves' by single homeless people was eight times higher than in the general population. The King's Fund Review of Health and Homelessness in London concluded that:

> 'Studies of single homeless people who are not statutorily homeless have indicated ... particularly high prevalence of mental health problems, especially among homeless women.'
>
> (Pleace and Quilgars, 1996)

In terms of mortality rates, a recent analysis of coroner's court records in Manchester, Bristol and London, UK conducted by the homeless charity CRISIS found that the life expectancy of someone who sleeps rough is now just 42 years, down from 47 years, just 4 years ago (the national average life expectancy is 76 years). Those who sleep rough are also 35 times more likely to kill themselves than the general population and four times more likely to die of unnatural causes such as murder, assault or accidents (CRISIS, 1996).

Causes of Ill health

The homeless population is not a homogeneous group, but rather a diverse population comprised of many individuals living in quite different environments. People sleeping rough are exposed to extreme weather conditions, and may have poor hygiene due to a lack of basic amenities. Difficulties in maintaining a balanced diet can lead to nutritional deficiencies, which coupled with stress may increase the risk of physical health problems.

Overcrowding and inadequate or unsanitary washing and cooking facilities characteristic of some Bed and Breakfast establishments predisposes homeless people to infectious diseases and respiratory infections, aggravated by cold and poor heating.

The lack of safety in the private rented sector is a serious health hazard:

> 'Most of the 30 deaths caused annually by faulty gas fires are in the private rented sector. 80% of bedsit properties have no satisfactory means of escape in case of fire. 150 people die each year in houses in multiple occupation fires.'
>
> (Cornwell, 1994)

There is a high possibility of accidents occurring due to tenants cooking in their bedrooms, and the accumulation of rubbish in houses of multiple occupation. Insanitary conditions and dampness in many private sector properties also increase the likelihood of such disorders as bronchitis and asthma (HPAS, 1994).

Wherever a homeless person is staying, be it an emergency shelter, on the streets or on a friend's floor, life is likely to be mentally as well as physically exhausting. The causes of mental health problems among homeless people are manifold. The kind of lifestyle which many homeless people inevitably lead is highly stressful. Drug and alcohol use may help to numb physical or emotional pain, but may consequently lead to other problems. Displacement from loved ones, constant relocation, marginalisation and loneliness can cause depression. At least 50% of homeless people have no social contacts and nobody with whom to talk over problems (Marshall, 1989, Weller, Weller and Coker, 1987).

Some people may initially have become homeless because they had a mental health problem. Others have become homeless after deinstitutionalisation without sufficient community-based services to help them, following the NHS and Community Care Act 1989 (Scott, 1993). For those who develop mental health problems as a result of being homeless, receiving treatment may address the symptom rather than the cause. They may have no option but to return to the stressful situation which could have caused mental health problems to develop in the first place.

Wolch and Akita (1988) observed a 'downward spiral' taking place, which had a negative effect on the mental, physical, and social well-being of a homeless individual:

'Unable to help themselves, refused aid and/or given inappropriate assistance, their difficulties accumulate, families break up, health and appearance decline, and victimisation increases.'

(Wolch and Akita, 1988)

Homeless women and health

Although many of the health problems already described affect both women and men, there are certain issues which are specific to women:

1. Mental health
2. Abuse
3. Health education

Mental health

Women in the general population are far more likely than men to present at their general practitioner (GP) surgery for reasons of mental or emotional ill health (Watson and Austerberry, 1986). Similarly, homeless women appear to suffer from higher levels of mental health problems than do homeless men (James, 1991; Johnson and Kreuger, 1989; Marshall and Reed, 1992; Scott 1991). Insecure or unsuitable emergency accommodation may exacerbate these problems.

Although women appear to retain their social networks more successfully than men, they may be suffering from acute anxiety and grief as a result of losing their children. Feelings of guilt may be overwhelming for those women who have fled the family home to escape violence, leaving children behind. Although there is a paucity of empirical evidence relating to homeless women and health, women appear to suffer more mental health problems and to be more alienated than homeless men (Dail and Koshes, 1992).

In 1992, Marshall and Reed conducted a study of 70 homeless women in London, and discovered very high levels of mental health problems among their sample. When tested for schizophrenia, 64% of women in the study fulfilled the criteria for schizophrenic illness. Crane's (1992) study of 50 older homeless people sleeping rough found that 65% of women interviewed seemed to experience thought disturbances compared with 17% of men in the sample.

Interestingly, in Johnson and Kreuger's (1989) study of 240 homeless women in St Louis, 40% of women without children had seen a mental health professional during the previous year, compared with only 13% of women with children.

Similarly, one-quarter of women without children reported a previous admission to a psychiatric hospital compared to 6% of those with children. Although there is no clear explanation for this, one could speculate as to the reasons. In a culture where motherhood is considered the natural desire of every woman and accorded great status, and single women without children are perceived as sad, barren or lonely, how easy is it for a woman alone to maintain a strong sense of self-esteem when she is also homeless? One wonders if indeed mental health professionals are more likely to view women without children as non-conformist or outside society in some way and thus more likely to admit them or diagnose them as mentally ill.

Abuse

Rape, childhood sexual abuse, physical attack on the streets and domestic violence are all issues impacting on homeless women's health in a unique way. CHAR's report of sexual abuse as a factor in women's homelessness concluded that four out of every 10 homeless women had become homeless as a result of fleeing sexual abuse (CHAR, 1992). A study of women living in emergency night shelters revealed that one-third had been abused during childhood (Bassuk, Rubin and Lauriat, 1986). Sexual and physical assault appear to be very common both preceding and also during periods of homelessness:

> 'homeless women *are* more vulnerable than their male counterparts. They tend to have a history of early and repeated child bearing, poor social relationships, childhood sexual abuse.'
>
> *(Dail and Koshes, 1992)*

As a result of being homeless, women may not gain access to counselling or support services able to assist them in tackling their feelings as survivors of physical or sexual abuse. Without the opportunity to share their experience, homeless women may internalise negative feelings, leading them to deliberately self-harm, or suffer from depression (CHAR, 1992).

Health education

Some women may lose out on preventative health care, such as breast and cervical screening as a result of being homeless and moving frequently. They may not receive sexual health education information such as safer sex or contraceptive advice:

> 'Research shows they are aware of the risks of HIV and AIDS, and other sexually transmitted diseases but they don't know where they can get free condoms.'
>
> *(Steele, 1991)*

Although homelessness impacts on the health of both women and men, certain issues affect homeless women in specific ways. The fear or experience of sexual or physical abuse, and the loss of children or family may have a significant effect on the mental health of homeless women. Lack of skills for employment, and social deprivation make them an acutely vulnerable group (Dail and Koshes, 1992).

Homeless people: access to primary health care

'Health and homelessness are linked together in three important ways. First, poor health ... is often a cause of homelessness ... second, poor health is often a consequence of homelessness ... finally, whatever the pathways of cause and effect, homelessness greatly complicates the delivery of adequate health care.'

(Wright, 1990)

The relationship between homelessness and ill health is complex. Irrespective of whether poor health is a consequence of homelessness, or homelessness a consequence of poor health, the problem is further compounded by the fact that homeless people experience difficulties in accessing primary health care services (Marshall and Reed, 1992; Pleace and Quilgars, 1996; Stern and Stilwell, 1989; Whynes and Giggs, 1992; Wright, 1990).

Access to mainstream services

GP registration levels can be used as a yardstick in measuring access to primary health care for different groups. The role of the GP is to provide a comprehensive, generalist service to the populace. The GP is also the linchpin of all other medical services and facilities, the coordinator of secondary care, and the first port of call when a person falls ill. Somebody who is not registered with a GP may find it difficult to access health services, except in cases of emergency.

GP registration among homeless people appears alarmingly low. A Brighton study found that out of a sample of 75 homeless people, only 21 were registered with a doctor, and of those who were not, 33 had been refused on repeated occasions (City and Hackney Community Health Council, 1989). In Manchester, research found that only half of the participants were registered with a GP within 3 miles of their current address. A further 19% of the sample had experienced problems registering with a doctor (Department of Social Security Health and Homeless Unit, 1990). More recently a *Shelter* survey suggested that 63% of homeless people are registered with a local GP compared to 98% of the general population (Shelter, 1996). A survey conducted by *The Big Issue* magazine in January 1997 found that nearly 50% of its magazine vendors were not registered with a doctor (Markey, 1997).

Where studies of homeless people have shown higher levels of registration, such registration is not necessarily appropriate. A significant proportion of homeless patients are only registered temporarily, or with surgeries situated several miles away from their current address (Clark and George, 1993).

As a consequence of poor registration with general practices, homeless people tend to make greater use of hospital Accident and Emergency (A & E) departments when compared to national levels, often using them as sources of primary care (Scheuer et al, 1991; Scott, 1993; Shelter, 1996). Not only is this a costly and inappropriate use of resources, but also it complicates the delivery of follow-up treatment after discharge.

Homeless people frequently miss out on health promotion information which may assist them in reducing their own health risks, and also early detection of disease through regular health checks (Pleace and Quilgars, 1996).

Late presentation to services may complicate or prolong treatment, or in the most extreme cases may render treatment ineffective and pointless.

Barriers to access

Homeless people encounter a variety of difficulties when attempting to access primary health care. Some of these result from prejudice and discrimination on the part of health care providers, and some from the inflexibility of National Health Service (NHS) procedures.

Service providers are sometimes reluctant to register homeless people because they believe that they will take up too much time and money (Dobson, 1990). The independent practitioner status of GPs and the framework of reimbursement allowance may not contain sufficient incentives to take on homeless people. Some doctors are under the misconception that they cannot claim for a patient who is of no fixed abode (Reuler, 1989). Others may believe that homeless people are likely to demand frequent 'home visits' and are unlikely to attend health promotion activities, thus adversely affecting targets. Fundholding practices may be afraid that homeless patients are simply too expensive, presenting in high-need emergency situations with immediate and manifold problems. The emergency may be further complicated by the lack of medical records and the patient disappearing before the treatment is complete:

> 'Homeless people are frequently viewed as 'difficult patients' who generate a lot of work for little medical or financial return.'
>
> *(Bower, 1994)*

Manchester Community Health Council reported that a number of GPs in the Manchester area appeared to have a policy of blanket refusal to register people who were homeless, or living in particular temporary accommodation (Manchester Metro News, 1995). It was unknown whether this 'policy' was more prevalent among fundholding than non-fundholding practices. Ultimately, GPs are under no obligation to accept any person. Homeless people who have a drug or alcohol problem are even more likely to be turned away (Markey, 1997). The following account of one single homeless woman's experience reflects the stark reality of the situation:

> 'Jane has suffered severe headaches and stomach pains for years but cannot find a doctor willing to examine her. She's been refused by numerous GPs in Manchester and West Yorkshire and has resorted to looking after herself: 'I've given up trying to get a doctor now. I go to pharmacists and ask for their advice or I just grin and bear it.'
>
> *(Markey, 1997)*

Some primary health care staff have internalised a stereotype of the homeless tramp who is dirty, drunk and even violent (Warner, 1992). Health care professionals argue that homeless patients frequently break appointments or fail to arrive at all. They also fear that the presence of homeless people in the waiting room may scare away other patients (McMillan, 1992). Staff may feel a general sense of impotence at the scale of health and social problems presented, and frustration with patients whose lifestyle makes appointment keeping difficult (Bower, 1994). GPs may also fear being swamped by a large proportion of the homeless population if they appear sympathetic.

In the current author's view, these problems may be further exacerbated by the fact that homeless people are a disempowered group, who may find it difficult to communicate with the staff or negotiate the system, or to stand up for themselves if treated unfairly. It has been argued that the NHS has developed according to the needs and values of middle class patients, overlooking those who are less articulate or have more complex needs (Townsend and Davidson, 1982). Official health care settings can be frightening and intimidating for people who are alienated from and mistrustful of society at large. Bureaucracy such as appointment systems or registration requirements may be off-putting. Previous experiences of hostility from staff or difficulty in registering may deter a homeless person's fresh attempts to register. Animosity from clerical staff is a frequently cited problem (Wright, 1990).

Health care may be a low priority for homeless people, especially if they perceive their current state of health to be good. Many remain registered with a previous GP, even though they are living outside the catchment area (Victor, 1992). Some may not realise where the GP surgery is located, or may decide to wait until they are rehoused before seeking a permanent doctor, not anticipating a long stay in temporary accommodation. Restricted access to a GP inevitably means restricted access to a whole range of health services, including preventive and continuous care.

COMMUNITY PARTICIPATION

This section concentrates solely on research as a means of facilitating homeless women's empowerment. As already discussed, women's homelessness is largely invisible, so it is perhaps unsurprising that the systematic study of homeless women's experience has been minimal, both in general and in relation to primary care. Very little is therefore known about how current models of care fit with the needs of homeless women.

Before homeless women can begin to participate in the design of appropriate health care services, a clearer picture must be constructed of their needs and experiences. For the research process to be empowering for homeless women rather than disempowering however, we must rethink traditional research theory and methodology. Rather than research *on* women it must be research *for* women. The following paragraphs will explain why traditional research is inappropriate, and shall introduce a more suitable framework.

Limitations of research

There are three main limitations of the body of work which exists in relation to homelessness and health.

First, the majority of research has been quantitative, involving large-scale surveys focusing largely on homeless men and usually examining a very specific and limited aspect of their experience. Studies appertaining specifically to homeless women are extremely scarce, thus homeless women tend to be 'lumped in' with homeless men by default, and very few gender-specific conclusions are drawn. Women tend to be omitted unless they are categorised by their role as a wife or mother. It is relatively rare for research to focus on women as individuals:

'Traditionally, concern about women's health has been justified in terms of their role within the family as the main care giver and the "producer" of future generations.'

(Orr, 1987)

As one might therefore expect, of the few researchers who have examined women's experience of homelessness, most have concentrated on women as the heads of homeless families. Studies have tended to include both women and children rather than women alone, and have usually perceived the women in the sample as 'mothers' (For examples see Drake, 1992; Hagen and Ivanoff, 1988; Wagner and Menke, 1992).

Those few studies which have addressed the predicament of women without children and homelessness have tended to focus on one specific aspect of health, rather than an all-encompassing investigation (Bunston and Breton, 1990; Marshall and Reed, 1992; Simons and Whitbeck, 1991). The approach has tended to be fragmented rather than holistic. Miller's study (1990) was exceptional in that it addressed issues of emotional, social and spiritual well-being.

Second, research concerning homelessness and health tends to be based on negative assumptions about homeless people, such as the manifestation of supposed 'problem' behaviour. One striking feature of much of the research into homelessness, irrespective of the sex of the participants, is that it is inclined to highlight a social 'problem' such as prostitution, criminal activity or drug use. This approach is reductionist and only serves to dilute and simplify the experience of homelessness. In some respects such research is a self-fulfilling prophecy. If one begins a study from a specific premise, such as an assumed link between homelessness and deviance, then it is surely not difficult to find instances of such a link.

Such research may lead to the labelling of homeless people as 'alcoholic' or 'schizophrenic', a status which scarcely reflects the complexity of an individual's life or acknowledges the existence of power in society and the consequent inequalities (For examples see Gelberg, Linn and Leake, 1988; Spinner and Leaf, 1991; Struening and Padgett, 1990; Welte and Barnes, 1992). This kind of research does not dispel myths about the homeless population. A more holistic and inductive approach needs to be taken, where the researcher approaches the project with an open mind rather than being weighed down with preconceptions.

Finally, there are methodological problems with most research into homelessness and health. The vast majority of studies are quantitative, involving large samples and invariably the use of a questionnaire or survey method. From the great quantity of literature available, only two pieces of qualitative research dealing with homeless women have come to light (Francis, 1992; Miller, 1990).

One of the drawbacks of quantitative, survey-based studies is that they tease out an 'average' picture, thus negating diversity and reducing people to numbers. As Ropers and Boyer conclude in their paper 'Perceived Health Status Among the New Urban Homeless' (1987):

'Understanding who the homeless are and where they come from must be the first step in proposing strategies to help them'.

While large quantitative studies are useful in gauging the prevalence of specific health problems, the need for small-scale, in-depth research in order to make sense of such data has not yet been addressed.

Feminist research framework

Feminist research is a means of recording women's experiences in such a way that the women involved are more likely to feel valued by the process. Before considering feminist methodology however, it is crucial to examine feminist theory. *How* we do something is inevitably influenced by *what* we believe.

Theoretical considerations

It is important for the feminist researcher to be clear about her theoretical standpoint if she is to successfully develop an appropriate research methodology.

The invisibility and 'non-existence' of women in the construction of knowledge is well documented (Rowbotham, 1973; Spender, 1985; Miles, 1988). Miles (1988) argues that historically, women's experiences have rarely been recorded, and have been frequently subsumed into men's experiences:

'Our view of history concentrates on men only, claiming a universal validity for the actions of less than half the human race.'

Scientific empirical research has tended to be the domain of men, who have defined and interpreted not only themselves, but also women:

'Civilisation has been created on male terms which have then been generalised as human and considered to be objective.'

(Callaway, 1981)

'Male' has often been perceived as the norm, and female as 'other', so that the subjective experience of women has largely been ignored or discredited (Callaway, 1981). As already noted in research into homelessness and health, findings from studies on men are usually merely extrapolated to include women. Callaway urges women to take:

'a critical stance against the dominant models of scholarship which place male at the centre and female as peripheral and which confer on males the powers to define and interpret not only themselves but females as well.'

(Callaway, 1981)

Reason and Rowan (1981) suggest that historically, research has been valued for its 'male' characteristics. Quantitative, detached, reductionist, the traditional scientist has tended to deal in numbers and variables, claiming to be objective and value free. People have been broken down into units of data, studied in isolation from their social contexts, thus providing a fragmentary and distorted view of the human experience.

Feminist researchers have begun to reject this positivist tradition. As the invisibility of women's experiences has been gradually recognised, women have begun to challenge the notion that a subjective, 'male' perspective is scientific or neutral. There is a new commitment to a research process where women participate as subjects rather than objects.

Methodological considerations

If the experience of homeless women is to be recorded in a meaningful way, it is important to maintain a strong sense of the underlying theoretical foundation when considering a suitable research method.

A qualitative approach

The aim of the feminist researcher must be 'to validate women's subjective experience' (Oakley 1981). A qualitative approach may well be the most appropriate method for recording and examining homeless women's lives, whilst also adhering to a feminist theoretical framework.

Qualitative research has emerged largely from the anthropological and sociological tradition. Methods include participation, observation, and semi-structured or unstructured interviews. Rather than seeking an overview, qualitative research explores the 'worm's eye view' of relationships, feelings, motivation and behaviour from the participants' perspective (Hakim, 1987). Qualitative studies do not set out to simplify, or to produce yes/no answers, but rather to illuminate the complexity of the human condition. While quantitative research aims to achieve detachment and objectivity, qualitative research accepts some personal interaction between the researcher and the participant, acknowledging that this will be reciprocal. Qualitative research:

> 'Seeks to understand and portray the social life of a particular group within its own physical, social, and cultural context.'
>
> *(Kielhofner, 1982)*

Where qualitative research is concerned, it may be necessary to accept and acknowledge the difficulty of achieving total detachment when presenting findings, and to make this explicit from the outset.

The interview process

The conventional interview poses problems for the feminist researcher hoping to interview homeless women in such a way that they can participate fully in the process and outcomes. First, the interviewer is traditionally the all-knowing expert, gleaning as much information as possible from the 'subject' (as the interviewee is generally known as), whilst maintaining a friendly detachment. The 'subject' is viewed as data, a static being who is uninvolved in the process:

> 'Objectives of the study are often not disclosed to them, all decisions are made unilaterally by researchers. Only token initial assent is gained from the individual under scrutiny.'
>
> *(Heron, 1981)*

Graham points out how easily women have been exploited over the years by researchers:

'The ease of access enjoyed by feminist and non-feminist researchers is a measure of the extent to which women have only their knowledge to lose.'
(Graham, 1984)

The personal interaction which takes place during an interview is traditionally considered insignificant. Any interest in the research from the interviewee is discouraged, as well as questions from her, which are evaded where possible. Power relations between interviewer and participant are obscured, although the interview establishes a hierarchy between the 'expert researcher' and 'naïve subject' (Oakley, 1981).

Techniques may be used which encourage interviewees to continue talking in order to reveal more personal information to the researcher. The participant may disclose more information than she means to, and may be left feeling distressed or 'used'. In the orthodox research interview, the interviewee is rarely in control. She may have no idea what she will be asked or what is expected of her (Malhotra, 1988). Some women may find it validating to talk about their experiences, while others may not. Although there is a power imbalance inherent in any 'interview' situation, feminist research should aim to minimise the exploitative aspects of the process.

In response to these problems feminist researchers have developed a different type of interview which attempts to be more equal. Attention is paid to the needs and privacy of those being interviewed. Confidentiality and anonymity are addressed at the beginning of the interview. Information about the objectives of the study is freely shared, so that there is no 'hidden agenda' unknown to the participant. There is recognition that the interview process will affect both the participant and the interviewer (and that this reciprocity will enhance the research experience). It may be appropriate for the researcher to share her own feelings during the conversation and both parties may experience an increase in self-awareness as a result of the interaction. Oakley (1981) states:

'The goal of finding out about people through interviewing is best achieved when the relationship is non-hierarchical and when the interviewer is prepared to invest her own personal identity in the relationship.'

By acknowledging a degree of subjectivity and taking an explicit theoretical stance from the outset, the values of the researcher are overt rather than implicit.

Ethical guidelines

In view of the ethical problems of interviewing women, which have already been noted, it may be useful for the researcher to devise some personal guidelines which are discussed fully with each participant at the beginning of the interview. These could include an explanation and reassurance of confidentiality and anonymity, and some information about the rationale for the study. The researcher may wish to make a personal disclosure about her life or interest in the area.

The feminist researcher may need to discuss permission to use a tape recorder, and issues relating to control of the interview process. For example, the researcher may wish to reassure the participant that she may terminate the interview at any time, switch off the tape recorder (if the interview is being recorded), or decline to answer any question if she so chooses.

The researcher will also need to give thought to how to answer personal questions from the participant and how to deal with requests for advice and help. For example, will the researcher refer a participant to an appropriate agency if requested, and/or accompany her there if the participant wishes it? What level of involvement will the researcher have with the participants after the study is complete? What level of involvement will the participants have in collating results or implementing research findings? Finally, the researcher must consider and be sensitive to each participant's social class, sexuality, age, ability, ethnicity, and so forth, and thus the diversity of her life experience.

Feminist research which fully involves participants in the interview process, 'data' analysis, research findings and implementation of consequent recommendations or strategies will begin to give homeless women a voice.

HEALTHY ALLIANCES

This part of the chapter will explain how the concept of 'healthy alliances' has emerged. It will outline some of the arguments for and against specialist vs mainstream primary health care provision for homeless people and move on to give examples of primary health care initiatives aimed at homeless people which demonstrate effective multi-agency working. Finally it will consider services for homeless women.

Health for all

In 1978, the World Health Organization (WHO) made the Alma Ata declaration, in which it challenged the countries of the world to attain 'health for all by the year 2000.' The World Health Assembly determined that:

'The main social target of governments and WHO in the coming decades should be the attainment by all citizens of the world by the year 2000 of a level of health that will permit them to lead a socially and economically productive life.'

(World Health Organization, 1985)

There are several key themes in *Health For All*, including equality, health promotion, community participation, and a focus on primary health care. The development of 'healthy alliances' so that agencies and communities work together to improve health is seen as a cornerstone of the strategy.

Health For All asserts that the health needs of each community should be met ideally through primary health care services which should be local, accessible and equally available to all. Primary health care is seen as the 'hub' of the health care system, with secondary and tertiary health care in support (World Health Organisation, 1985). The UK is a signatory to this declaration, and is thus committed to the pursuit of *Health For All*.

In February 1998, the Green Paper *Our Healthier Nation* (DoH, 1998) set out a new national strategy to improve the nation's health. Very sensibly this document acknowledged a correlation between decent housing, environmental quality and good health and also accepted that some groups of people are 'socially excluded' in terms of psychological, economic and social isolation.

Specialist vs mainstream provision

As previously discussed, primary health care services are not currently accessible for homeless people. There is an urgent need for a coordinated approach to primary health care in order to tackle the existing discontinuity of care experienced by many homeless people.

There are three main models of primary health care provision for homeless people. These are as follows:

1. Specialist (separate) services designed to cater solely for homeless people, which do not attempt to integrate them back into mainstream care
2. Generalist or mainstream services which already exist and should arguably be improved to become more accessible for homeless people
3. A combination of the two models above, where homeless people are provided with specific services in order to integrate them back into mainstream care in the longer term.

The schools of thought in relation to these three models will be discussed in turn.

Specialist services

Specialist services are clinics operated within a hostel or day centre setting, or direct-access medical centres where homeless people can walk in off the street without an appointment. A range of facilities may be on offer, including medical treatment, dental care, chiropody, counselling, advice and information on housing, health, contraception, welfare benefits and so on.

Such services have been criticised as further marginalising care for homeless people by categorising them, thus increasing discrimination, and ultimately creating a two-tier system. They have been accused of allowing mainstream services to 'wash their hands' of homeless people, absolving them from their responsibility to provide health care to all sections of the community (Oldman, 1994). Homeless people are rarely homeless for their entire lives and will at some stage move back into the mainstream of medical care. Specialist provision could complicate the transfer of medical records. There are also fears that homeless women will lose out in such a system, as they may not feel comfortable receiving health care in settings which are likely to be predominantly male (Connelly and Crown, 1994).

However, specialist provision also has obvious advantages. Specialist services tend to treat homeless people in a more holistic manner, addressing the full range of problems with which they present, and treating patients as people (Reuler, 1989). Appointment systems and facilities tend to be more flexible than mainstream services, offering a far wider range of support and attending to emotional or social problems as well as those of a physical/medical nature.

Staff are more likely to be motivated to provide a high standard of care to homeless people, and to understand the difficulties that they are experiencing. Specialist provision also allows more continuity of care, as medical records can be kept for each patient, and a full picture built up over time. Perhaps one of the most convincing arguments for such services is that homeless people themselves prefer them to mainstream services. They do not have to disclose the fact of their homelessness to staff, and need not fear hostility and prejudice

(Connelly and Crown, 1994). In one recent study, all eight women interviewed stated that they would prefer specialist services (Ibbitson, 1995). They felt that such services would be more welcoming, accessible, flexible and holistic.

Mainstream services

Arguments in favour of fully integrating homeless people into mainstream services are that these services already exist and have a duty to provide a service to all sections of the population, including the homeless population. Indeed Virginia Bottomley (then Secretary of State for Health) stated in *The Patient's Charter*:

> 'The National Health Service is a service for everybody ... a comprehensive service available to all on the basis of clinical need.'
>
> *(Rt. Hon. V. Bottomley, 1995)*

One might argue that primary health care teams would become more accessible and sensitive to the needs of homeless people if they were provided with training to raise their awareness and help them understand the issues involved. This might include examining some of the causes of homelessness and some of the reasons why homeless people suffer greater ill health than other population groups.

Criticisms of this model however are that although few would disagree that mainstream services ought to become more accessible, this is not going to be achieved in the near future. Rigid, inflexible procedures may take years to change and in the meantime homeless people are not receiving appropriate care. Moreover, primary health care staff are already overburdened with training and may simply not have the time, or may not identify such training as a priority within the practice.

Although this is a desirable long-term goal, focusing on this model alone is no immediate solution for those many people who need appropriate health care right now.

Combined services

Alternative strategies aimed at facilitating access to primary care have focused on the gradual re-integration of homeless people back into mainstream services. Such strategies tend to combine specialist services to homeless people with training to mainstream health service staff to improve their skills. Their focus is neither solely on mainstream services nor on specialist services, but a mixture of both. Homeless people may be encouraged by specialist workers to attend specific services as an interim measure, with the intention of transferring them back to mainstream care in the longer term. A peripatetic health care professional may act as a link worker, accompanying a homeless person when registering with a doctor, advocating on their behalf with primary care staff, and perhaps assisting with other general matters such as negotiating the benefits system.

Criticisms of this model of care are that it may be confusing or distressing for homeless people to begin to develop a relationship with health care staff at a specialist centre only to be referred somewhere else yet again. Some schemes currently in operation have also experienced difficulty finding a GP who will register the homeless person when the time comes (Connelly and Crown, 1994).

Models of good practice

Encouragingly, there are examples from around the country where targeted services have been established in an effort to improve delivery of care to the homeless population. Their success demonstrates the importance of integrated planning and cooperation between statutory agencies and voluntary groups. The Royal College of Physicians' report on homelessness and ill health (1994) noted:

> 'The few examples of good practice ... emphasise the importance of improved communication and better joint planning and working practices between health, housing, social services, and voluntary agencies.'

As one might expect, many of these initiatives are based in London, but there are others in the UK in, for example, Leeds, Sheffield, Nottingham, Bristol and Newcastle. Box 8.1 details three such schemes.

BOX 8.1	*Models of good practice*

■ In Nottingham, a multi-agency group has been organised to coordinate services for homeless people. The Nottingham Community Health Team for the Homeless is part of this strategy, providing walk-in clinics, offering health education, treatment, counselling and support. Two nurses liaise between statutory and voluntary service providers, accelerating referral procedures and working alongside health staff, challenging and exploring attitudes and practices (CHAR, 1994).

■ The Hannover and Devonshire Street General Practices in Sheffield have set up a 'homelessness team' incorporating an outreach service to local hostels with a 'non-judgemental holistic approach' towards homeless patients who are referred to the surgery (Practice Nurse, 1994). It aims to integrate homeless people into mainstream care and involves six GPs, three practice nurses, two health visitors, a community psychiatric nurse (CPN), alcohol counsellor, general counsellor, social worker, psychiatrist and chiropodist (Connelly and Crown, 1994).

■ Great Chapel Street Medical Centre in London, established in 1978, is the largest and probably the oldest primary care medical centre for homeless people in the country, providing a walk-in clinic and outreach sessions in hostels and day centres. Its staff include several GPs, a dentist, optician, consultant psychiatrist and practice nurse (Pleace and Quilgars, 1996). It collaborates closely with a number of statutory and voluntary agencies. In addition to the direct-access clinic, it has opened Wytham Hall, a 14-bed sick bay where homeless people can be admitted as inpatients, a facility which it admits: 'blurs the sharp divisions between primary and secondary care.' (Great Chapel Street Medical Centre, 1991).

Services for homeless women

Although there are some similarities between homeless women and homeless men, as discussed earlier there are also important differences, some of which render women more vulnerable. For example, it may be very important for women that they have the choice of being seen by a female doctor, particularly when discussing sexual health. They may have different emotional or mental health needs or may feel threatened or frightened using mixed services. There is some evidence to suggest that homeless women are indeed reluctant to use services which are predominantly male (Connelly and Crown, 1994). In a recent review of services conducted by The King's Fund (1996) providers expressed concern that they were not reaching certain groups, namely women, younger people and ethnic minority groups.

In a survey of homeless women conducted in 1992, 73% of respondents stated that they would like to see a women-only session at a local specialist medical centre. Potential reasons for attending included contraceptive advice, cervical smear tests, immunisation, advice about sexually transmitted diseases, drug and alcohol information, general medical care, help with menopausal or menstrual problems, housing advice, antenatal and postnatal care and family problems (Bridge Medical Centre, 1992).

If services for homeless people are to become more coordinated, organisations must endeavour to work within a multi-agency framework. In the White Paper *The New NHS. Modern, Dependable* (DoH, 1997) the Government stresses the importance of the NHS working together with others not only to improve health but also to reduce health inequalities. The new primary care groups will be working in partnership with local authorities and others to identify how local action on economic and social issues will impact on the health of local people. A new statutory duty of partnership has also been placed on local NHS bodies to work together for the common good. Although working in a spirit of shared responsibility may prove challenging for some agencies more accustomed to working in isolation or even competing against others, one would hope that they will rise to the challenge and that these changes will lead to more coordinated services for homeless people.

STRATEGIES AND EVALUATION

This final section will look at ways in which health promotion could address the problems facing homeless women and men, as explored in this chapter.

Role of health promotion

The main thrust of health promotion is to reduce inequalities in health and champion the rights of disempowered groups. It therefore has an important role to play in addressing the needs of the homeless population.

As a key aim of health promotion is to enable people to take more control over their lives, it has 'a clear philosophical basis of self-empowerment' (Ewles and Simnett, 1992). Health promotion is in the unusual position of working with diverse agencies in both the statutory and voluntary sector. Its broad scope encompasses the bottom-up approach of community development as well as the 'top-down' approach of policy development. Health promotion is thus uniquely placed for working with the homeless community.

One of the myriad activities of health promotion is to conduct research. This may be in the form of a needs assessment into the particular health needs of a client group in order to develop appropriate care. Research into homeless women and health as outlined in this chapter could fall within the remit of health promotion.

Since the purchaser/provider dichotomy occurred in the (now) market-led National Health Service (NHS) many health promotion departments have been transferred out of health authorities (purchaser) and into local health care trusts (provider). Despite this however, many departments have maintained a close relationship with commissioners of services and have thus been able to influence some purchasing decisions. Since the publication of the White Paper, *The New NHS. Modern, Dependable* (DoH, 1997) commissioning of services will gradually move away from the health authorities towards the new primary care groups. Health authorities will draw up a 3-year health improvement programme which will inform purchasing decisions and may be an opportunity for health promotion to push the health of homeless people up the agenda.

Strategies

Box 8.2 lists some strategies to improve the health of homeless people.

BOX 8.2	*Strategies for health improvement of homeless people*
	■ Conducting research and consultation with homeless people ■ Providing information for homeless people ■ Taking measures to target primary health care teams ■ Lobbying Government ■ Providing portable record cards *Research and consultation* As has been discussed in some depth, little is known about the predicament of homeless women without children and their specific health care needs. *Perceived* needs may be different from *actual* needs. Before appropriate services can be planned, it is imperative that homeless women are consulted through method-ologically robust research. In many ways this research must be a precursor to the development of further strategies. Research must be ethically sound as already discussed so that women participate at every stage of both the process and the outcomes. Health promotion is in an important position from which to exhort purchasers to include homeless women and men in service planning at all levels. *Information for homeless people* Information for homeless people would equip them with knowledge of primary health care structures and procedures. A clear and jargon-free leaflet or 'flyer' written in conjunction with homeless people could be distributed to all places of temporary accommodation, such as day centres, women's refuges and organisa-tions in contact with homeless people. It could also be available in Social Security Departments, Citizens' Advice Bureaux and so on. Information might include details of local GP surgeries, how to register, services available at each surgery,

and the right of each homeless person to be registered with a doctor. This would be a local version of the national leaflet *Why Bother?* distributed by CHAR (1994).

Measures targeting primary health care teams

This strategy would be designed to improve mainstream service provision and would involve a two-pronged approach consisting of an information pack combined with a training programme.

The dissemination of a resource pack written in conjunction with homeless people would provide GPs with information about housing, homelessness and health. It would include a section explaining the particular problems facing women who are homeless and some of the causes of women's homelessness. It would also aim to challenge the myths about homelessness. It would give clear guidance to GPs addressing their concerns regarding, for example, registering somebody who cannot provide an address.

In addition, regular training could be offered to all primary health care staff on a rolling programme. This would need to be flexible to fit in with the time commitments of the primary care team. Training could be delivered in consultation with homeless people and address the issues of homelessness, discrimination and labelling, and gender awareness as outlined in Box 8.3.

BOX 8.3	*Training topics for the primary care team*

- Homelessness – providing practical information and advice, including causes of homelessness, particular health needs of homeless people etc.
- *Discrimination and labelling* – including anti-discriminatory practice, how to make services more welcoming of, for example, lesbians and gay men, minority ethnic communities. The diversity of the homeless population.
- *Gender awareness* – considering the health needs of homeless women, causes of women's homelessness, dispelling myths and stereotypes, the heterogeneity of homeless women.

Further work could be carried out with the primary health care team, such as encouraging the team to review to what extent their services are accessible and flexible (covering topics such as reception areas, waiting lists, appointment systems, opening hours, information on display, interpreting facilities). The idea of assigning several team members to monitor the numbers of homeless patients, and to continually reappraise services could be suggested. A user group could be set up including homeless patients to air their views on the service received.

Lobbying government

As health promotion is a politically sensitive strategy, it is important that it supports organisations in political lobbying. It may be unrealistic and ultimately self-defeating for health promotion to be at the forefront of any campaign. However, independent organisations which counsel government as to the deleterious effects of current housing policy and encourage a redirection of policy away from home ownership and back into the rented sector should be supported. In the long term such a change in policy would improve the health of homeless people. There is little point to improving health care services to homeless people if once treated they are forced back to the situation which caused their ill health in the first place. Further lobbying might urge the Government to fund more women's refuges and to change the homelessness legislation so that women who are victims of violence do not have to show evidence of injury.

Portable record cards

Health promotion could be instrumental in liaising with the necessary bodies in order to initiate hand-held record cards for homeless people. This could go part way to improving the discontinuity of care experienced by homeless people at present. Portable records would be kept with the homeless person to alleviate the problem of medical records going astray or never catching up.

Monitoring and evaluation

In line with the *Health For All* key theme of multisectoral collaboration, a multidisciplinary working group could be established to monitor and evaluate the above initiatives, with representation from homeless people, local housing and homelessness agencies (both statutory and voluntary), the health authority, Social Service departments, GPs and general practice staff.

In order to evaluate the strategy, clear targets should be set, which should be specific and measurable. Some thought must be given as to what will be measured and how. What would be the best means of evaluating the training for primary health care teams for example? Would it be more useful to ask homeless people if they perceived an improvement in staff attitudes or to ask staff if they thought that their practice had changed as a result of attending? Would the ultimate aim be to increase uptake of services by homeless people to the practice? Structures would need to be in place to monitor the developing research, thus ensuring that it was ethical. Monitoring the involvement of homeless people themselves in the strategy as a whole must be rigorous and ongoing.

CONCLUSION

Although the measures proposed in this chapter may ameliorate accessibility of current services, most will inevitably address the symptoms of homelessness rather than the cause. Ultimately, no matter how accessible and appropriate the services, and no matter how assertive and empowered homeless women and men become, the root cause must be confronted.

There is deep public concern about housing and homelessness in the general population. In a MORI opinion poll, housing and homelessness were ranked above both health and education in importance, and the majority of people wished to see an increase in council house building (Roof, 1993). As the Royal College of Physicians concluded in their 1994 study of homelessness and ill health:

'The central thrust of Government housing policy – has been to encourage the erosion of the subsidised rented sector in favour of wider home ownership. If homelessness is to be tackled effectively, there must be a restatement of the need for an affordable, acceptable and secure rented sector.'

DISCUSSION QUESTION

- What steps might you take to involve homeless women in the research process from start to finish?
- How would you design a 'code of ethics' for interviews with women?
- In lobbying government, what sort of demands might organisations make in terms of the direction of housing policy?
- What kind of temporary accommodation would be most suitable for homeless women and why?
- How would you evaluate the information leaflet for homeless people?

REFERENCES

Bassuk, E.L., Rubin, L. & Lauriat, A.S. (1986) Characteristics of sheltered homeless families. *American Journal of Public Health*, 76: 1097–1101.

Big Issue (1996/1997) (139): 30 December 1996–5 January 1997.

Bines, W. (1994) *The Health of Single Homeless People*. York: Centre for Housing Policy, University of York.

Bottomley, V. (1995) *The Patient's Charter & You*. pp. 2–3. London: HMSO.

Bower, H. (1994) Homeless equals healthless. *Practice Nurse*, 15 February: 136–139.

Bridge Medical Centre (1992) *Survey of Homeless Women*. Newcastle on Tyne: Single Homeless on Tyneside.

Bunston, T. & Breton M. (1990) The eating patterns and problems of homeless women. *Women and Health*, 16(1): 43–62.

Burns, G. (1996) A hope in hell. *The Pink Paper*, 9 September: 10.

Callaway, H. (1981) Women's perspectives: research as re-vision. In *Human Inquiry. A Sourcebook of New Paradigm Research* Reason, P. & Rowan, J. Chichester: John Wiley.

CHAR (1991) *Women and Housing: What Do We Want?* Report of a seminar held in Manchester on 6 March.

CHAR, (1992) *4 in 10*. A Report into the Relationship between Young Women's Homelessness and Sexual Abuse.

CHAR (1994) *Campaign News*. January (All CHAR reports available from CHAR, 5–15 Cromer Street, London WC1H 8LS).

City and Hackney Community Health Council (1989) *Homeless and Healthless*. Hackney: Hackney Community Health Council.

Clark, C. & George, C. (1993) Accessible, acceptable, appropriate. *Health Service Journal*. 25 March: 28–29.

Connelly, J. & Crown, J. (1994) *Homelessness and Ill Health*. Report of a Working Party of the Royal College of Physicians. London: Royal College of Physicians.

Connelly, J. Roderick, P. & Victor, C. (1990) Health service planning for the homeless population: availability and quality of existing information. *Public Health*, 104: 109–116.

Cornwell, P. (1994) The Private Rented Sector. *Housing Projects Advisory Service News*, March: 2.

Crane, M. (1992) Elderly, homeless and mentally ill: a study. *Nursing Standard*, 7(13).

CRISIS (1996) *Still Dying For A Home*. London: CRISIS. (Available from CRISIS, Challenger House, 42 Adler Street, London, 1E 1EE).

CRISIS (1996) *The Big Issue* (143): 27 January–2 February 1997.

Dail, P.W. & Koshes, R.J. (1992) Treatment issues and treatment configurations for mentally ill homeless women. *Social Work in Health Care*, 17 (4).

Department of the Environment (1993) *Single Homeless People*. London: HMSO.

Department of Health (DoH) (1997) *The New NHS. Modern, Dependable*. London: HMSO.

Department of Health (DoH) (1998) *Our Healthier Nation: A Contract for Health*. Consultation Paper. London: HMSO.

Department of Social Security Health and Homelessness Unit (1990) *Final Report*. Manchester: DSS.

Dobson, J. (1990) Boxed out. *New Statesman and Society*, **3** 22.

Drake, M.A. (1992) The nutritional status and dietary adequacy of single homeless women and their children in shelters. *Public Health Report*, **107** (3): 312–319.

Ewles, L. & Simnett, I. (1992) *Promoting Health: A Practical Guide*. 2nd edn. London: Scutari.

Fischer, P.J. & Breakey, W.R. (1986) Homelessness and mental health: an overview. *International Journal of Mental Health*, **14** 6–41.

Francis, M.B. (1992) Eight homeless mothers' tales. *Image: Journal of Nursing Schools*, **24**(2): 111–114.

Gelberg, L., Linn, L.S. & Leake, B.D. (1988) Mental health, alcohol and drug use, and criminal history among homeless adults. *American Journal of Psychiatry*, **145**: 191–196.

George, S.L., Shanks, N.J. & Westlake, L. (1991) Census of single homeless people in Sheffield. *British Medical Journal*, **302** 1387–1389.

Graham, H. (1984) Surveying through stories. In *Social Researching: Politics, Problems, Practice*. eds. Bell, J. & Roberts, H. Ch. 6. Routledge & Kegan Paul.

Grant, L. (1997) Romance of the road. *The Guardian Weekend*. 15 February: 12–17.

Great Chapel Street Medical Centre (1991) *Annual Report 1990–1991*. London: Great Chapel Street Medical Centre. (Available from the Great Chapel Street Medical Centre, London W1)

Guardian (1993) Housing. *Education Supplement*, 23 November: 10–11.

Guardian (1996) 22 January.

Guardian (1996) Homelessness. *Education Supplement*, 5 March: 10–11.

Hagen, J.L. & Ivanoff, A.M. (1988) Homeless women: a high risk population. *Affilia*, **3**(1): 19–33.

Hakim C. (1987) Qualitative research. In *Research Design: Strategies and Choices in the Design of Social Research*, Ch. 3. London: Unwin Hyman.

Heron, J. (1981) Philosophical basis for a new paradigm, Ch 2. In *Human Inquiry. A Sourcebook of new Paradigm Research*. eds Reason, P. & Rowan, J. Chichester: John Wiley.

Housing Projects Advisory Service (HPAS) (1994) *HPAS News*, March.

Ibbitson, M. (1995) *Homeless Women and Primary Health Care: A Study of Eight Women's Experiences*. MSc Thesis. Manchester: University of Manchester.

James, A. (1991) Homeless women in London: the hostel perspective. *Health Trends*, 23: 80–83.

Johnson, A.K. & Kreuger, L.W. (1989) Toward a better understanding of homeless women. *National Association of Social Workers*, November: 537–540.

Keyes, S. & Kennedy, M. (1992) *Sick to Death of Homelessness*. London: CRISIS.

Kielhofner, G. (1982) Qualitative research: Part one. Paradigmatic grounds and issues of reliability and validity. *Occupational Therapy Journal of Research*, **2**(2): 67–79.

King's Fund (1996) *Health and Homelessness in London: A Review*. London: King's Fund.

McMillan, I. (1992) Down and out in New York. *Nursing Times*. **88**(50): 45–46.

Malhotra, V.A. (1988) Research as self reflection: a study of self, time, and communicative competency. In *Nebraska Sociological Feminist Collective. A Feminist Ethic for Social Science Research*. Ontario: Edwin Mellen.

Manchester Metro News (1995) 24 March.

Markey, K. (1997) Doctor In The House? *The Big Issue* (145): February 10–16: 8–9.

Marshall, E.J. & Reed, J.L. (1992) Psychiatric morbidity in homeless women. *British Journal of Psychiatry*, **160**: 761–768.

Marshall, M. (1989) Collected and neglected: are Oxford hostels for the homeless filling up with disabled psychiatric patients? *British Medical Journal*, **299**: 706–709.

Miles, R. (1988) *The Women's History of the World*. London: Paladin Grafton.

Miller, M. (1990) *Bed and Breakfast: Women and Homelessness Today*. London: Women's Press.

Morrisey, J. & Levine, I. (1987) Researchers discuss latest findings, examine needs of homeless mentally ill persons *Hospital and Community Psychiatry*, **38**: 811–812.

Oakley, A. (1981) Interviewing women: a contradiction in terms. In *Doing Feminist Research*. ed. Roberts, H. Ch. 2. London: Routledge & Kegan Paul

Oldman, J. (1994) Integration or ghetto-isation? *Practice Nurse*, 15 February: 140–141.

Orr, J. (1987) *Women's Health in the Community*. Chichester: John Wiley.

Pickin, C.A. & Ramsell, P.J. (1991) *A Profile of Single Homeless People in Manchester:*

Their Health Status and Access to Health Care. (Study available from North West Regional Health Authority).

Platt, S. (1989) The forgotten army. *New Statesman and Society.* 3 November: 12–15.

Please, N. & Quilgars, D. (1996) *Health and Homelessness in London.* A Review. London: King's Fund.

Practice Nurse (1994) *Public Health, 5* February: 140–142.

Reason, P. & Rowan, J. (1981) *Human Inquiry. A Sourcebook of New Paradigm Research.* Chichester: John Wiley.

Reuler, J.B. (1989) Health care for the homeless in a national health program. *American Journal of Public Health,* 79(8): 1003–1035.

Roof (1994) *Politicians Caught Napping.* November December: 9.

Ropers, R.H. & Boyer, R. (1987) Perceived health status among the new urban homeless. *Social Science and Medicine,* 24(8): 669–678.

Ross, M. (1990) *Counting Women – A Summary of Research Into Women and Homelessness.* London: London Housing Unit.

Rowbotham, S. (1973) *Woman's Consciousness, Man's World.* Middlesex: Penguin.

Royal College of Physicians (1994) *Homelessness and Ill Health.* London: Royal College of Physicians.

Scheuer, M.A., Black, M., Victor, C., Benzeval, M., Gill, M. & Judge, K. (1991) *Homelessness and the Utilisation of Acute Hospital Services in London.* Paper 4. London: King's Fund.

Scott, J. (1991) *Resettlement Unit or Asylum?* Paper presented at the Royal College of Psychiatrists, Brighton 3 July.

Scott, J. (1993) Homelessness and mental health. *British Journal of Psychiatry,* 162: 314–324.

Shelter (1990) *Homelessness: What's The Problem?* London: Shelter.

Shelter (1996) *Go Home To Rest.* London: Shelter.

Simons, R.L. & Whitbeck, L.B. (1991) Sexual abuse as a precursor to prostitution and victimisation among adolescent and adult homeless women. *Journal of Family Issues,* 12(3): 361–379.

Spender, D. (1985) *Man Made Language.* London: Routledge & Kegan Paul.

Spinner, G.F. & Leaf, P.J. (1991) Homelessness and drug abuse in New Haven. *Hospital*

Community Psychiatry, 43(2): 166–168.

Steele, A. (1991) A question of contraception. *Social Work Today,* August.

Stern, R. & Stilwell, B. (1989) *From the Margins to the Mainstream: Collaboration in Planning Services with Single Homeless People.* London: West Lambeth Health Authority

Struening, E.L. & Padgett, D.K. (1990) Physical health status, substance use and abuse, and mental disorder among homeless adults. *Journal of Social Issues,* 46: 65–81.

Townsend, P. & Davidson, N. (1982) *Inequalities in Health – The Black Report.* Harmondsworth: Penguin.

Vergare, M.J. & Aarce, A.A. (1986) Homeless adult individuals and their shelter network. In *The Mental Health Needs of Homeless Persons: New Directions for Mental Health Services.* ed. Bassuk, E.L. San Francisco: Jossey Bass.

Victor, C. (1992) Health status of the temporarily homeless population and residents of North West Thames Region. *British Medical Journal,* 305: August 15.

Wagner, J.D. & Menke, E.M. (1992) Case management of homeless families. *Clinical Nurse Specialist,* 6: 65–71.

Warner, L. (1992) Access to health. *Nursing Times.* 88(50): 42–44.

Watson, S. & Austerberry, H. (1986) *Housing and Homelessness: A Feminist Perspective.* London: Routledge & Kegan Paul.

Weller, B., Weller, M., Coker, E. et al (1987) Crisis at Christmas 1986. *Lancet,* 553–554.

Welte, J.W. & Barnes, G.M. (1992) Drinking among homeless and marginally housed adults in New York State. *Journal of Studies on Alcohol,* 53(4): 303–315.

Whynes, D.K. & Giggs, J.A. (1992) The health of the Nottingham homeless. *Public Health,* 106(4): 307–314.

Wolch, J.M. & Akita, A. (1988) Explaining homelessness. *American Psychological Association Journal,* (1): 447.

World Health Organisation (1978) *Declaration of Alma Ata.* Adopted at the International conference on Primary Health Care, Alma Ata, USSR, 6–12 September 1978 (document). Copenhagen: WHO.

World Health Organisation (1985) *Targets For Health For All.* Copenhagen: WHO.

Wright, J.D. (1990) Poor people, poor health: the health status of the homeless. *Journal of Social Issues,* 46: 49–64.

9 Mental health promotion

Phil Keeley

KEY ISSUES

- Identification of need for mental health promotion
- Influence of health and social policy
- Examples from practice
- Autonomy and empowerment
- Critique of available evidence

INTRODUCTION

It has been estimated that 25% of the population are at risk of mental illness in any one year (DoH, 1994) and this figure alone gives an indication of the numbers of individuals who are vulnerable to, or perceived to have, mental health problems. The scale of the demand for mental health services is also highlighted by the estimate that there are 60–80 service contacts per 1000 people in the population (DoH, 1993). These figures indicate that mental health problems are a major cause of illness and disability. The costs to the health service and industry are significant with mental illness accounting for an estimated 14% of National Health Service (NHS) inpatient costs and 14% of certificated absences from work (DoH, 1993).

Any chapter which considers mental health promotion must address conceptual questions such as: What is mental health?, What is health promotion?, and whilst some discussion does take place, essentially a pragmatic approach is adopted. A broad definition of mental health promotion is embraced here, which includes examples of how interventions are employed for populations through to work targeted at individuals who have severe and enduring mental illness. Discussion concerning who has the role of health promoter and which target groups should be prioritised unfolds and the impact of health and social policy on the promotion of mental health practice is contemplated.

Issues concerning empowerment and advocacy are explored. The tensions between the desire to promote autonomy whilst ensuring the welfare of vulnerable individuals and the public in particular are considered.

It is acknowledged that the word limit of this chapter means that there has had to be necessary selectivity in the issues discussed. However emphasis has been placed on the use of examples in practice to illustrate points being made.

A critique of the quality of evidence about the effectiveness of the identification of need, establishing target groups and evaluation of mental health promotion interventions is offered, with some recommendations for the way forward.

This chapter focuses on the mental health promotion of adults and older people.

CONCEPTS OF MENTAL HEALTH, HEALTH PROMOTION AND ILLNESS PREVENTION

In the absence of critical thought it may appear that consideration of the concepts of mental health and health promotion would lead to an uncomplicated development to mental health promotion. Unfortunately this is not the case! Whilst it is not the primary purpose of this chapter to spend too long clarifying concepts, it is necessary to engage in some analysis of terminology prior to moving forward. Concepts of mental health, mental illness, health promotion, mental health promotion and mental illness prevention need to be clarified.

Definitions of mental health vary. Authors highlight capability for growth and development (Chwedorowicz, 1992), the ability to lead a purposeful life (Neumann et al, 1989) and the need for inner psychological health (Maslow, 1968). Caplan (1961) perceived mental health as the ability of an individual to address problems in a manner acceptable to the prevailing tradition or culture whilst retaining a realistic viewpoint. A common theme here is the subjective nature of the concept.

More specifically the factors associated with mental health have been highlighted by Tudor (1996) and Tilford, Delaney and Vogels (1997). These include:

- The development of coping skills, which includes the ability to identify stressors and effect a constructive response. This may include either the alteration of perception of the stressor (cognitive approach). These skills help individuals to be adaptable to cope with life changes.
- The development of a 'self' concept and its impact on the self-esteem of the individual. This includes the individual's perceived sense of worthiness and ability to influence life events.
- The degree of social support available is also seen as useful in providing a buffering effect to stresses associated with life changes.

The concept of mental illness is even more problematic in terms of its definition and causation. More radical authors such as Szasz (1964) challenge the existence of mental illness whilst other authors acknowledge the existence of mental illness but highlight different causes. The importance of cultural factors in mental health have been acknowledged, for example gender issues (Busfield, 1988; DHSS, 1986) and ethnicity (Littlewood and Lipsedge, 1982; Harrison et al, 1988). Biological factors, such as genetic predisposition, family dynamics, environmental factors and social factors such as class and mental illness are highlighted by a number of authors (Brown and Harris, 1978; Lieberman, 1982; WHO, 1992; Zubin and Spring 1977). In short, there are numerous factors which are viewed as the potential cause or contributor to mental illness.

Given the lack of consensus about the definitions and causation of mental illness and, indeed, what constitutes mental health we now arrive at a situation where the challenge is to promote mental health. In other areas of health care the cause of a particular problem may be clearly established leading to appropriate health promotion strategies, for example the development of a vaccine against infectious diseases or reduction of pollution in the case of respiratory problems. With mental health promotion the selection of interventions is less clear. Should biological, social and/or environmental factors be addressed?

A variety of views on the concept of health are evident in the literature. The World Health Organisation (WHO, 1985) adopt a positive stance stating it is a state of well-being whilst Blaxter (1990) uses a more negative definition and writes about the absence of illness and a healthy lifestyle. Again, definitions are not clear cut, the view of health is multi-faceted and open to interpretation.

Dennis et al (1982) consider that health promotion concerns all activities that improve the health status of individuals and communities. They include health education, and attempts to improve public health through environmental and legislative change. This chapter embraces all these perspectives and includes them in the discussion which follows.

Hodgson et al (1996) adopt a view that:

'Interventions to promote mental health can be applied to the population at large, to those at risk of mental health problems, and to those with a mental health problem ranging from mild to severe illness.'

(p55)

This provides a pragmatic working definition which is adopted for the purpose of this chapter, though it is acknowledged that this definition blurs the boundaries between mental health promotion and mental health prevention.

The prevention of mental illness is fraught with difficulty. It has been argued that the cause of mental illness is not agreed and in view of this there is a tendency to focus narrowly on the medical perspective (which has strong ties with the illness model). In contrast, mental health promotion is concerned with the promotion of positive mental health and can be studied from the perspective of individuals, groups and communities. The next section considers the impact of health and social policy on the promotion of mental health.

HEALTH AND SOCIAL POLICY

The incorporation of mental illness as one of the five key areas included in *The Health of the Nation* document (DoH 1992a) highlights the importance given to mental health issues by the Department of Health (DoH).

The primary objective outlined in *The Health of the Nation, Key Area Handbook, Mental Illness* (DoH, 1993) was to reduce ill health and death caused by mental illness, with the targets listed in Box 9.1.

BOX 9.1	*Targets to reducing ill health and death by mental illness*

- To improve significantly the health and social functioning of mentally ill people.
- To reduce the overall suicide rate by at least 15% by the year 2000 (From 11 per 100 000 in 1990 to 9.4 per 100 000 in the year 2000).
- To reduce the suicide rate of severely mentally ill people by at least 33% by the year 2000 (From 15% in 1990 to no more than 10% in the year 2000).

The strategy to address the targets listed in Box 9.1 identified three major areas which needed to be addressed (Box 9.2).

BOX 9.2	*Needs identified in the Key Area Handbook, Mental Illness*

1. The improvement of information and understanding of mental health problems through the development of more extensive national and local data collection, use of standardised assessment procedures and clinical audit of service delivery
2. The development of comprehensive local services through the adoption of local joint purchasing and planning arrangements to ensure continuity of health and social care
3. The development of good practice by health care providers with the provision of education and training, and the establishment of protocols to enhance the standards of good practice

The publication of the Green Paper entitled *Our Healthier Nation. A Contract for Health* (DoH, 1998) acknowledges the progress made since the publication of *The Health of the Nation* (DoH, 1992a) and makes a continuing commitment to the promotion of mental health. As one of four priority areas, there is a call for promotion of mental health through enhanced public health intervention and evidence-based interventions. The acknowledgement of the many factors which contribute to mental health problems is evident in the Paper, for example:

- Genetic factors
- Social and economic factors (poverty, employment, social exclusion)
- Lifestyle
- Access to services (education, health, transport, leisure)
- Environment.

The proposal for addressing the many perceived causes of mental health problems encompasses the role of all major stakeholders, for example, individuals, commissioners and providers of services and the Government.

The continuing prioritisation of mental health problems in the national strategy is justified in view of the impact on the population in terms of the numbers affected and the expenditure on service provision. It has been estimated that in England 20% of women and 14% of men have experienced mental illness (Prescott-Clarke and Primatesta, 1998) and the total expenditure on services related to mental health and social care was more than £5 billion in the year 1992/1993 (DoH, 1996). These 'costs' of mental health problems outlined do not account for the unpaid work of carers and the impact on industry of days lost through certificated mental illness.

The main target proposed by the Government in the Green Paper *Our Healthier Nation* (DoH, 1998) is:

'To reduce the death rate from suicide and undetermined injury by at least a further sixth (17%) by 2010, from the baseline at 1996.'

(p78)

This figure represents a reduction in the number of deaths of approximately 800 per year.

The Paper also recognises the need to make progress within the group of clients experiencing serious mental illness if targets are to be addressed. The next section considers strategies to address the concerns about the suicide rate.

The use of suicide as an indicator of mental illness can be criticised. The main flaw is the implicit assumption that suicide is a reliable and valid indicator of mental illness. The premise is that effective management, treatment or interventions with individuals deemed to have mental health problems will correspond with a reduction in suicide rate. However, there is an implicit acknowledgement that suicide rates offer a narrow view of mental health gain and the Paper invites ideas for alternative measures.

Early developments in community mental health care involved community psychiatric nurses (CPNs) working with individuals with severe mental illness, though as the number of CPNs increased in the 1980s Wooff, Goldberg and Fryers (1988) highlighted the tendency for CPNs to work with clients presenting in the primary health care sector. This coincided with an emphasis on clients with 'minor' mental health problems rather than individuals with severe and enduring mental health problems. The response of the Government to this trend was to introduce policy intended to guarantee a minimum standard of care for individuals referred to the specialist psychiatric services. This included the allocation of a key worker responsible for planning of a care programme (DoH, 1990). Further, the DoH (1992b) emphasised the need to secure provision of care for clients with severe and enduring mental illness as a priority when considering the extension of GP fundholding into mental health services.

FOCUS ON SUICIDE

It has been acknowledged that two of the three targets for mental health outlined in the *The Health of the Nation* document relate to suicide prevention (DoH, 1992a). The justification for targeting suicide prevention is evident when population statistics are reviewed. Suicide is a major cause of death accounting for 1% of deaths annually and the true figure may be higher as some 'undetermined deaths' may be inappropriately recorded (NHS Advisory Service, 1994).

The rate of suicides for England and Wales over the last 10 years is approximately 11 per 100 000 people per year (Office of Population Censuses and Surveys, 1995). However this figure masks the fact that there are regional variations and differences within gender, age and ethnic groupings. Manchester, for example, has an annual suicide rate of 17–20 per 100 000 people per year with the rate for young males (aged 15–24 years) increasing by 75% since 1982. Indeed, the rate for male suicide is two, three or four times higher than females dependent on age and region (NHS Advisory Service, 1994; Suicide Prevention Sub-group, 1996). Another vulnerable group which has been identified is young Asian women (Soni Raleigh, Bulvsu and Balarajan, 1990).

The value of gathering evidence about the trends within populations is the opportunity to devise strategies to address the concerns of vulnerable individuals and to effectively target resources for health promotion initiatives. The work by Charlton et al (1992), which highlights the rise in the use of car fumes to commit suicide by young men, provides a justification for the policy initiative of a reduction in exhaust emissions. Another policy initiative which is informed by evidence is the reduction in availability of medicines, for example the restriction on the number of paracetamol that can be sold over the counter (Hawton et al, 1996).

Value of evidence-based practice

It is argued that there is a need to compile evidence about the incidence of mental health problems, the identification of vulnerable groups, effective assessment and intervention strategies. The 'thematic review' which presented an evidence-based guidance for purchasers and providers of health care who are addressing the issue of suicide prevention is an excellent example of how research can inform practice. Once this information is in the public domain then a strategic approach to the provision of effective care can be adopted. Consideration needs to be given to which agency is responsible for planning, training and delivery of services (see Box 9.3).

HEALTH EDUCATION

Whilst health education is dealt with in a discrete section here, it is perceived as an integral part of all aspects of health promotion.

Given the difficulty in establishing a concept of mental health and differing views of causation, the consideration of health promotion strategies is fraught with difficulty. The challenge is to establish a focus when causes are deemed to be multifactorial. Ferguson (1993) argues that teaching people to be mentally healthy may be questioned in view of the difficulty targeting education appropriately and concern that education does not necessarily lead to changes in lifestyle.

However, despite the concerns identified Ferguson (1993) goes on to argue for including education in programmes of care for patients and their carers. The justification for inclusion is informed by the notion that patients and carers have a right to information and the emerging evidence that education can be effective in the reduction of relapse rate, compliance and patient satisfaction.

MIND, the mental health charity has taken an initiative in the promotion of mental health through education. Their 'Mental Health Promotion' series of booklets is aimed at users and carers. Their booklet 'How to look after yourself' emphasises the identification of factors which influence physical and/or mental health, including environmental factors, relationships, activities and situations. Following this there is consideration of the changes that need to be made, minimising events which are unhealthy and increasing constructive activity such as the expression of emotions when grieving follows bereavement and loss. 'Exercise and mental health' focuses on the mental health benefits of exercise, relaxation, diet, sleep and rest. Another booklet 'What is mental distress?' provides a clear overview of the topic area including:

- Recognising the first signs
- Early recognition and support
- Triggers to mental health problems, for example bereavement, relationship breakdown, abuse, depression/childbirth
- Media view of mental distress
- Less emphasis on perceiving mental distress exclusively as an illness as

there is a view taken that there are is a range of solutions to mental health problems (not just medical treatment).

All the booklets are eminently readable and readily accessible jargon-free publications. They are targeted at service users, relatives and carers with a view to empowering individuals through education.

| **BOX 9.3** | *Health professionals' roles* |

Health authority

- Identifies local health needs and targets interventions appropriately, for example setting up a local initiative to target young, vulnerable men. One such initiative is the Campaign Against Living Miserably (CALM), a high profile advertising campaign offering a telephone service to young men who perceive themselves as low in mood
- Promotion of the use of short-term prescriptions by general practitioners (GPs) for vulnerable individuals
- Audit the effectiveness of health services
- Funding of training for key staff regarding assessment and effective interventions for clients with low mood associated with skills for the assessment of suicide risk

Mental health service provider

- Reviews critical incidents (for example suicide or deliberate self-harm) to learn from any events with a view to improving preventive health strategies
- The provision of an individualised care plan managed by a key worker for individuals considered a high risk. This is in accordance with the principles of the care programme approach (DoH, 1990). This is particularly important in the first 3 months following discharge when the risk of suicide is high (Morgan and Priest, 1991)
- Follow up individuals who do not attend the service but have a clearly identified need

General practitioner

- Adopt the practice of providing short term prescriptions for vulnerable individuals, for example when prescribing antidepressants
- Early referral of elderly clients to local, specialist old age psychiatry teams for clients who have committed deliberate self-harm

(Adapted from Suicide Prevention Sub-group, 1996)

PRIMARY PREVENTION

Primary prevention concerns the reduction of risk that people in the community will become mentally ill and considers the promotion of the ability of individuals to look after their own mental welfare (DoH, 1993).

Caplan (1961) proposed that primary preventative strategies included:

- Assessment or screening of populations to determine health needs
- Identification of at risk groups
- Early intervention.

Primary prevention of mental illness is not solely the remit of the health and social services. The Samaritans already play an important role in the promotion of mental health by attending schools to discuss lifestyle issues in addition to their telephone service activities.

In principle the prevention of risk of illness is a laudable ideal to strive for. The Mental Health Nursing Review Team (DoH, 1994) viewed primary prevention as work targeted at vulnerable people or those at risk of mental illness. The aim was identified as the reduction of incidence of mental illness with an estimate of 250 per thousand people per year at risk. The Team advocated the need for health visitors, district nurses, school nurses and practice nurses to target vulnerable individuals and groups whilst having access to the specialist support of mental health nurses.

An important question to arise from this discussion is: are psychiatrists and trained nurses in mental health the most appropriate providers of mental health primary promotion strategies? Perhaps counsellors are more effective and have the more appropriate perspective, i.e. they have a health perspective rather than an ill-health perspective. A concern which may be raised is the classification of mental health problems as mental illness if professionals focusing on mental illness become involved. It is tentatively suggested that intervention at this early stage can be left to other more appropriate groups whilst the expertise of the specialist workers can be focused on the more needy. In addition the specialist mental health workers could provide more strategic input to the primary preventative strategies, for example helping to clarify the routes of referral for people who require secondary or tertiary preventative services.

Examples of primary prevention in practice

Whilst there have been few examples of major investment in primary prevention in the UK, there are examples from the USA which can be considered. During the Carter Administration, the move to establish Community Mental Health Centres accompanied the shift from hospital to community-based interventions for individuals with mental health problems. Nationally 2000 centres were established. Their role was to offer both an alternative to hospital care for patients with mental illness and to promote mental health to the wider population. The premise for the establishment of the service was the notion that mental health problems were caused and exacerbated by social and environmental factors (Rogers and Pilgrim, 1996). The establishment of the centres did not lead to a subsequent reduction in the incidence of mental health problems recorded within the population. Wagenfield (1983) highlighted the lack of clear evidence of a clear relationship between social factors as a cause of mental health problems as a flaw in the strategy. Ironically, the Green Paper *Our Healthier Nation* (DoH, 1998) includes emphasis on social problems without a clear evidence base for interventions.

A development of the policy in the USA was the move away from tackling the broad social issues, which had proved difficult to target, and an increased emphasis on the life events which were stressors likely to lead to mental health problems. The new focus was to identify stressors and eliminate or minimise their effect by initiating appropriate interventions.

Working with populations

Abbott and Raeburn (1989) describe a study in New Zealand designed to compare the effectiveness of an information-based health education programme with a programme which included both educational *and* behavioural elements (including goal setting and relaxation exercises). The programme was designed for any member of the public rather than targeting vulnerable groups or people with identified mental health problems. The results indicated that the programme which included behavioural elements was twice as effective at achieving gains in physical, mental health, happiness and stress management skills than the information-only programme. Both groups however demonstrated health gains greater than the control group. The study was encouraging for informing the development of an effective low-cost health education and promotion programme for the population.

Workplace interventions

The promotion of mental health is not merely the concern of health care professionals and agencies specifically set up to deal with health issues. Industry is adversely affected by the impact of the workforce suffering both mental and physical health problems. One study commissioned by the World Health Organisation (WHO) suggested that billions of dollars were being lost on an international scale as long ago as 1982 (Kalimo, El-Batawi and Cooper, 1987) and it has already been stated that 14% of certified sickness absence is attributed to mental health problems.

Cooper (1994) writes about the workplace as a cause of mental health problems and a place where health promotion can be delivered. He also highlights the motives for employers becoming more interested in the promotion of health for employees which go beyond the concerns about loss of productivity. First, in the USA, the cost of employee health care financed by the employer is rising and therefore the incentive to reduce costs is in place. Ironically however the UK system of funding health care through direct taxation may provide a disincentive for UK employers to implement health promotion strategies. Second, the incidence of employees suing employers for stress-related problems in the workplace in the USA is rising. Cooper (1994) reports that 3000 cases are being brought each year in the State of California! There are early indicators of litigation increasing in the UK with the recent case of a social worker who successfully sued his local authority employers for work-related stress.

When addressing workplace stress more than one approach can be used. One approach is to focus on the individual in terms of reduction of stressors, management of stress and helping employees deal with problems. Other approaches consider the role of the organisation in the contribution to employee stress and consider how the organisation can change to accommodate the needs of employees.

Factors identified as contributing to stress in the workplace include: work overload, repetitive and boring work which does not fulfil the individual, and shift work. Lack of clarity of role and expectations, lack of security and unfulfilled ambition also contribute to stress in the workplace. Women are over represented in the group of people stressed at work due to the impact of discrimination, difficulty in gaining promotion and relative lack of investment in training when compared to men. Organisational factors can also play a part in creating stress for individuals. A work culture which restricts employee consultation and involvement in decision making can adversely affect health, particularly stress-related problems (Cooper, 1994).

Whilst it may be tempting to target interventions aimed at individuals because they are easier to change than organisations (Ivancevich et al, 1990), an opportunity to significantly affect health promotion gains may be missed if organisational issues are not addressed. Cooper (1994) asserts that the way forward is to identify sources of workplace stress and then intervene with a view to moving from treatment to preventative action. It seems that the focus of promotion of mental health in the workplace is a grossly under-utilised approach. Large numbers of individuals can be targeted and health concerns pre-empted and dealt with quickly and efficiently. This would involve a shift away form the reactive response of the health services to a more proactive strategy. The role of health care professionals such as occupational health nurses could be enhanced by the incorporation of workplace health needs assessment, development of evidence-based interventions and effective evaluation.

Working with vulnerable groups

An example of a study which targets a vulnerable group is described by Elliott, Sanjack and Leverton (1988). The study focused on first- and second-time mothers with a higher risk of postnatal depression due to, for example, lack of social support and/or previous history of mental health problems.

The intervention, by a psychologist and a health visitor, included monthly meetings which commenced once pregnancy was confirmed. The programme comprised of providing information and giving social support sessions, augmented with individual counselling sessions according to need. The benefits attributed to the programme 3 months following delivery included reduced levels of anxiety, especially in first-time mothers. The potential for integration of this cost-effective initiative into existing pre-natal provision was highlighted.

Use of the media to promote mental health

The World Mental Health Day is promoted by the Health Education Authority. In 1997 the theme was 'Promoting Positive Mental Health' and the identified aims of the day are listed in Box 9.4.

BOX 9.4	*Aims of the World Mental Health Day on 'Promoting Positive Mental Health'*

- To reduce fear, misunderstanding and stigma surrounding mental health problems
- To raise awareness that mental health problems concern everyone
- To provide resources and expertise to support local initiatives
- To raise the status and the profile of mental health promotion

The initiative, which was highlighted in professional journals, encouraged local initiatives to raise the profile of mental health promotion. However, despite the laudable aims, there does not seem to be any available evidence of effectiveness.

SECONDARY PREVENTION SECTION

Secondary prevention involves the early detection and intervention with individuals with most work carried out in the primary health care setting. The number of people at risk has been estimated at 100 per 1000 year (DoH, 1994). The recommendation of the Review Team was that health visitors, district nurses, school nurses and practice nurses would be the primary workers whilst specialist mental health nurses provide some case work and maintain close contact with primary nurses.

The dilemma for service providers concerns how to establish priorities between those who may have the potential for mental illness and provision of care for individuals with severe and enduring mental illness (tertiary prevention).

Secondary preventative approaches are designed to reduce both the severity and duration of presenting mental health problems. Strategies adopted to respond to the challenge include rapid community psychiatric nurse follow-up to prevent hospitalisation and provide support in the community; however, it is debatable whether this reduces severity/duration or whether it is merely a more cost-effective way of delivering care. In reality hospitalisation does not necessarily equate with severity and/or duration of illness but may reflect the quality and flexibility of service provision available.

Screening for mental illness

The arguments for mental health screening, especially for identified vulnerable groups, includes the positive effect mental health has on the quality of life and the potential for prevention of further deterioration. However, the following questions must be addressed:

- Can better therapeutic benefits be gained through early detection of mental health problems and vice versa?
- Are the screening tools sensitive and specific enough?
- Is there an effective, evidence-based method of treatment available?

The policy initiatives in the UK have led to the involvement of general practitioners (GPs) and primary health care services in the delivery of secondary preventative services. Positive elements of this arrangement are the accessibility of

GPs and the move to employ counsellors, CPNs and psychologists to facilitate delivery of the service made possible with the resources at the disposal of GP fundholders (Ferguson and Varnam, 1994)

The ability to diagnose mental health problems effectively is enhanced by the development of standardised tools for assessment, for example the mini mental state examination, Beck's Depression Inventory (Falloon and Fadden, 1993).

Working with vulnerable groups

Families of patients, especially those involved in a carer role are often perceived as a group vulnerable to stress and anxiety. The impact of caring for individuals with physical and mental illness cannot be underestimated. Concern about carers has led to initiatives to help them to cope. Some of the findings of studies are now outlined.

Caring for an individual who has severe and enduring mental health problems presents many challenges and relatives have been identified as a vulnerable group. Brooker (1993) evaluates the impact of the CPN's role in educating relatives about schizophrenia and recommends that CPNs are ideally placed to engage relatives, to ascertain their perceptions and beliefs about schizophrenia and then tailor an education package to meet their needs. The outcome of the study is a recommendation that a more systematic approach to the professional support of relatives is required to facilitate understanding, management of stress and avoidance of unhelpful behaviour which may exacerbate the mental health problems of the individual with schizophrenia. Indeed, the beneficiaries are both the relatives and the individual with a diagnosis of schizophrenia.

The establishment of support groups have been evaluated. A small-scale study by Halm (1990) found that working with families of patients requiring surgical intensive care had a significant impact in decreasing anxiety levels and was positively received by attendees.

In the USA, Greene and Monahan (1989) evaluated the impact of a series of workshops for care givers held over 8 weeks and targeted individuals caring for an elderly relative who were considering moving the patient into an institutional care setting. The course included discussion of feelings, education about the nature of health care problems and relaxation training. Whilst the benefits in terms of perceived reduction in stress and burden were noted following the course of eight meetings, the 6-month follow-up showed no significant reduction in perceived burden. The implication seems to be that whilst brief interventions may be helpful in the short term, there is a need to consider how the benefits of intervention can be sustained when carers have long-term responsibilities and commitments. Haley (1989) embarked upon a longitudinal study of a group of care givers looking after individuals with dementia, which received information and emotional support, and looked at problem-solving strategies. In the long term, no changes in depression ratings were detected, though satisfaction was expressed about the value of the group. In summary, the interventions were valued by individuals, but the studies did not provide an objective measure of benefit.

Toseland et al (1990) explored the impact of brief interventions targeted at individuals vs groups of family carers; a control group received respite care only. The interventions included either 1 hour of individual counselling or 2 hours of group work over a period of 8 weeks. Both the individual counselling and socially supportive group work was seen as beneficial compared to the control group in terms of decrease in psychiatric symptoms. However, the group work was seen as offering more social support whilst the individual work offered more psychological support.

Schultz et al (1993) carried out a long-term follow-up of a brief intervention which addressed the promotion of understanding, coping through problem solving and skill development. Targeted at carers of older people with health problems, the programme involved nine 2.5-hour meetings. Whilst the participants valued the programme, there was little evidence of long-term benefit in terms of mental health. The need for a replication study using a larger sample was indicated.

Hill and Balk (1987) conducted a study in the USA into the effects of a brief educational programme with families of individuals with severe and enduring mental health problems. Whilst there were perceived benefits in terms of stress and anxiety at the end of the 9-week course, questions need to be raised about the sustainability of health gains. Although there are early indications of the potential benefits derived from brief interventions with carers, there is a need to set up larger studies to explore whether the benefits can be sustained in the long term.

In a Scottish study (Holden, Sagovsky and Cox, 1989), women identified as depressed 6 weeks following childbirth were referred to health visitors for eight weekly visits of a minimum length of 30 minutes. The main approach included non-directive counselling with a view to the facilitation of decision-making skills of the mothers. The impact following the intervention was statistically significant. Of the mothers included in the study, 69% showed no sign of depression 13 weeks following the intervention compared to a control group, where only 38% recovered. The health visitors received a brief training course to enhance their counselling prior to the study and therefore did not require a major investment in resources.

Another study by Gerrard et al (1993) concerned a more in-depth training of health visitors to prepare them for their role in the detection, treatment and prevention of postnatal depression. The content of the training addressed non-directive counselling, information about postnatal depression, use of assessment tools and prevention strategies. Whilst the resource implications of the extra training were acknowledged, the outcomes were promising. Following the interventions, the health visitors managed to effect a statistically significant reduction in the incidence of postnatal depression for the mothers in the group when assessed 6 months after the study. The study provides some evidence to back up the notion that health visitors should develop their role in this area.

Maynard (1993) studied the effectiveness of structured group interventions for women who perceived themselves as depressed. Following a brief series of meetings held in a community setting over 12 weeks the short-term benefits included less depression and feelings of hopelessness and raised self-esteem for the participants. This study produced encouraging results for a relatively modest investment in the time of the mental health worker. Replication of the study is required to establish whether the benefits could be sustained over a longer period of time.

Given the emphasis on suicide prevention in *The Health of the Nation* document, the Canadian study by de Man and Labrèche-Gauthier (1991) provides interest. The community-based intervention involved the provision of social support alongside work to improve self-esteem and stress management skills. The target group included individuals who expressed suicidal ideas. Although this was a small-scale study, there were encouraging signs of increased self-esteem and a reduced incidence of stress and suicidal ideas for participants following the intervention.

A Swedish study has examined the impact of providing an educational programme for GPs with a view to enhancing their role in the prevention and treatment of depression (Rutz et al, 1989). After an initial increase, the referral rates to consultant psychiatrists decreased and the prescription patterns of anti-depressants increased to therapeutic levels. The major outcome was the more effective treatment of individuals in the primary care setting with a reduction of hospitalisation. Furthermore, there was no change in the incidence of suicide. Whilst a larger study is required to inform future service development, these findings could be relevant in the UK.

The impact of environmental factors, specifically housing, was explored by Elton and Packer (1986). The study targeted individuals who perceived that their mental health problems were adversely affected by their housing circumstances. The findings indicated that individuals in the group who were rehoused showed significantly reduced scores for anxiety and depression. The study provides an impetus for the broadening of the view of what constitutes health promotion interventions. The strategic importance of the role of the housing policy and the promotion of mental health is highlighted here. In Manchester this idea has been embraced by the establishment of 'Creative Support' services which focus on meeting the housing needs of vulnerable individuals and the strategic planning in the development of new housing stock to address the needs of individuals with health problems.

Psychological interventions for individuals with physical problems

In the hospital and community setting there is an increasing recognition of the need to meet the mental health needs of clients presenting with physical illness (Royal College of Physicians/Royal College of Psychiatrists, 1995). Findings include recognition that 15% of inpatients on medical wards have mood disorders which are associated with low patient satisfaction with the service and extra health care costs related to extended hospitalisation.

Strategies are emerging to meet the needs of clients. They include the establishment of a liaison psychiatry service, i.e. the provision of a mental health worker to work effectively with clients. Other strategies include the development of training programmes for 'general' nurses to enable accurate assessment of psychological needs and effective implementation of care or referral if appropriate. This highlights the fact that mental health promotion is relevant to everyone and should not be left to mental health workers.

Conclusions

There is emerging evidence of the effectiveness of secondary preventative strategies though some evidence is methodologically flawed and there remain question marks against the long-term effectiveness of brief interventions. It is clear that a wide range of professionals are involved in this work and not just dedicated mental health professionals. The evidence seems to indicate that it is easier to target interventions to vulnerable groups rather than whole populations.

TERTIARY PREVENTION

Tertiary prevention is based on the principle of providing intervention for the most vulnerable individuals with persistent or enduring mental health problems. Their needs indicate the requirement for the input of specialist health care professionals who work with the client to reduce the risk of relapse. It is estimated that there are 24 people per 1000-year at risk (DoH, 1994).

Brooker (1990) highlights the social, economic and emotional costs to individuals and families of severe and enduring mental illness. With an estimated 100 000 people diagnosed with schizophrenia in Britain, there is a clear need to identify strategies for the promotion of health and prevention of further deterioration.

Evidence is being accrued to support the notion of psycho-social interventions for clients with severe and enduring mental illness informed by the stress and vulnerability model of schizophrenia proposed by Birchwood, Hallett and Preston (1989). The stress vulnerability model introduced by Zubin and Spring (1977) and Lieberman (1982) has provided much of the theoretical drive and clinical focus for psycho-social interventions. The factors considered by the model include genetic vulnerability and environmental stressors, and therefore embrace psychological, sociological and biological factors.

In tackling the issue of environmental stress, the work of Vaughn and Leff (1976) on the impact of expressed emotion within families has led to several researchers recommending that family intervention is a way forward for working. This involves working with the individual who has a severe and enduring mental health problem and their family. Work by Leff et al (1989), Falloon et al (1987) and Hogarty et al (1986) support this approach. The Camberwell study (Brown and Rutter, 1966) was key to the exploration of expressed emotion in families and the authors highlighted the impact of family hostility, criticism and emotional overinvolvement as an indicator of increased probability of relapse.

The use of psycho-social interventions is intended to promote the quality of life of individuals with severe and enduring mental health problems and their families through the promotion of a positive and constructive environment (Barrowclough and Tarrier, 1992). This can lead to work with family members to deal with feelings of anger, frustration and guilt which may be directed at the 'ill' family member. Indeed a strategy that is proving beneficial is the reduction in face-to-face contact between clients and their family, especially where high levels of expressed emotion is identified.

Whilst medication is still advocated for some clients with mental health problems, it is clear that the medication alone does not provide all the answers. It has been estimated that 40–50% of clients with severe and enduring mental health problems still experience positive symptoms, for example delusions and hallucinations, anxiety and/or depression, despite receiving neuroleptic medication (Tarrier, 1987). Falloon and Talbot (1981) highlight the high suicide rates for this client group.

In order to meet the challenges presenting by this client group, an active initiative, the THORN course, aims to ensure that health and social care professionals are trained effectively to meet the needs of individuals with enduring mental illness. Course participants develop relevant clinical skills and explore the evidence for psycho-social interventions with a view to promote effectiveness of care. The THORN course development has been informed by the emerging research evidence about effectiveness of interventions and policy initiatives. As a result, the course involves training in cognitive-behavioural therapy, effective use of standardised mental health assessment tools, working with families and working as a case manager.

The problems experienced at present in the effective implementation of tertiary prevention relate specifically to the lack of investment in training. Until 1998, there has been a restriction on the number of courses available, however, the accumulation of evidence to support the value of the course may persuade commissioners of education to fund an expansion of the course.

AUTONOMY, ADVOCACY AND EMPOWERMENT

The WHO recognise the value of empowerment in health promotion by emphasising the importance of enhancing health status by helping individuals to have control over their life (WHO, 1984). Whilst it may be deemed desirable to maximise the autonomy and actively support the notion of empowering individuals to take control of their own health status, clients with mental health problems may present unique dilemmas to health care professionals. Health promotion initiatives discussed elsewhere in this book include an element of choice however individuals with mental health problems may find themselves in a situation where non-compliance with treatment may be interpreted as deviant behaviour (Playle and Keeley, 1998).

A fundamental concern is for the welfare of the individual and the safety of others. The Report of the Confidential Inquiry into Homicides and Suicides by Mentally Ill People (Royal College of Psychiatrists, 1996) highlights the tragic consequences of failure to meet the health care needs of mentally ill people. The cases of Ben Silcock and Christopher Clunis, who received psychiatric care in the community and subsequently engaged in anti-social and dangerous behaviour, raised public concern and highlighted the need to ensure that vulnerable individuals are monitored effectively and treated in the community. The Mental Health Act (1983) has been amended to include clearer guidelines for discharge planning and the supervision of individuals in the community has been implemented (Section 25). The implementation of the Care Programme Approach (DoH, 1990) has clarified the obligations and accountability of keyworkers. Alongside this has been the focus of resources to clients with severe and enduring illness.

The justification for treating an individual against his or her will is usually based on the notion that the individual is a risk to themselves or others and competence is called into question. This means that empowerment is difficult to achieve, especially when the individual is deemed to be incompetent. The situation then arises whereby the health or social care professional has to make a clinical judgement about the intervention required. Too little intervention may ascribe autonomy to an individual who is not competent whilst too much intervention may serve to undermine autonomy and lead to well-meaning but paternalistic interventions. The complicating factor is the duty of the professional to the wider society as well as to the individual with mental health problems.

The legal mechanism of the Mental Health Act (1993) governs how health and social carers can intervene; however, the ethical principle that is appealed to is beneficence, where the aim is to achieve a 'good' outcome for the client informed by a professional perspective of what is in the 'best interests' of the client (and the wider society).

Whilst it has been argued that treatment of individuals against their will can be justified where there is a risk to themselves or others, there are initiatives which have been developed with a view to increasing the voice of the client and promoting participation individually or collectively. A joint report from the Confederation of Health Service Employees (COHSE) and the mental health charity MIND provides a concrete suggestion (Read and Wallcraft, 1992). The document acknowledges the encouragement of user groups to become involved in the management of mental health services by the Government. In essence the guidance proposes user involvement in staff recruitment, short listing and interviewing.

To increase the participation of clients, ex-users and advocates, a more consumer-orientated approach is proposed, in which these individuals are actively involved in decision making. Brown (1985) describes this as a rights-based system. However, the implications are that there would need to be a move away from the current system where health care professionals dominate. To effect the change, the professional hierarchy would need to be challenged and more emphasis placed on self-help.

The pursuit of participation and the promotion of autonomy seems morally sound as it strives to empower users. However, on a cautionary note, pursuit of this idea may place at risk the view that the Government needs to fund the welfare provision for this group. Further, concern may be voiced about the ability of relatively vulnerable individuals to argue with health care professionals to influence care, especially as confidence may be low and knowledge of the system may be limited (Dalley, 1988). If this notion is pursued then resources need to be released to provide advocates and develop the knowledge and assertiveness skills of users.

The pursuit of participation can also promote integration of people with mental health problems into the community by the involvement of clients in the practical organisation of the service. Both changes to the mental health system and attitudes in society are required to ensure a policy of integration. If the proposed values are upheld, then welfare and beneficent acts will be available when an individual is vulnerable, to show respect for the person, yet at the earliest opportunity the intervention will be minimised to promote autonomy. This requires members of the mental health service to constantly question involvement in care and promotion of the value of minimum intervention.

When facilitating autonomy by the promotion of user groups, it is valuable to encourage them to be free of professional involvement (unless a contribution is invited by users). From this position of strength the users should be offered representation on service planning and development groups. This seems an appropriate approach to encourage participation; dealing with the system as an individual may prove daunting, but as a group users can and should be empowered to coordinate collective action within a locality. To facilitate this health care, professionals need to be proactive despite conflict with their professional status. MIND (1990) also believes that the promotion of self-help groups will facilitate self-advocacy, reveal personal preferences and inform service developments.

On a practical level, the promotion of a user-centred approach could involve clients in the development, management, and operation of the services, including assessment of need. However, the question must be raised about who the user interacts with? With the advent of the mixed economy of welfare, the question is difficult to answer. Interaction may take place between the local authority or the providers, but given the fact that there may be a large number of providers, the latter option may not prove feasible. Further, the question: 'Who are the users?' must be addressed. It is suggested that individuals with mental health problems, their carers and ex-clients may be appropriate and, where necessary, vulnerable individuals could be represented by independent advocates.

The preceding discussion leads to the following suggestion. There is a need to give the clients, carers and ex-users a legal right to be involved rather than continuing with the present discretionary arrangement. This should be done to ensure there is a genuine participation between clients and carers. The aim would be to enable informal carers to feel supported, clients to receive appropriate care and to ensure cost-effective use of resources.

To enable all these changes to take place would need a shift in government policy and training and development for clients, carers and advocates to ensure they can make informed choices and have the appropriate skills to make effective representation. Otherwise, Croft and Beresford (1990) assert that without the resources and skills, there will be a possibility of lack of genuine progress due to lack of confidence and ability to deal with professional groups.

To facilitate the change, there would also need to be a shift in the relationship between professional and client, in particular, the problem of the professional dominating the relationship. There is a need for the professional to cooperate more and enter into a partnership with service users. This requires a challenge to the traditional professional status and the facilitation of the more informed user. To accommodate the shift in focus towards a partnership in care, there is a need for health care professionals to change their role from autonomous expert to facilitator of informed choice (Walker, 1993).

There is an opportunity in the NHS and Community Care Act (1990) to increase user involvement and empowerment, though the option of containing costs and the reduction in emphasis on public services for economic and ideological reasons may undermine the initiatives in reality.

Enhancing the involvement of service users and carers is a priority identified by the Government for both health and social service delivery. The aim is to involve individual and group representatives in the development of local services. At a national level, views are to be sought about the development of NHS policy (NHSE, 1995). The opportunity to translate these ideas to the development of health promotion strategies is worthy of note here, rather than keeping to the narrow confines of treatment and care delivery.

The nursing profession has placed user involvement as a high priority with the Review of Mental Health Nursing Team (DoH, 1994) highlighting how user involvement can be effective in determining future service development and improvement of service outcomes. Following recommendations by the Review, the English National Board (ENB) for Nursing, Midwifery and Health Visiting has published *Learning from each other* (ENB, 1996). This publication is intended to highlight and promote the involvement of users and carers in the planning, delivery assessment and evaluation of education provision, thus ensuring that their views can ensure that health care professionals can be influenced as they prepare for their role as service deliverers and planners.

For involvement to be a positive and active process, rather than a token gesture, consultation, negotiation, partnership and mutual respect all need to be addressed. Especially if the top-down paternalistic approach of professionals is to be replaced by a more collaborative, shared approach to decision making. Rodgers (1994) asserts that users and carers must be empowered to work with professionals.

CONCLUSIONS

At a time when evidence-based practice has a high priority in the commissioning and delivery of services, it is clear that more research is required into the effectiveness of mental health promotion. Whilst this is easy enough to state, there are some historical obstacles to be overcome. The lack of evaluation studies in the UK is a poor starting point though there are studies from other countries, notably the USA, which may offer ideas for future research. However, the review of the literature by Tilford, Delaney and Vogels (1997) is an excellent text which highlights the limited evidence in support of mental health promotion interventions. The methodological problems of measuring health gains have already been alluded to, both in terms of the difficulty in defining mental health and the complexity of causative factors.

It is envisaged by the author that research into mental health promotion lends itself to a long-term strategic approach as many mental health interventions are long-term investments. The exceptions to this are brief interventions targeted at specific problems as they arise, for example bereavement counselling and working with individuals who have or are susceptible to postnatal depression.

Decisions relating to the targeting of resources must be considered, for example whether to address the whole population or to target specific groups. In addition, decisions must be taken regarding who should deliver services, for example voluntary sector, school teachers, health and social care professionals. Though the studies described in this chapter support the idea that a wide range of individuals from the statutory and non-statutory sectors have a role to play.

The major conclusion, therefore, is to emphasise the need for a strategic approach to the evaluation of mental health interventions with the use of longitudinal studies to reflect the long-term investments that are required. Whilst acknowledging the need to identify and measure the effectiveness of interventions, the author would not wish to infer that only quantitative designs are the way forward but rather that a qualitative approach that takes into account the experiences and perceptions of individuals should also be adopted.

DISCUSSION QUESTIONS

- Is the emphasis on the prevention of suicide in health policy documents justified?

■ Can you propose and justify any alternative measures of the mental health of the population?

■ Are health care professionals ever justified when they forcibly promote the mental health of an individual by invoking the Mental Health Act (1983)?

REFERENCES

Abbott, M.W. & Raeburn, J.M. (1989) Superhealth: A community-based health promotion programme. *Mental Health in Australia*, **2**(1): 25–35.

Barrowclough, C. & Tarrier, N. (1992) *Families of schizophrenic patients: cognitive behavioural interventions*. London: Chapman & Hall.

Birchwood, M. Hallett, S.E. & Preston, M.C. (1989) *Schizophrenia: an integrated approach to research and treatment*. New York: New York University.

Blaxter, M. (1990) *Health and Lifestyles*. London: Tavistock/Routledge.

Brooker, C. (1990) The health education needs of families caring for a schizophrenic relative and the potential role for community psychiatric nurses. *Journal of Advanced Nursing*, **15**(9): 1092–1098.

Brooker, C. (1993) Evaluating the impact of training community psychiatric nurses to educate relatives about schizophrenia: implications for health promotion at the secondary level. In *Research in Health Promotion and Nursing*. eds Barnett, J. & Macleod Clark, J. Basingstoke: Macmillan.

Brown, P. (1985) *The Transfer of Care*. London: Routledge.

Brown, G.W. & Harris, T.O. (1978) *Social Origins of Depression*. London: Tavistock.

Brown, G.W. & Rutter, M. (1966) The measurement of family activities and relationships: a methodological study. *Human Relations* **19**: 241–263.

Busfield, J. (1988) Mental illness as a social construct: a contradiction of feminist's arguments? *Sociology of Health and Illness*, **10**: 521–542.

Caplan, G. (1961) *An Approach to Community Mental Health*. London: Tavistock.

Charlton, J. Kelly, S. Dunnell, K. Evans, B., Jenkins, R. & Walis, R. (1992) Trends in suicide deaths in England and Wales. *Population Trends*, **69**: 10–16.

Chwedorowicz, A. (1992) Psychic hygiene in mental health promotion. In *Promotion of Mental Health*. ed Trent, D.R. Vol. 1. Aldershot: Avebury.

Cooper, C. (1994) Finding the solution – Primary prevention (Identifying the causes and preventing mental ill health in the workplace). In *Mental Health in the Workplace*. London: HMSO.

Croft, S. & Beresford, P. (1990) *From Paternalism to Participation*. London: Open Services Project.

Dalley, G. (1988) *Ideologies of Caring: Rethinking Community and Collectivism*. London: Macmillan.

Dennis, J., Draper, P., Holland, S., Shipster, P., Speller, V. & Sunter, J. (1982) *Health Promotion in the Reorganised NHS*. London: Unit for Study of Health Policy.

de Man, A. & Labrèche-Gauthier, L. (1991) Suicide ideation and community support: an evaluation of two programs. *Journal of Clinical Psychology*, **47**(1): 57–60.

Department of Health (DoH) (1990) *The Care Programme Approach for People with a Mental Illness Referred to the Specialist Psychiatric Services*. HC (90) 23. London: HMSO.

Department of Health (DoH) (1992a) *The Health of the Nation: A Strategy for Health in England and Wales*. London: HMSO.

Department of Health (DoH) (1992b) *Extension of GP Fund-holding to Include Mental Health Services*. EL (92) 48. London: HMSO.

Department of Health (DoH) (1993) *Key Area Handbook: Mental Illness*. London: HMSO.

Department of Health (DoH) (1994) *Working in Partnership: A Collaborative Approach to Care*. A Report of the Mental Health Nursing Review Team. London: HMSO.

Department of Health (DoH) (1996) *NHS Executive. Burdens of Disease: a Discussion Document*. London: HMSO.

Department of Health (DoH) (1998) *Our Healthier Nation*. A Contract for Health. London: HMSO.

Department of Health and Social Security (DHSS) (1986) *Health and Personal Social Services Statistics for England 1986s*. London: HMSO.

Elliott, S.A. Sanjack, M. & Leverton, T. J. (1988) Parents' groups in pregnancy: a preventative intervention for post natal depression? In *Marshalling Social Support: Formats, Processes and Effects.* ed. Gottlieb, B.D. Newbury Park, CA: Sage.

Elton, P.J. & Packer, J.M. (1986) A prospective randomised trial of the value of rehousing on the grounds of ill health. *Journal of Chronic Disorders*, 39(3): 221–227.

English National Board for Nursing, Midwifery and Health Visiting (1996) *Learning From Each Other.* London: ENB.

Falloon, I., Boyd, J., McGill, C. et al. (1987) Family management in the prevention of morbidity in schizophrenia: clinical outcome of a two year longitudinal study. *Archives of General Psychiatry*, 42(9): 887–96.

Falloon, I. & Fadden, G. (1993) *Integrated Mental Health Care.* Cambridge: Cambridge University.

Falloon, I. & Talbot, R. (1981) Persistent auditory hallucinations: coping mechanisms and implications for management. *Psychological Medicine*, 11: 329–339.

Ferguson, B. & Varnam, M. (1994) The relationship between primary care and psychiatry: and opportunity for change. *British Journal of General Practice*, 44: 527–530.

Ferguson, K. (1993) Meeting mental health education needs of patients: the potential role of the psychiatric nurse. In *Research in Health Promotion and Nursing.* eds Barnett, J. & Macleod Clark, J. Basingstoke: Macmillan.

Gerrard, J., Holden, J.M., Elliott, S.A., McKenzie, P., McKenzie, J. & Cox, J.L. (1993) A trainers' perspective of an innovative programme teaching health visitors about the detection, treatment and prevention of post natal depression. *Journal of Advanced Nursing*, 18: 1825–1832.

Greene, V.L. & Monahan, D.J. (1989) The effects of a support and education program on stress and burden among family caregivers to frail elderly persons. *Gerontologist*, 29: 472–477.

Haley, W.E. (1989) Group intervention for dementia family caregivers: a longitudinal perspective. *Gerontologist*, 29: 478–480.

Halm, M.A. (1990) Effects of support groups on anxiety of family members during critical illness. Heart and lung. *Journal of Critical Care*, 19(1): 62–71.

Harrison, G., Owens, D., Holton, A., Neilson, D. & Boot, D. (1988) A prospective study of servere mental disorder in Afro-Carribbean Patients. *Psychological Medicine*, 18: 643–657.

Hawton, K., Ware, C., Mistry, H. et al. (1996) Paracetamol self-poisoning: characteristics, prevention and harm reduction. *British Journal of Psychiatry*, 168: 43–48.

Hill, D. & Balk, D. (1987) The effect of an education program for families of the chronically mentally ill on stress and anxiety. *Psychosocial Rehabilitation Journal*, 10(4): 25–40.

Hodgson, R.J., Abbasi, T. & Clarkson, J. (1996) Effective mental health promotion: a literature review. *Health Education Journal*, 55: 55–74.

Hogarty, G.E., Anderson, C.M., Reiss, D.J. et al. (1986) Family psychoeducational social skills training and maintenance chemotherapy in the aftercare treatment of schizophrenia. *Archives of General Psychiatry*, 43: 633–642.

Holden, J.M., Sagovsky, R. & Cox, J.L. (1989) Counselling in a general practice setting; controlled study of health visitor intervention in treatment of postnatal depression. *British Medical Journal*, 298: 223–226.

Ivancevich, J.M., Matteson, M.T., Freedman, S.M. & Phillips, J.S. (1990) Worksite stress management intervention. *American Psychologist*, 45(2): 252–261.

Kalimo, R., El-Batawi, M. & Cooper, C. (1987) *Psychosocial Factors at Work and Their Relation to Health.* Geneva: WHO.

Leff, J., Berkowitz, R., Shavit, N., Strachan, A., Glass, I. & Vaughn, C. (1989) A trial of family therapy versus a relative's group for schizophrenia. *British Journal of Psychiatry*, 154: 59–66.

Lieberman, M.A. (1982) The effects of social supports in response to stress. In *Handbook of Stress: Theoretical and Clinical Aspects.* eds Goldborger, L. & Breznetz, S. New York: The Free Press.

Littlewood, R. & Lipsedge, M. (1982) *Aliens and Alienists: Ethnic Minorities and Psychiatry.* Harmondsworth: Penguin.

Maslow, A.H. (1968) *Towards a Psychology of Being.* New York: Van Nostrand.

Maynard, C.K. (1993) Comparison of effectiveness of group interventions for depression in women. *Archives of Psychiatric Nursing*, 7(5): 277–283.

MIND (1990) Advocacy. *Different Forms of Empowerment.* London: MIND.

Morgan, H.G. & Priest, P. (1991) Suicide and

other unexpected deaths among psychiatric inpatients. *British Journal of Psychiatry*, **15**: 368–374.

NHS Advisory Service (1994) *Suicide Prevention. The Challenge Confronted*. A manual of guidance for the purchasers and providers of health care. London: HMSO.

National Health Service Executive (NHSE) (1995) *Priorities and Guidance for the NHS*. 1996/1997 (EL(95)68). Leeds: NHSE.

Neumann, J., Schroeder, H. & Voss, P. (1989) *Mental Health and Well-being in the Context of the Health Promotion Concept*. Copenhagen: WHO.

Office of Population Censuses and Surveys (1995) *Mortality Statistics 1993*. London: HMSO.

Playle, J.F. & Keeley, P. (1998) Non-compliance and professional power. *Journal of Advanced Nursing*, **27**: 304–311.

Prescott-Clarke, P. & Primatesta, P. (1998) *Health survey for England 1996: findings*. London: HMSO.

Read, J. & Wallcraft, J. (1992) *Guidelines for Empowering Users of Mental Health Services*. London: COHSE/MIND.

Rogers, A. & Pilgrim, D. (1996) *Mental Health Policy in Britain*. Basingstoke: Macmillan.

Rodgers, J. (1994) Power to the people. *Health Service Journal*, **104**: 24–29.

Royal College of Physicians/Royal College of Psychiatrists (1995) *The Psychological Care of Medical Patients: Recognition of Need and Service Provision*. London: Royal College of Physicians/Royal College of Psychiatrists.

Royal College of Psychiatrists Steering Committee of the Confidential Inquiry into Homicides and Suicides by Mentally Ill People (1996) *Report of the Confidential Inquiry into Homicides and Suicides by Mentally Ill People*. London: Royal College of Psychiatrists.

Rutz, W., Wålinder, J., Eberhard, G. et al. (1989) An educational program on depressive disorders for general practitioners on Gotland: background and evaluation. *Acta Psychiatrica Scandinavica*, **79**: 19–26.

Schultz, C.L., Smyrnios, K.X., Schultz, N.C. & Grbich, C.F. (1993) Longitudinal outcomes of psychoeducational support for family caregivers of dependent elderly persons. *Australian Psychologist*, **28**(1): 21–4.

Soni Raleigh, V., Bulusu, L. & Balarajan, R. (1990) Suicides among immigrants from the Indian sub-continent. *British Journal of Psychiatry*, **156**: 46–50.

Suicide Prevention Sub-group (1996) *A Health Service Strategy for Suicide Prevention in the North West Region*. Warrington: North West Regional Health Authority.

Szasz, T.S. (1964) *The Myth of Mental Illness*. New York: Harper and Row.

Tarrier, N. (1987) An investigation of residual psychotic symptoms in discharged schizophrenic patients. *British Journal of Clinical Psychology*, **26**: 141–143.

Tilford, S., Delancey, F. & Vogels, M. (1997) *Effectiveness of Mental Health Promotion Interventions: A Review*. London: HEA.

Toseland, R.W., Rossiter, C.M., Peak, T. & Smith, G.C. (1990) Comparitive effectiveness of individual and group interventions to support family caregivers. *Journal of the National Association of Social Workers*, **35**(2): 209–217.

Tudor, K. (1996) *Mental Health Promotion: Paradigms and Practice*. London: Routledge.

Vaughn, C.E. & Leff, J.P. (1976) The influence of family and social factors on the course of psychiatric illness. A comparison of schizophrenic and depressed neurotic patients. *British Journal of Psychiatry*, **129**: 125–137.

Wagenfield, M. (1983) Primary prevention and public mental health policy. *Journal of Public Health Policy*, **4**(2): 168–180.

Walker, A. (1993) Community care policy: from consensus to conflict. In *Community Care: A Reader*. eds Boronat, J., Pereira, C., Pilgrim, D. & Williams, F. London: Macmillan.

World Health Organisation (WHO) (1984) *Health Promotion. A discussion document on the concepts and principles*. Copenhagen: WHO.

World Health Organisation (WHO) (1985) *Targets For Health For All*. Copenhagen: WHO.

World Health Organisation (WHO) (1992) *Health for all*. Copenhagen: WHO.

Wooff, K., Goldberg, D. & Fryers, T. (1988) The practice of community psychiatric nursing and mental health social work in Salford. *British Journal of Psychiatry*, **152**: 783–792.

Zubin, J. & Spring, B. (1977) Vulnerability: a new view of schizophrenia. *Journal of Abnormal Psychology*, **86**(2): 103–126.

FURTHER READING

Tilford, S., Delaney, F. & Vogels, M. (1997) Effectiveness of mental health promotion interventions: a review. London: HEA.

An invaluable text which critically reviews the evidence (or lack of it) to support the implementation of health promotion interventions.

Tudor, K. (1996) *Mental Health Promotion: Paradigms and Practice*. London: Routledge.

A detailed text which considers the philosophical and practical aspects of mental health promotion.

NHS Health Advisory Service (1994) *Suicide Prevention: The Challenge Confronted*. A manual of guidance for purchasers and providers of health care. London: HMSO.

This publication outlines the policy initiatives and proposes practical responses to fulfil the targets set out in The Health of the Nation.

10 Men's health: concepts, criticisms and challenges

Timothy Simon Faltermeyer and Steven Pryjmachuk

KEY ISSUES

- Men's health from a biological, socio-cultural and masculinity point of view
- Gender-specific aspects of morbidity and mortality
- Lifestyle risk factors
- Promoting men's health
- Screening and 'well-man' clinics
- Differences amongst men
- Empowering men

INTRODUCTION

As society strives towards equal opportunities for all, there appears to be a paradox where health is concerned. As an issue, women's health has received much coverage, in both the scholarly and popular press. Most of the national newspapers carry a women's section at least once a week (where health issues are given regular consideration), and there are a plethora of women's magazines on the market. In contrast, there is a dearth of information concerning men's health. Though men's health has received some popular consideration in recent times – the publication of *The Which? Guide to Men's Health* (Carroll, 1995) and *Men's Health Matters* (Bradford, 1995), and the launch of the magazine *Men's Health* being notable examples – there has been little scholarly discussion of the issue. As far as service provision is concerned, it is much the same story. 'Well-woman' clinics are an established part of primary care, as is screening for female-specific diseases such as breast and cervical cancer. There have been some attempts to establish comparable services for men (see, for example, Williamson, 1995; McMillan, 1995), but these have been few and far between. Furthermore, of the well-man programmes that have been established, few have been formally evaluated (Robertson, 1995).

Framed within a historical perspective, this disparity is readily explainable by advances in the women's movement and the growth of feminist scholarship over the past few decades (Sabo and Gordon, 1995). In addition, the fact that the health professionals with the greatest responsibility for health promotion – nurses and health visitors – are predominantly female, may also go some way to explaining why there have been greater strides in the establishment of women's health as an issue.

There is an irony here, however. This irony is at its most striking when you consider that, whilst men generally die at an earlier age than women, it is women who make greater use of primary health care services (Office for National Statistics, 1997).

MEN'S HEALTH AS A SPECIFIC ISSUE

Attempting to define men's health formally would serve no real purpose given the scope of this book. Some exploration and critical examination of the concept of men's health is, however, necessary.

Though each of us is different whether these differences are defined by gender, race, culture, socio-economic status, age and so on 'health' (and to some extent illness) is an essential characteristic of all of us. It is legitimate to ask, therefore, whether there is a real need to consider health in terms of the specific differences between us. In particular, the reader may ask whether there is a need to consider health in gender-specific terms.

What are the advantages and disadvantages of having 'special' health services for specific population groups? Contrast for example, services for 'ethnic minorities', lesbians and gay men, and people with human immunodeficiency virus (HIV) and acquired immune deficiency syndrome (AiDS) with services for children, older people and mentally ill people.

Do these advantages and disadvantages differ when primary health care, in particular, is considered? From a primary health care point of view, what are the advantages and disadvantages of having gender-specific services?

The arguments for a gender-specific approach to health follow several lines of reasoning. Perhaps the most simple is the 'tit-for-tat' argument: because there is a movement for women and women's health, there has to be, for the sake of equality, a parallel movement for men so that men too may have their fair share of access to health services.

The academic arguments, however, are more complex. The case for men's health as a separate, specific issue is based on three perspectives (For examples, see Sabo and Gordon, 1995; Royal College of Nursing (RCN) 1996):

1. Biological perspective;
2. Socio-cultural perspective;
3. Masculinity perspective.

Biological perspective

At first sight, the adoption of a biological framework for exploring men's health seems logical. It is an inescapable fact that men and women differ biologically; ultimately, it is our genes (genes are *biological* entities after all) which determine, at least physically, our gender. The biological framework, however, has its limitations. Whilst it easily accounts for gender-specific illnesses (only men can suffer from testicular cancer, impotence or prostate enlargement; similarly, only women can suffer from cervical cancer and pre-menstrual syndrome), it founders when trying to account for some of the gender-specific differences found in the morbidity and mortality data to be discussed later. Nor is the biological framework a particularly suitable framework for the advancement of health promotion and empowerment strategies.

Socio-cultural perspective

This framework acknowledges that, as well as biological differences, there are important social and cultural differences between men and women. The socio-cultural perspective brings into play issues such as:

1. Roles of men and women in society
2. Societal influences
3. Socialisation process
4. Socio-economic status
5. Education
6. Religion
7. Race.

Despite the advances in equal opportunities over the last few decades, Western society remains largely patriarchal. Men still dominate most social, political, cultural and economic institutions: it is men who wield power in business (most company directors are men), in health care (most doctors and senior executives in the National Health Service (NHS) are men), in government and politics (most politicians and senior civil servants are men), and in religion (most religious leaders are men).

One central theme running through the socio-cultural perspective is exposure to *risk* (see, for example, RCN, 1996). In other words, societal and cultural demands expose men to a set of risks different to those of women. Within this framework, it is *lifestyle* which forms the cornerstone of any conceptualisation of men's and indeed women's health.

The sorts of risks which men are exposed to include the risks associated with employment. For example, the workforce in the heavy industries, such as oil and chemicals, mining and construction, is predominantly male. Likewise, the majority of managers and high-profile sales personnel are men. Contrast these occupations with the occupations dominated by women: caring, retailing, and administrative and clerical work.

To what extent do you think changes in the availability of paid employment opportunities over the last decade or so have influenced the traditional employment roles of men and women? More men may be entering traditional female occupations (such as nursing), but is the reverse true?

Social lifestyles also differ between men and women. Men are more likely to spend their leisure time engaged in activities such as watching sports, betting, gardening, fishing or going to the pub; women, on the other hand, are more likely to spend their leisure time watching TV, visiting friends or relatives or reading a book or women's magazine (Central Statistical Office 1995a). Furthermore, despite the strides that have been made towards equal opportunities, there is still a general expectation that a man's role in life is that of 'breadwinner', whereas a women's role is that of 'wife', 'mother' or 'carer'.

Masculinity

The third perspective sees 'masculinity' as the most important factor in defining men's health. Though there are many academic interpretations of masculinity, in this context the concept is best seen as 'what it takes to be a man'. This interpretation obviously incorporates the socialisation process; it also includes related issues such as gender role/identity and societal expectations. (To this extent, a consideration of masculinity takes into account socio-cultural factors and could, perhaps, be seen as merely one aspect of the socio-cultural perspective. The reader should be aware, however, that there is some overlap between the three perspectives and that, to a great extent, they are not mutually exclusive.)

In looking at 'what it takes to be a man', it is worth considering the seminal work of the psychologist Bem. Bem's 'sex-role inventory' (1974) lists a number of traits deemed to be masculine', some of which are listed in Box 10.1

BOX 10.1	*Masculine traits*	
■ Aggressive	■ Ambitious	
■ Assertive	■ Athletic	
■ Competitive	■ Dominant	
■ Forceful	■ Self-reliant	
■ Self-sufficient	■ Strong	
■ Willing to take risks.		

These traits are, by and large, incompatible with being ill. Moreover, not showing one's emotions, keeping a 'stiff upper lip' and not crying are part and parcel of being masculine. As the saying goes: 'big boys don't cry'.

Although these three perspectives overlap, it is the biological perspective (perhaps because it is the simplest to understand) that has dominated most of the advances in men's health.

Nearly all of the scant literature available on men's health is concerned with testicular self-examination, prostate cancer and sexual health (and sexual health issues seem to be primarily targeted at gay men). This is reflected in the writings of *The Men's Health Trust* – 'the UK registered charity concerned only with health problems which just affect men' (Men's Health Trust, 1998) – an organisation that seems to be exclusively concerned with problems of the male reproductive system.

The concept of women's health developed in much the same way. In the early stages of its development, women's health was concerned merely with reproductive and sexual health issues. It is only in more recent times, following challenges from the radical feminists in particular, that women's health has encompassed a much broader range of issues.

Similar challenges can be made to the current position on men's health. The biomedical approach to men's health is not necessarily the most efficacious way of promoting the health of men and, as the reader will discover, its continuing dominance may actually be selling the health of men short.

GENDER, LIFESTYLE, MORBIDITY AND MORTALITY

Before proceeding any further with this chapter, speculate on the reasons why men generally die at an earlier age than women and why men are less likely than women to make use of primary health care services.

Garman (1996) notes a 'paradox' in the official statistics on gender, morbidity and mortality: that whilst women have greater morbidity rates than men, they have lower mortality rates. It is worth noting however that, as Robertson (1995) points out, the morbidity rates in men are probably much higher than reported, but remain 'hidden'. This is perhaps because men are more likely than women to keep their problems to themselves; Harrison, Chin and Ficarrotto (1992) claim it is the 'stiff upper lip' which may be responsible for this observation – men would rather not share their problems with spouses, friends, peers or health care professionals. The Central Statistical Office (1996; 1993–1994 data for England) reinforce this argument by reporting that the proportion of men and women self-reporting good health is almost equal. Moreover, Verbrugge (1989) suggests that men's morbidity may actually be higher than women's if the different lifestyle risk factors affecting men and women are taken into account.

Leaving aside the debate on whether morbidity rates are, in actuality, higher in women than in men, a simple explanation for the lower mortality rates in women may well lie in the fact that women are more likely than men to consult a health care professional if they feel they have a problem. Although this explanation is backed up by the statistics, some caution has to be exercised: the main reason women consult their family doctors is for contraceptive management (Central Statistical Office, 1995b). This is hardly a health problem per se, though it could be argued that the very fact that women visit, and talk to, health care professionals on a more regular basis than men suggests that there are more opportunities for women to discuss, and for health care professionals to investigate, the general state of their health.

As with women's health, and as the reader will be aware, there are some diseases that are unique to men, specifically, diseases associated with the male reproductive system. Furthermore, there are some diseases common to both men and women but which affect men and women differently. According to the Central Statistical Office (1996; UK age-adjusted data for 1994), more men than women die from ischaemic heart disease (mortality rate 23% higher) and more men die from bronchitis and allied conditions (mortality rate 55% higher). With cerebrovascular accident (stroke), the picture is reversed: the mortality rate is 64% higher for women. The suicide rate for men is more than three times higher than the corresponding rate for women, and twice as many men than women die in road traffic accidents. In addition, more men are involved in non-fatal accidents and more men than women consume alcohol above the 'safe' limits (1996 data for England; DoH, 1998a). Given these statistics, it seem that although society may be dominated and led by men, as far as health is concerned, men are failing to set their own agenda.

Verbrugge (1989) argues that biology may indeed be a key determinant in health; Verbrugge adds however that a biological explanation alone is insufficient to explain the disparities in the mortality and morbidity data. Naidoo and Wills (1994) also suggest that there is a definite link between mortality in men and the conforming or socialisation process. To this extent, the gender differences in the morbidity and mortality data are best explained by the socio-cultural perspective and by a consideration of masculinity. In other words, it is an adherence to the traditional male role and not just biological factors that affect a man's life chances. As Harrison, Chin and Ficarrotto (1992) comment: '... the price paid for belief in the male role is shorter life expectancy' (p282).

Lifestyle risk factors

Some of the factors influencing mortality and morbidity amongst men (Browne, 1998; Jones and Siddel, 1997; DoH, 1995a, 1995b) are listed in Box 10.2.

BOX 10.2	*Factors affecting mortality and morbidity amongst men*
	■ Men generally eat less healthy diets than women ■ Blood pressure tends to be higher in men ■ When high blood pressure is identified, men tend to ignore it ■ Men tend to sleep less than women ■ Men are more likely to be involved in criminal activity ■ Social networks for men are smaller than for women ■ Social networks that men have tend to be less intimate

Whilst some of these factors may have a biological basis (men tending to have higher blood pressure and sleeping less, for example), only the socio-cultural and masculinity perspectives can account for the others.

Doyal (1997) points out that one of the major risk factors in the health of men is employment: traditional male jobs carry more risks of injury, disablement and damage to health than traditional female jobs. At the same time, Doyal reports that unemployment can also be seen as a risk factor, particularly where the mental health of the individual is concerned. Socio-economic status appears to play some role too: the mortality rate for men in the lowest social class (class V) is three times greater than for men in the highest social class (class I) (Office for National Statistics, 1997). In addition, men in the lower socio-economic classes are 50% more likely to die of coronary heart disease than men overall (DoH, 1998b).

It is well established that there are links between cigarette smoking and circulatory diseases, respiratory diseases and cancers, especially lung cancer (HEA, 1996a; Scientific Committee on Tobacco and Health, 1998). The proportion of men and women who smoke is roughly equivalent at 30% and 27%, respectively (1996 data for England; DoH 1998a). Smoking is as such a lifestyle risk factor in both men's and women's health. Although the proportion of women who smoke appears to have remained stable since 1993, there has been over the same period an increase in the proportion of men who smoke, particularly young men aged 16–34 (DoH, 1998a).

Alcohol is also seen as a lifestyle risk factor (HEA, 1996b). Whilst 30% of men drink more than the recommended 'safe' weekly limits of alcohol, this figure has remained stable since 1993 (DoH, 1998a) and men are three times more likely to become dependent on alcohol than women (Central Statistical Office, 1995b). Women are significantly less prone to drink more than the safe weekly limits (only 15% of women exceed these limits), though this figure has risen since 1993 (DoH, 1998a).

There is some evidence that companionship appears to have an effect on health, for both men and women (Blaxter, 1990). As far as men are concerned, married or co-habiting men report fewer perceived symptoms of illness and better psycho-social health than single men, perhaps because these men have the support of a partner or cohabitee.

Think about your own lifestyle. What are the risk factors in your own life? Do you conform to the 'typical' lifestyle for your gender?

MEN'S PROBLEMS

By now, it should be clear to the reader that some health problems affect men to a greater degree than they do women. To explore these disparities further, this section considers first the health problems that affect only men by virtue of their biological make up (i.e. health problems concerned with the male reproductive system). Second, the health problems considered important by the Department of Health (DoH, 1998b) in the Green Paper *Our Healthier Nation* will be considered: circulatory diseases (heart disease/stroke), accidents, cancer and mental health. Given the focus on the male reproductive system in men's health issues, the need to consider the former is obvious; the need to consider the latter arises because, as the DoH point out, these health problems are significant causes of premature death and poor health.

Reproductive system issues

With regard to the male reproductive system, the two issues interesting health professionals the most appear to be prostate and testicular cancer. Cancer of the prostate is the most common cancer affecting British men. It is also the second biggest cause of cancer mortality after lung cancer (DoH, 1998b). The risk of developing prostate cancer is 1 in 12 and around 8500 men die each year from this cancer (Prostate Cancer Charity, 1997).

Though the incidence of testicular cancer is relatively rare, the RCN (1996) point out that significant interest in this issue has arisen in recent times because of a rising incidence rate, the fact that it affects predominantly young men and the fact that it is preventable.

It is surprising that health professionals appear to have targeted these two issues in particular, given that there are other, perhaps more worthy, issues concerning the male reproductive system. Infertility, for example, affects one in 12 men (Bradford, 1995). Impotence is also a significant problem for men: as many as one in four men have erectile problems and around one in 20 men suffer permanent erection difficulties (Bradford, 1995).

 Consider the popular 'soap' programmes on the television. Can you think of any episodes where issues to do with the female reproductive system (such as breast cancer, hysterectomy, female infertility/fertility treatments) have been considered? What about similar issues for men? Have prostate cancer, testicular cancer, impotence or male infertility been considered by the soaps?

Our healthier nation issues

Coronary heart disease

As the reader will be aware, men are more likely to die from coronary (ischaemic) heart disease than women, whilst women are more likely to die from a cardiovascular accident. Heart disease accounts for one-third of deaths in men and stroke one-fifth of deaths in women under the age of 65 (DoH, 1998b). Whilst both these diseases are circulatory diseases, it is interesting to speculate why men should succumb to heart disease rather than stroke.

 An analysis of the risk factors explored earlier reveals significant gender differences when diet, alcohol consumption and work (consider the role of occupational stress) are considered. How might these lifestyle factors account for the increased risk of heart disease in men and the increased risk of stroke in women?

Accidents

The DoH (1998b) define an 'accident' as an incident sufficiently severe to require attention at hospital or from a GP, though there are problems with this definition (Gould, 1998a). Men generally have more accidents than women: 21% of men compared to 15% of women. When road traffic accidents are considered, men, as has already been noted, are twice as likely to be killed. Alcohol, with its ability to impair judgement and coordination, is clearly one risk factor when (fatal and non-fatal) accidents are considered. According to a report by Gould (1998a), 75% of those attending the Accident & Emergency department of Birmingham City Hospital after 10 p.m. had had a significant amount of alcohol. Bear in mind that men generally 'overconsume' alcohol to a greater extent than women. Couple this with the fact that the physical nature of traditional male employment is probably a significant contributor to the accident statistics too and it is easy to understand why there is a higher risk of accidents amongst men. Often these two risk factors coexist: consider, for example, a man who has a couple of pints at lunchtime and who then returns to work to operate heavy machinery (or, indeed, drive).

Cancer

Overall, the cancer mortality rates for men and women are similar, though there are significant differences between men and women when specific cancers are considered. With regard to the mortality rates for cancers, breast cancer is the biggest killer amongst women (accounting for 18% of deaths from cancer), followed closely by lung cancer (17% of deaths from cancer). In men, the biggest killer is lung cancer (28% of deaths from cancer), with prostate cancer the second biggest killer (though deaths from prostate cancer, at 12%, are roughly half of those from lung cancer). The third biggest killer for both men and women (with almost equal mortality rates of 11% and 12%, respectively) is colorectal cancer (1996 data for England; DoH 1998b).

From a men's health point of view, the cancers most worthy of discussion are prostate and lung cancer. As prostate cancer has already been given some consideration, this section will focus on lung cancer. Death rates from lung cancer are falling generally (DoH 1998b), but rising for women. At first sight, there appears to be a paradox here when smoking – the biggest single risk factor in lung cancer – is considered. As the reader will be aware, the proportions of men and women who smoke are roughly equal. However, the reader has to bear in mind that lung cancer often takes decades to materialise and that the current mortality statistics reflect the position of many years ago when more men were much more likely to smoke than women (Central Statistical Office, 1995b). In a few decades time, the mortality rates from lung cancer may well balance out, reflecting the current position regarding smoking.

Stress and mental health

Defining 'stress' is fraught with difficulties and it is beyond the scope of this chapter to enter into a debate about its meaning. Perhaps the most useful view of stress in relation to health care, is that of Lazarus and Folkman (1984), who argue that stress occurs when an individual sees the interaction between the environment and him- or herself as taxing, exceeding his or her resources or detrimental to his or her well-being.

Stress has been implicated in a wide variety of illnesses such as hypertension, coronary heart disease, cancer and infectious diseases (Edelmann, 1996); there is also some evidence that stress has an adverse effect on the immune system (Atkinson et al, 1996). What is deemed 'stressful' varies from individual to individual. Some jobs are clearly more stressful than others: Karasek et al, (1982) report that having a high-stress job (one that is highly demanding and where the employee has little control over these demands) is a risk factor in coronary heart disease for both men and women. Whilst men have been, and to a great extent still are, employed in occupations that can be detrimental to health on the grounds of the physical input involved, it seems that a stressful 'white collar' occupation such as in sales, finance and management does not necessarily offer a health advantage.

Robertson (1995) suggests that many of the other risk factors affecting men's health (risks associated with alcohol consumption, smoking and diet, for example) might, in actuality, be responses to stress rather than habits. Stress as such may be a significant determinant of men's morbidity and a significant factor in men's mortality.

As well as links between stress and physical health, there are established links between stress and mental health. The mental health of men is considered elsewhere in this book (Ch. 9), but it is worth a brief mention here. According to the DoH 1995 data for England (1998b), 20% of men suffer from mental illness compared with 14% of women. Note that these figures refer specifically to 'mental illness'. If one views a mental health–mental illness continuum, mental illness represents merely one extreme. The figures cited are likely to be considerably higher if the right-of-centre part of the health–illness continuum, which might be called 'mental health problems', is considered.

Whilst men are three times more likely to commit suicide than women, women are more likely to suffer from anxiety and depression (DoH, 1998b). A possible explanation for these observations may be that whilst stress manifests itself as anxiety and depression in women, it manifests as aggression in men, which when focussed on the self leads to self-harming or suicidal acts. Though suicide rates are generally falling, there has been a steady increase in the number of young men committing suicide (Office for National Statistics, 1997). Doyal (1997) presents arguments suggesting that these increases in male suicide may be due to the number of women entering the employment market and leaving men without a traditional role. It seems, therefore, that both employment and unemployment are factors that can influence the health of men.

Eating and body-image disorders

Whilst on the subject of psychological health, it is worth considering eating and other body-image disorders, primarily because eating disorders such as anorexia nervosa and anorexia bulimia, are generally seen as a women's health issue. Think of famous people with eating disorders and it is nearly always women who come to mind. Increasingly, men are suffering from eating disorders and current statistics indicate that around 0.3% of men aged 16–35 suffer from an eating disorder, compared with around 3% of women of similar age (Button, 1993).

Interestingly, there has been speculation (Klein, 1995) that there is an equivalent body-image disorder in men: bodybuilding. This is a body-image problem spurred on by media presentations of 'ideal' (i.e. fit, muscular) men in much the same way as the media, through idealised presentations of women as sylph-like beauties, is thought to play a role in anorexia in women.

Obesity can also be viewed as an eating disorder. Again, obesity is seen as a women's issue (most of the many magazines directed at slimming are aimed at women), although the rates of obesity (defined as a body-mass index (BMI) of more than 30 kg/m^2) for men and women are roughly equivalent at 16% and 18%, respectively (DoH, 1998a). Remarkably, more men than women are overweight (defined as a BMI of between 25 and 30 kg/m^2): 45% of men and 34% of women are overweight (DoH, 1998a) and the prevalence of obesity is increasing in men at a faster rate than women.

A conclusion that can be drawn, therefore, is that whilst eating disorders may be seen as a women's issue, if body-image disorders are considered, then it is an issue that affects both men and women. Moreover, if we count obesity and 'overeating' as eating disorders, there are clear implications for men's health given the statistics cited.

HEALTH PROMOTION

The three perspectives on men's health: biological, socio-cultural and masculinity, are not mutually exclusive. Any health promotion strategy must, therefore, take into account all three perspectives. Robertson (1995), for example, argues that there is a strong case for men's health promotion, based on the following three observations:

1. High levels of mortality in men
2. 'Hidden' levels of morbidity in men
3. Male-specific health problems.

It is clear from Robertson's third observation that the biological perspective has to be included when the health of men is being considered; indeed Verbrugge (1989) claims that biology may play a significant role in determining a man's health status. However, the first two observations cannot be interpreted by means of biology alone; health promoters have to, when considering why there are high levels or mortality and morbidity amongst men, examine socio-cultural and masculinity issues too.

Political demands

Any health promotion strategy has to be subject to the political demands of the time. At the current time, the Government's Green Paper *Our Healthier Nation* (DoH, 1998b) is likely to play a role in determining a health promotion strategy for men. Although this consultation paper makes no specific reference to men, it does make specific comments about inequalities in health. It is clear from the discussion presented thus far that there are inequalities when it comes to the health of men and women. Moreover, there are implicit references to men's health in *Our Healthier Nation*, especially when the four target areas of (1) coronary heart disease/stroke, (2) cancer, (3) accidents and (4) mental health are considered.

In what ways are the four *Our Healthier Nation* target areas of (1) coronary heart disease/stroke, (2) cancer, (3) accidents and (4) mental health, relevant to a discussion on men's health? Is inequality an issue when these four target areas are considered?

'Well-man' clinics

A major movement in health promotion has been the call for the establishment of 'well-man' clinics to parallel clinics set up for women. This could be seen as a challenge, particularly since '[i]n requiring men to be passive, compliant and submissive, well-men clinics clash with the characteristics normally associated with masculinity' (Piper, 1997, p49). Piper also points out that well-man clinics which focus on the biomedical framework ignore gender, socio-economic and cultural influences. Given Piper's comments, it is interesting to note that the two men's health initiatives cited in the introduction to this chapter (see McMillan 1995; Williamson 1995) – initiatives that appear to have had some degree of success – are initiatives that can hardly be described as well-man clinics: McMillan describes a men's health project in a underprivileged area of Glasgow, and Williamson discusses a men's health network in the East Midlands/Trent region.

Is there a specific need for 'well-women' and 'well-man' clinics? Would 'well-person' clinics suffice?

What advantages might men's health *projects* or *networks* have over a well-man clinic?

Screening

Screening has played a major role in the prevention of certain cancers, particularly breast and cervical cancer. However, colorectal cancer (the third biggest cause of death from cancer in men) has 23% more fatalities than breast cancer (Kadar, 1994) and prostate cancer (the second biggest cause of death from cancer in men) can be treated fairly effectively (Prostate Cancer Charity, 1997). These observations imply that screening might be a useful strategy in primary care for men. However, screening for these two cancers would involve a rectal examination and the question has to be asked whether men would embrace screening given that a rectal examination could well be seen as an affront to their masculinity. There is also little evidence to suggest that a rectal examination is efficient at detecting prostate cancer (RCN, 1996). Interestingly, the UK National Screening Committee, a semi-governmental organisation, have recently advised the Secretary of State for Health that a national screening programme for prostate cancer would be of no benefit to men and could cause considerable harm (DoH, 1998c).

Given that lung cancer is the biggest cause of death from cancer in men, it is worth questioning why men – particularly male smokers – are not called for regular chest examinations. Such an examination might include a chest X-ray; chest X-rays are, after all, standard procedure in the diagnosis of lung cancer. Of course the costs of these examinations and the dangers of repeated exposure to X-ray radiation have to be considered; however, similar considerations must have been made when breast screening was introduced. Regular chest examinations (whether an X-ray is included or not) may also help reduce the number of men suffering from bronchitis, another disease that has a greater incidence in men.

With regard to testicular cancer, 'self-screening' in the form of testicular self-examination (TSE) has been given some attention in the nursing press. Koshti-Rickman (1996) points out that nurses are in an ideal position to advise on TSE; TSE could, as such, easily form part of any health promotion strategy for men. However, the value of TSE has been questioned. Morris (1996), for example, argues against TSE on the grounds that testicular cancer is a rare disease. She writes:

'In the unlikely event that testicular self-examination reduces the mortality by half, half a million men aged 15–34 would need to carry out monthly testicular self-examinations for 1 year in order for one death to be prevented.'

(p41)

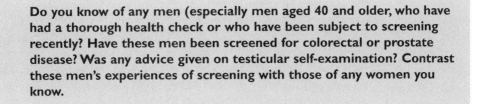

Do you know of any men (especially men aged 40 and older, who have had a thorough health check or who have been subject to screening recently? Have these men been screened for colorectal or prostate disease? Was any advice given on testicular self-examination? Contrast these men's experiences of screening with those of any women you know.

Mental health promotion

Mental health promotion is considered in detail in Chapter 9 of this book. A brief consideration of approaches to mental health promotion is warranted however given the suicide statistics for men. The highest suicide level for young men in the UK is in the Manchester area (Gould, 1998b). As such, the local health authority, in a bid to tackle the rise in suicides in young men, launched a DoH pilot scheme in December 1997, called the *Campaign Against Living Miserably* (CALM). A major part of the campaign involved advertising hoardings. The posters erected on these hoardings displayed statistics relating to the deaths of young men from depression in comparison to other well-publicised health issues such as heroin and ecstasy misuse, as well as a freephone helpline number. The figures were surprising: far more men die as a result of depression than drug misuse, yet depression hardly ever gets a mention in the media. The campaign appears to have had some success: over 1000 calls per week have been received, 75% of which were from men in the target under-35 age group (Gould, 1998b).

Mental health is one of the target areas in *Our Healthier Nation*, and it is interesting to note that Manchester, along with two of its neighbouring boroughs, Salford and Trafford, was one of the successful bidders for the first wave of health action zones, an initiative (discussed in more detail in the next section) closely linked to the Green Paper and to the new White Paper *The New NHS* (DoH, 1997). The Manchester-Salford-Trafford bid 'will take a holistic approach to mental health, with programmes to provide employment and training opportunities to people with serious mental illness problems alongside improving mental health services' (DoH, 1998d).

Differences amongst men

Williamson (1985) points out that men are not a homogenous group and that 'subsets' of men must be examined when considering health promotion strategies. Men who are interested in promoting their own health appear to be one of these particular subsets. In addition, there appears to be a confusion amongst some men between health and physique (see Klein, 1995) in that some men see 'health' – and especially 'fitness' – as equivalent to a muscular, powerful body.

The readership of *Men's Health* gives some indication of the sort of men interested in their own health. Whilst the authors have no figures as to the readership of this magazine, it is highly likely that the typical reader will not be the unemployed labourer, [who may spend what little money he has on cigarettes, a few beers and take-away food.] More likely they will be young (i.e. below the age of 40), white, middle-class professionals. This group of men are also more likely to attend health promotion events (Robertson, 1995). These same individuals are also likely to be in positions of responsibility and control within society, and therefore are more likely to be those who are able to influence the health care service that they wish to have.

Gay men: a special case?

One 'subset' of men for whom health appears to play a significant role is gay men. On the surface, there does appear to be a move towards promoting health with organisations such as 'Healthy Gay Manchester', 'Rubberstuffers', 'Body Positive' and the Terence Higgins Trust active in health promotion. The primary focus of these organisations however appears to be the promotion of sexual health. This focus, though relatively unsurprising given the recent impact of HIV and AIDS on the gay community, gives out the message that for a gay man, 'health = sexual health', which it clearly does not. It is interesting to note that whilst HIV/AIDS and sexual health were one of the five target areas for the previous government's *The Health of the Nation* initiative (DoH, 1992), these issues do not feature in its successor, *Our Healthier Nation (1998b)*.

Given the spotlight on health (even though it may be limited to sexual health) amongst gay men, there is an irony when gay lifestyles are considered. As Taylor and Roberston (1994) summarise, depression is common amongst gay men and gay men are more likely to attempt suicide than heterosexual men. Taylor and Roberston also report that gay men are also more likely to misuse alcohol and illicit drugs than their heterosexual counterparts. Given that alcohol and drugs are commonly associated with risk taking – especially where sexual activity is concerned (see Plant, 1996 for a review) – one might have thought that the health promotion activities of gay men's organisations would also have included some focus on other activities associated with health (For a more detailed discussion on gay men's health, see Ch. 12)

Openly gay men may not necessarily be subject to the demands of the traditional male role. Do you think they might as such be more susceptible to health promotion activities?

In what ways might a gay men's health group differ from a men's health group?

EMPOWERING MEN

When it comes to promoting the health of men, Roberston (1995) claims the most effective way is to use client-centred and social change approaches to health promotion. In particular, if we look at how a health professional might *empower* men, then these two approaches offer the best hope (Ewles and Simnett, 1995).

According to Tones (1997), health promotion is about enabling, not coercing, individuals to foster their own good health and the health promotion process should be about cooperation rather than compliance. This is in direct contrast to the medical model, which generally sees patients as the passive recipients of care. Tones also argues that empowerment is the key to health promotion; it is the link between two widely accepted aspects of health promotion: health policy and health education. (An analysis of the concept of 'empowerment' is unwarranted here as it is discussed in Ch. 2.) According to Tones, empowerment:

> '... helps to resolve an important dilemma in health promotion: the need, on the one hand, to prevent disease and safeguard the public health while, on the other hand, respecting individual freedom of choice – including the freedom to adopt an 'unhealthy' lifestyle.'
>
> *(p.33)*

How does the health professional set about empowering men? Tones argues that there are two aspects to empowerment:

1. *Individual* (or *self*) empowerment (cf. Ewles and Simnett's 'client-centred' approach)
2. *Collective* (or *community*) empowerment (cf. Ewles and Simnett's 'societal change' approach)

As such, any strategy for empowering men must encompass these two aspects.

Individual empowerment

When it comes to individual empowerment, traditional health education models have been woefully inadequate. Merely informing people of, for example, lifestyle risks will not lead to changes in behaviour. Vernon (1996) argues that more can be gained by asking the following questions than by attempting to coerce of frighten individuals into changing their behaviour:

- Which specific individuals adopt unhealthy behaviours?
- What makes them adopt these behaviours?
- Why do some people adopt these behaviours while others do not?

Attempting to understand the barriers to health promotion should also help increase the chances of a successful behavioural change.

Can you think of any barriers to a successful health promotion campaign for men?

One of the major challenges to the empowerment of men concerns those responsible for the facilitation of empowerment. By and large, those best placed from a health point of view to empower men are women; this in itself is a fundamental barrier to the empowerment process. One suggestion for overcoming this hurdle is to employ men as facilitators. However, men who hold traditionally female jobs (such as nursing) are likely to be viewed suspiciously by men (Fitzgerald and Cherpas, 1985). If health promoters are to help facilitate empowerment in men, what skills and qualities might they possess? Some ideas are set out in Box 10.3.

BOX 10.3	*Aids for health promoters in empowering men*

- *Consider the uniqueness of every man.* Every man is unique. Each man has a differing set of values, beliefs and opinions relating to his own health, based upon his life experiences, the socialisation process and interactions with the world around him. Some men are knowledgeable about healthy lifestyles and are motivated to change. Others neither know about a healthy lifestyle nor are motivated to change. Some men, though perhaps wanting to change, may believe that change is beyond their control, and some (particularly those in the lower social classes) may not have the resources to adopt a more healthy lifestyle. The health promoter must take the individual circumstances, attitudes and beliefs of each individual man into account.

- *Understand where men are coming from.* Health promoters working with men must consider how the socialisation process affects men. For example, one might ask whether there is any point to discussing healthy eating with men if cooking is the domain of women in the household? Is there any point informing a man he is drinking too much alcohol per week when he is convinced his alcohol intake is acceptable because his drinking pals drink far more than he does? These are questions health promoters must consider if there is to be any hope of behavioural change amongst men.

- *Understand the circumstances under which men live.* By virtue of their occupation, health promotion specialists are essentially members of the middle class. From the statistics discussed in this chapter, it is clear that the group most likely to benefit from health promotion are men in the lower social classes. Some health promotion specialists may, as such, have difficulty conceptualising the circumstances under which men live. To many underprivileged men, smoking, going to the pub and betting may be the only pleasurable activities in their lives, especially if they are unemployed or money is restricted. One suggestion here is for health promoters to visit men in their own environments so that they can obtain a degree of empathy for the circumstances under which they live. This approach also fits in with a community-based approach to health promotion; asking men to come to a health centre or clinic merely perpetuates the biomedical approach to health promotion.

- *Be a skilled communicator.* Any health professional seeking to empower men must not only be knowledgeable about the subject matter, they must also possess an understanding of human behaviour, both individually and within groups. In other words, the health promoter has to be a skilled communicator. The skills and qualities identified by Carl Rogers (see, for example, Rogers, 1970) as essential to the counselling process (which is, after all, a communication process) are as pertinent to health promotion as to any other communication process. A 'non-judgmental approach' forms part of Rogers' approach and, given the wide variety of men and circumstances health promoters have to confront, it should be obvious why they too need to adopt such an approach. Rogers also talks of 'warmth', 'genuineness' and 'empathy'. Warmth is essential for establishing trust; no-one would expect a health promoter to be anything but genuine (though the 'scare tactics' used in some recent health promotion campaigns might lead one to question this expectation). The essence of good communication frequently involves empathy (Burns, 1990).

- *Take advantage of men's attributes.* Men are commonly seen as aggressive, assertive, dominant, competitive and achievement-orientated; women on the other hand are commonly seen as anxious, timid, compliant and sociable (see, for example, Lloyd and Archer, 1976). A skilled health promoter would not see these attributes as barriers, but as a foundation on which to frame a particular health promotion strategy. In other words, these attributes should be seen as a challenge rather than an obstruction.

Given that health promoters must consider the uniqueness of men and understand where men are 'coming from', does this mean that the individuals responsible for health promotion with men should be men themselves?

What difficulties can you envisage with this client-centred approach? Is it possible for a health promoter to be non-judgemental, warm and empathic towards men who, for example, become aggressive or abusive?

Suppose, as a health promoter, you were invited by two large organisations – a bank and a steelworks – to implement strategies for improving the health of the two organisations' male workforce.

How would the forum differ between the two organisations? What factors need to be analysed and employed if the health promotion strategies are to stand any chance of working? (Consider, for example, the vocabulary of the health professional, body language, the style and quality of the delivery, an awareness of the unique circumstances of the men involved, the lifestyles of the men, how the men perceive their roles to be within society, and the reality of how these strategies may be internalized by those men and their families.)

Collective empowerment

Carey, in Chapter 2, points out that there is a tautology in the term 'self-empowerment', in that the 'self' is redundant – empowerment can only come from within, from the self. As such, Carey argues that to effect empowerment, health promoters must look beyond the individual and embrace collective action. To some extent, this view makes the discussion about individual empowerment redundant; however, if the reader bears in mind that the role of the health promoter is to facilitate rather than teach or instruct, the suggestions listed in the box still have relevance.

Collective – or community – empowerment is also at the heart of The Ottawa Charter (WHO, 1986). Given its importance, how might health promoters foster community empowerment?

One aspect of health promotion requiring consideration is health education. Education plays a key role in empowering individuals (Friere, 1972), and education is, after all, a collective action. Health education too must, therefore, be seen as a collective, not individual, act. For health education and indeed health promotion to be seen as a collective act, health promoters must allow any particular client group – in this case, men – to set the agenda. This could prove difficult given that it is the Government which, by and large, sets health promotion agendas.

In what ways does the Goverment influence health promotion agendas? Do health promoters need to take heed of gorverment suggestions and directives?

There have been some recent moves by the Government towards collective action. Health action zones are a new initiative discussed briefly earlier in this chapter and it is claimed they 'will bring together local partnerships of NHS organisations, local authorities, community groups and businesses to better organise services and improve ... public health' (DoH, 1998e). This 'what would you as a community like?' approach is a big leap forward in health service provision; the traditional approach has been very much 'here's what we're offering; take it or leave it'. This 'bottom-up' approach is also much more likely to succeed in effecting change (the ultimate goal of health promotion) than traditional 'top-down' approaches (Pryjmachuk, 1996). If they are to be effective, health promoters must play a key role in these health action zones.

Our Healthier Nation also makes explicit reference to community influences when its four target areas are considered. For each of the four target areas, the Government has set a 'national contract', the three 'stakeholders' in this contract being the Government and other 'national players', 'local players' and communities, and the individual.

Health professionals can also influence collective action in a number of other ways. The most obvious way is via the ballot box (Tones, 1997). Almost every health professional has a vote and, as such, has the opportunity to change the political landscape at both a local and a national level. However, health professionals are much more powerful when they act together: it is by no means inconsequential that some of the professional bodies – the British Medical Association (BMA) and the RCN, for example – are also powerful lobby groups.

CONCLUSION

Men's health is an evolving issue that is subject to a number of influences, most notably those arising from a consideration of biological, socio-economic and masculinity issues. Throughout this chapter, the reader will have observed that there are a number of challenges facing health promoters when the issue of men's health is considered. Perhaps the most significant challenge, however, is the challenge to society itself.

Sabo and Gordon (1995) write: '... if aspects of ... masculinity are dangerous to men's health, then they ought to be changed, abandoned, or resisted ... more men ought to refuse to be men' (p16). This is a bold but somewhat unrealistic statement. For more men to refuse being men implies that there has to be a major change at societal level. This will be a long and arduous process – if it ever occurs – particular since, as Doyal (1997) points out, men may well have to surrender some of their power in society if men are to achieve better health.

Whilst health professionals can play a role in effecting this change (via the ballot box or by being part of an active lobbying organisation, for example), a far more pragmatic approach would be to examine the situation of men in the 'here and now' and attempt to incorporate into their health promotion strategies what they know and understand about men's lives. This, coupled with an eagerness to allow men to set their own health agendas may prove to be a particularly fruitful way to effect some degree of behavioural change amongst men and, perhaps, result in some reduction in the mortality and morbidity statistics for men.

REFERENCES

Atkinson, R.L., Atkinson, R.C., Smith, E.E., Bem, D.J. & Nolen-Hoeksema, S. (1996) *Hilgard's Introduction to Psychology*. 12th edn. Fort Worth, Texas: Harcourt Brace.

Bem, S.L. (1974) The measurement of psychological androgyny. *Journal of Consulting and Clinical Psychology*, 42: 155–162.

Blaxter, M. (1990) *Health and Lifestyles*. London: Routledge.

Bradford, N. (1995) *Men's Health Matters: The A–Z of Male Health*. London: Vermilion.

Browne, K. (1998) *An Introduction to Sociology*, 2nd edn. Cambridge: Polity.

Burns, D.D. (1990) *The Feeling Good Handbook*. New York: Plume/Penguin.

Button, E. (1993) *Eating Disorders: Personal Construct Therapy and Change*. Chichester: John Wiley.

Carroll, S. (1995) *The Which? Guide to Men's Health*. Revised edn. London: The Consumers' Association.

Central Statistical Office (1995a) *Social Trends*. London: HMSO.

Central Statistical Office (1995b) *Social Focus on Women*. London: HMSO.

Central Statistical Office (1996) *Regional Trends*. London: HMSO.

Department of Health (DoH) (1992) *The Health of the Nation*. London: HMSO.

Department of Health (DoH) (1995a) *The Health of the Nation. Fit for the Future*. London: HMSO.

Department of Health (DoH) (1995b) *The Health of the Nation. Key Areas Handbook, Coronary Heart Disease and Stroke*. London: HMSO.

Department of Health (DoH) (1997) *The New NHS: Modern, Dependable*. London: HMSO.

Department of Health (DoH) (1998a) *Health Survey for England '96. vol 1. Findings*. London: HMSO.

Department of Health (DoH) (1998b) *Our Healthier Nation: A Contract For Health*. London: HMSO.

Department of Health (DoH) (1998c) *First Report of the National Screening Committee Published*. Press Release 98/147; 21 April.

Department of Health (DoH) (1998d) *Frank Dobson Gives the Go-ahead for the First Wave of Health Action Zones*. Press Release 98/120; 31 March.

Department of Health (DoH) (1998e) *Health Action Zone Bids Focus on Improving Elderly, Children's and Mental Health Services*. Press Release 98/054; 9 February.

Doyal, L. (1997) Gendering health. In *Debates and Dilemmas in Promoting Health: A Reader*. eds Siddell, M., Jones, L., Katz, J. & Peberdy, A. London: Macmillan.

Edelmann, R.J. (1996) Stress. In *Behavioural Sciences for Health Professionals*. eds Aitken, V. & Jellicoe, H. London: W B Saunders.

Ewles, L. & Simnett, I. (1995) *Promoting Health: A Practical Guide*. 3rd edn. London: Scutari.

Fitzgerald, L.F. & Cherpas, C.C. (1985) On the reciprocal relationship between gender and occupation: rethinking the assumptions concerning masculine career development. *Journal of Vocational Behaviour*, 27: 109–122.

Friere, P. (1972) *Education of the Oppressed*. Harmondsworth: Penguin.

Garman, S. (1996) Gender and health. In *Behavioural Sciences for Health Professionals*. eds Aitken, V. & Jellicoe, H. London: W B Saunders.

Gould, M. (1998a) Cutting edge. *Health Service Journal*, 8(5594): 12–13.

Gould, M. (1998b) Better network. *Health Service Journal*, 8(5592): 12–13.

Harrison, J., Chin, J. & Ficarrotto, T. (1992) Warning: masculinity may be damaging to your health. In *Men's Lives*. eds Kimmel, M. & Messner M. New York: Macmillan.

Health Education Authority (HEA) (1996a) *Smoking: The Facts*. London: HEA.

Health Education Authority (HEA) (1996b) *Think About Drink: There's More to a Drink Than You Think*. London: HEA.

Jones, J. & Sidell, M. eds (1997) *The Challenge of Promoting Health: Exploration and Action*. Basingstoke: Macmillan.

Kadar, A.G. (1994) The sex-myth bias in health care. *Atlantic Monthly*, 274 (2): 66–70.

Karasek, R.A., Theorell, T.G., Schwarz, J.,

Pieper, C. & Alfredson, L. (1982) Job, psychological factors and coronary heart disease: Swedish prospective findings and US prevalence findings using a new occupation inference method. *Advances in Cardiology*, 29: 62–67.

Klein, A.M. (1995) Life's too short to die small: steroid use among male bodybuilders. In *Men's Health and Illness: Gender, Power and the Body*. eds Sabo, D. & Gordon, D.F. London: Sage.

Koshti-Rickman, A. (1996) The role of nurses in promoting testicular self-examination. *Nursing Times*, 92(33): 40–41.

Lazarus, R.S. & Folkman, S. (1984) *Stress, Appraisal and Coping*. New York: Springer.

Lloyd, B. & Archer, J. (1976) *Exploring Sex Differences*. London: Academic Press.

McMillan, I. (1995) The life of Riley. *Nursing Times*, 91(48): 27–28.

Men's Health Trust (1998) *The Men's Health Trust*. World Wide Web: http://freespace.virgin.net/mens.health/ [Retrieved: 1998, 10 April].

Morris, J. (1996) The case against TSE. *Nursing Times*, 92(33): 41

Naidoo, J. & Wills, J. (1994) *Health Promotion – Foundation for Practice*. London: Bailliére Tindall.

Office for National Statistics (1997) *Health Inequalities: Decennial Supplement*. London: HMSO.

Piper, S. (1997) The limitations of well men clinics for health education. *Nursing Standard*, 11(30): 47–49.

Prostate Cancer Charity (1997) *The Prostate Cancer Charity*. http://www.prostate-cancer.org.uk/ [Retrieved: 1998, 10 April].

Pryjmachuk, S. (1996) Pragmatism and change: some implications for nurses, nurse managers and nursing. *Journal of Nurse Management*, 4: 201–205.

Robertson, S. (1995) Men's health promotion in the UK: a hidden problem. *British Journal of Nursing*, 4(7), 382: 399–401.

Rogers, C.R. (1970) *On Becoming a Person: A Therapist's View of Psychotherapy*. London: Constable.

Royal College of Nursing (RCN) (1996) *Men's Health Review*. [Prepared on behalf of the Men's Health Forum.] London: RCN.

Sabo, D. & Gordon, D.F. (1995) Rethinking men's health and illness. In *Men's Health and Illness: Gender, Power and the Body*. eds Sabo, D. & Gordon, D.F. London: Sage.

Scientific Committee on Tobacco and Health (Department of Health, Department of Health and Social Services Northern Ireland, The Scottish Office Department of

Health and The Welsh Office) (1998) *Report of the Scientific Committee on Tobacco and Health*. London: HMSO.

Taylor, I. & Robertson, A. (1994) The health needs of gay men: a discussion of the literature and implications for nursing. *Journal of Advanced Nursing*, **20**: 560–566.

Tones, K. (1997) Health education as empowerment. In *Debates and Dilemmas in Promoting Health: A Reader*. eds Siddell, M., Jones, L., Katz, J. & Peberdy, A. London: Macmillan.

Verbrugge, L.M. (1989) The twain meet: empirical explanations of sex differences in health and morbidity. *Journal of Health and Social Behavior*, **30**: 282–304.

Vernon, L. (1996) Health promotion in practice. In *Behavioural Sciences for Health Professionals*. eds Aitken, V. & Jellicoe, H. London: W B Saunders.

Williamson, P. (1995) Their own worst enemy. *Nursing Times*, **91**(48): 25–27.

World Health Organisation (WHO) (1986). *Ottawa Charter for Health Promotion: An International Conference on Health Promotion*. Geneva: WHO.

FURTHER READING

Bradford, N. (1995) *Men's Health Matters: The A–Z of Male Health*. London: Vermilion.

Carroll, S. (1995) *The Which? Guide to Men's Health*. Revised edition. London: The Consumers' Association.

Two popular books on men's health – both designed as a 'handbook' for men.

Royal College of Nursing (1996) *Men's Health Review*. [Prepared on behalf of the Men's Health Forum.] London: RCN.

The state of men's health from a nursing perspective.

Sabo, D. & Gordon, D.F. (1995). Rethinking men's health and illness. In eds Sabo, D. & Gordon D.F. *Men's Health and Illness: Gender, Power and the Body*. London: Sage.

The foremost academic text on the subject (American).

11 Health promotion and ethnic minority groups

Abbie Paton and Julie A. Higgins

KEY ISSUES

- Approaches to health education with ethnic minority groups
- Recent health policy changes and ethnic minority groups
- Community development for health
- Alliances with community groups
- Interagency collaboration

INTRODUCTION

This chapter will start by exploring the social policy background from which various approaches to health promotion with ethnic minority communities have grown. The assimilationist, integrationist and anti-racist approaches to this field are outlined. It will then move on to explore the health service changes of the late 1980s onwards, discussing their implications on the health of ethnic minority groups.

Community development for health is investigated next and this section begins with an exploration of the principles of this field and then provides real-life examples of working with ethnic minority communities. Interagency collaboration is discussed next. Once again, some basic principles are outlined and then specific real-life examples relating to ethnic minority groups are provided.

The chapter concludes with a section which brings together the various strands discussed earlier and provides direction for health promotion work with ethnic minority communities.

CONTEXT

This section provides background to the issue of health education/promotion with ethnic minority communities. It starts with an analysis of three approaches to ethnic minority health education based on differing outlooks on the health influences on the UK's ethnic minority populations. These are discussed within a framework of dominant social policies. The implications for health education/promotion initiatives of each will be considered. This section will then move on to outline changes to UK health service policy and the impact of these changes on ethnic minority groups.

Approaches to health education with ethnic minority groups

The approaches taken to health education within minority ethnic communities are intrinsically linked to the social policy framework from which they grew. This section will examine the assimilationist, integrationist, and anti-racist frameworks, exploring the health education approaches built upon each of these ideological perspectives.

Assimilation

The economic boom following the Second World War and the resultant labour shortage brought about a major influx of immigrants from the New Commonwealth (Smaje, 1995). The predominant view was that assimilation of these groups was desirable. The focus of discussion on health matters relating to ethnic minority groups at this time was on exotic diseases and cultural differences. The philosophy was that individuals coming to live in Britain should adhere to the 'British way'. Cultural and lifestyle diversity within Britain was frowned upon.

Health education efforts during this time were underpinned by notions of control and focused on behaviour seen as deviant and in need of changing to fit in with the rest of British society. Examples of topics addressed are tuberculosis and family planning. It has been suggested that tuberculosis was viewed as important largely in context only of the threat to the ethnic majority rather than the high levels of the disease among the ethnic minority population (Smaje, 1995). Family planning initiatives were arguably underpinned by a philosophy of State control of the growth of non-white populations (Bryan et al, 1985, cited in Smaje, 1995).

Integration

In the mid- to late-1960s, the assimilationist approach was replaced by pluralist notions of integration which recognised that ethnic minority groups would not, in the foreseeable future, loose their individual sense of cultural identity as different to that of the ethnic majority (Douglas, 1991).

Government policies, developed as a result of downward trends in the economy, were introduced to reduce immigration (Popple, 1995). The Commonwealth Acts of 1965 and 1968 and the Race Relation Acts of 1965 and 1968, however, aimed to enhance integration and prevent the racial disharmony seen in the USA. These policy shifts sent out two somewhat conflicting messages: people from ethnic minority groups were a problem and should be kept out, but at the same time, tolerance and recognition of cultural differences was promoted.

During the mid- to late-1960s, 'culture' became an increasing focus of 'race' discourse. The culturalist perspective emphasised cultural practices, drawing comparisons between those of ethnic minority groups and those of the ethnic majority. These comparisons frequently had undertones of disapproval and a lack of respect for practices different from those engaged in by the white majority. Culturalist philosophy views illness in terms of the differences in family organisation, knowledge and practices, with those of ethnic minority groups seen as less favourable to those of the ethnic majority. As a result, health education efforts were focused on issues seen to be associated with these 'problematic' cultural practices.

Aside from its inherent ethnocentricity, this approach has a number of other problems. Firstly, it is apparent that the topic areas emphasised by this outlook are grounded purely on the views of health professionals, and reflect neither the perceptions of need within the communities themselves nor the epidemiological data (Bhopal and White, 1993). The 'culturalist' approach has also been criticised for failing to acknowledge the broad range of social and economic factors influencing health. Many British ethnic minority communities experience higher levels of deprivation, for example than the population as a whole (Modood et al, 1997). These structural concerns are, therefore, arguably of particular importance in this context. The de-emphasis on the broader influences on health is illustrated in the work of the Department of Health and Social Service's 1981 Stop Rickets Campaign. Rickets had been identified as particularly prevalent within the UK South Asian population. The Government's response was to establish an information-giving campaign to parents about diet and skin exposure to sun. In contrast to this individualistic approach, rickets in the white population during the Second World War had been perceived as a problem associated with poverty. A structuralist solution was found when commonly eaten foods were fortified with vitamin D (Smaje, 1995).

The Stop Rickets Campaign was criticised for making inaccurate and ethnocentric assumptions about ethnic minority communities (Douglas, 1995), while ignoring the major influence that poverty and socio-economic factors have on health. The victim-blaming philosophy illustrated by the rickets campaign acts to reduce the responsibility of decision makers to deal with the high levels of poverty found within these communities. It also serves to encourage notions of 'black pathology' (Smaje, 1995) by identifying these groups as problems exhibiting pathological behaviours.

With its focus on 'culture', the culturalist framework has emphasised the need for health professionals to build up their knowledge of customs, traditions and religions of ethnic minority communities in order to promote 'ethnic sensitivity' in their practice. A large selection of books and training materials (e.g. Henley, 1983) have been produced for the purpose of educating professionals about the 'cultural practices' of ethnic minority cultures. While this approach arguably does acknowledge the validity of a multitude of ethnic groups in Britain, it could be said to promote a stereotyped view of ethnic minority lifestyle. Leaflets and educational materials such as those described earlier are often based on a view of homogeneity within a single ethnic minority group. In fact, as with social groups of all sorts, any ethnic minority community will, of course, have individuals adhering to varying degrees of religion, traditional dress and other practices.

The 1980s saw the start of considerable criticism of the culturalist perspective on ethnic minority health. It was argued that differences in cultural practices between groups could not convincingly explain the variations in health experience of these groups. A fuller picture of the UK ethnic minority health experience needed to consider the socio-economic and structural factors at play. Included within this are the issue of discrimination in employment, housing etc. and the experience of racial harassment (Nazroo, 1997).

Anti-racism

As Stubbs (1993) points out, anti-racist perspectives take as their starting point notions of racism and power differentials rather than those of cultural difference. The ethnic minority health experience is viewed as largely a consequence of structural factors:

> 'General inequalities within a society have a racialised dimension ... [which] ... is of central importance in understanding black people's health needs.'
>
> *(Stubbs, 1993 p41)*

It is important, however, that this focus on racial inequality does not lead to a view of ethnic minority communities as the passive victims of white racism. The anti-racist analysis of health policy highlights black self-help and the important achievements of this movement.

The move from integrationist and culture-focused views of health to an anti-racist perspective has been typified by a shift in emphasis from 'cultural awareness' training to 'anti-racist' or 'anti-discriminatory practice' training. The former concentrates on information giving about cultural practices and difference between groups. The latter, on the other hand, aims to explore attitudes and challenge professionals to explore their own practices in relation to different client groups.

An anti-racist approach to health promotion focuses on structural and power issues in relation to 'race' and discrimination. It combines the emphasis on these broader issues with encouraging and involving the communities in identifying and addressing need.

Recent health policy changes and ethnic minority groups

This chapter will now turn to describe the growth of the field of 'ethnic health' within the NHS and examine how the NHS reforms of late 1980s and early 1990s impacted on this area.

It was not until 1989 that the first public health consultant with specific responsibility for ethnic minority groups was appointed. The field mushroomed from then, both in terms of national developments and volume of material published. The Department of Health (DoH) appointed their first special advisor on ethnic minority health in 1989. In 1991, the King's Fund and DoH set up the first national database of ethnic health matters. The chief medical officer devoted a chapter to the health of ethnic minority populations for the first time in his 1992 Annual Report. In 1993, The DoH's Ethnic Health Task Force was established to review services for those from ethnic minority groups. This led to the establishment of the Ethnic Health Unit.

Parallel to these developments, were the NHS reforms heralded by the 1989 White Paper, *Working For Patients* (DoH, 1989). Once in place, this legislation paved the way for massive organisational change within the National Health Service (NHS), with the separation of the providers of services (soon to become trusts) and the service purchasers (health authorities). This division resulted in the formation of the health service internal market. The health authority's new role was to assess health need across their district and commission services accordingly. This move, it is argued, brought about an increased 'consumer' orientation within the NHS, with the need to take into account all groups across a district (Rathwell, 1991).

This philosophical shift within the NHS was given further momentum by the 'Local Voices' movement. In 1992, the then National Health Service Management Executive published a document entitled *Local Voices: The Views of Local People in Purchasing for Health* (NHS Management Executive, 1992). It stated that the area of working to make health services responsive to local people was central to the role of district health authorities. This was to be achieved with the ongoing involvement of local people in purchasing activities. *The Patient's Charter* (DoH, 1991) was also published around the same time and has become the route for the rights of patients, as 'consumers' of health care, to certain quality standards (Jamadagni, 1996). Both *Local Voices* and *The Patient's Charter* highlighted the need for the health service to be responsive to local need, taking into account the views and requirements of the range of population groupings across a district.

The national policy developments outlined earlier point towards one of the reasons for the increased interest in ethnic minority health issues within the NHS. Community health and black self-help initiatives have also played an important part in pushing these issues up the national health agenda, although it is argued that this type of work has all too often been forgotten (Stubbs, 1993).

COMMUNITY DEVELOPMENT FOR HEALTH

This section examines community development for health as an approach to working with ethnic minority groups. It starts with an overview of the principles underpinning community development and outlines a model of community development. The section concludes with real-life examples of community development within ethnic minority communities.

Community development with a focus on health is the process of 'enabling and empowering disadvantaged communities to take action' in improving their own health (Curtice, 1991, p258). In community development for health, health is seen within a very broad context, focusing on well-being and not purely on absence of disease. An important emphasis is placed on Friere's philosophies with reference to redistribution of power from those who have plenty (Government, statutory bodies, etc.) to those who have little (marginalised and decentralised communities) (Carley, 1991). This empowerment is a dynamic process during which individuals or groups gradually change the power or influence in their favour without oppressing others (Cranidge, 1996).

Community development seeks to enable communities to understand their position and role in the past, present and future of society, and how their lives are controlled and influenced by society itself (Carley, 1991). That is, communities are enabled to understand their 'social reality'.

The process is one of collective participation (Curtice, 1991), pooling resources and enhancing the capacity of community members so they can take political action to change issues that impact on their health. The process of participation in itself is seen as contributing to the well-being of individuals and communities.

Bringing these points together, the Standing Committee for Community Development Charter describes community development for health as enabling people to gain more power by tackling inequality and discrimination so they can overcome factors that have a negative effect on their health and well-being (Harris, 1994). Community development for health workers facilitate communities to assess their needs, share them and develop skills to organise and meet these needs (Webster, 1991; Harris, 1994). In doing this, communities can take action to shape their wider social, political and economic conditions and bring about greater opportunities for health choices. This process has been described as community capacity building, i.e.:

'... development work that strengthens the ability of community organisations and groups to build their structures, systems, people and skills so that they are better able to define and achieve their objectives and engage in consultation and planning, manage community projects and take part in partnerships and community enterprises.'

(Skinner, 1997, p1)

Specifically, the role of the community development for health workers is to enable and support local communities to organise around self-identified health issues, by undertaking the tasks in Box 11.1.

BOX 11.1	*Role of the Community Development for Health Workers*

- Providing practical support in facilitating groups
- Arranging premises and funding
- Establishing networks
- Exchanging information and training
- Assisting in building alliances with voluntary and statutory sectors

(Webster, 1991)

Through this process, the community can set up groups for information sharing, gaining skills or addressing issues that impact on their health. Furthermore, through development, they can gain access to political structures and organisations that influence their health (Sidell, 1997).

A previous section in this chapter highlighted the disadvantaged position of many ethnic minority communities in the UK, both with regards to discrimination and levels of poverty. Health cannot be separated out from such issues which directly and indirectly impact on their health (Douglas, 1991) and therefore broad methodologies such as community development for health will have the greatest impact.

Beattie (1986) developed a simple model to illustrate the levels of community participation and position of power that takes place in community-based health initiatives (Fig. 11.1). This model contextualises community development and helps to identify the continuum from community-based initiatives to improve health to a situation in which communities are involved directly in changing the social context affecting their health.

Beattie describes the 'focus' of the intervention as either individual or collective and the 'mode' of the intervention as either 'top down' (authority led) or 'bottom up' (community led). These two 'dimensions' are laid across one another to form a model with four different approaches:

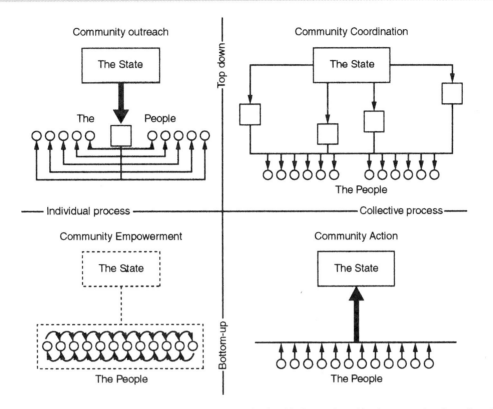

Figure 11.1 Four approaches to community development for health. Reproduced with permission from Beattie, A. Community development for health: from practice to theory. *Radical Health Promotion*, 1986, Summer: 12–18

1. Community outreach
2. Community coordination
3. Community empowerment
4. Community action.

Within the different approaches, the relationship of power and participation are fundamental. Top-down approaches, where a worker carries out activities to engender community spirit, suggest management or manipulation. Examples of this approach include community-orientated health promotion initiatives and community consulation processes in planning health services. Although both of these types of work often include community development techniques, they have limited potential for improving the health of ethnic minority groups when used in isolation. This is because participation is generally low and there is limited scope for community capacity building. As a result, the processes of enablement and empowerment are restricted, and change in power distribution or in existing structures is likely to be negligible.

Community coordination is also a top-down approach, but is considered a collective process. An example of this approach is found where the workers link individuals and communities with the services and agencies impacting on their health. Again, the process is limited in community capacity building and little changes are made in redistribution of power.

Community empowerment is a bottom-up approach. Here the process is non-directive and the people identify health needs themselves, either with or without facilitation by a worker. Self-help occurs, but within the constraints of existing structures and without placing the issues in a broader context (Adams, 1986). In contrast, community action is confrontational. Either alone or facilitated by a worker, the community directly attacks state structures and policies to overcome the inequality impacting on their health.

In work with ethnic minority groups, the model most often followed is one of community empowerment to bring about self-help. Due to the context of poverty and deprivation within which many ethnic minority communities live, a community action approach is also often adopted in the form of protest groups. An example of this is the Sickle Cell Anaemia Campaign, where community organisations lobbied for better NHS services (Douglas, 1991).

As is often found in community development for health, many ethnic minority health projects have a pre-identified agenda rather than working from community-led objectives. A common example is coronary heart disease. Within this context, the approach is not true community development but the community identifies pertinent issues that it believes to relate to the pre-identified agenda.

Projects which use community development techniques but have a pre-identified agenda, give the opportunity of working with ethnic minority communities on narrow health issues as well as broader concerns relating to associations between racism, poverty and health. Narrow issues can be used to raise trust with communities so that broader concerns can be addressed at a later stage (Sidell, 1997).

An example of this is the Ashton Asian Health Development Project (1996). This project was set up to promote the health and well-being of local Asian communities but with a specific agenda related to coronary heart disease (CHD). Following a community development for health philosophy, it aims to increase the opportunities for local people to make informed decisions about the issues affecting their lives. The project activities are guided by local need, initially closely linked to CHD prevention. In collaboration with local people acting as researchers, the project started by carrying out an in-depth assessment of local need. A range of activities and programmes were set up in attempt to address some of these expressed needs.

Recognising the social context of high unemployment, low self-esteem and poor access to health services (indirectly linked to the low employment in health services of people from ethnic minority communities), the project takes a broad perspective. One example of this is the Connect 4 Health Training Programme. The aim of this training programme is to increase the skills and confidence of participants and thus better equip them to access further training, education, employment and voluntary opportunities in health-related fields.

With reference to Beattie's Model of Community Development for Health, the project is an example of the community empowerment approach. Initially within the pre-identified agenda, local health needs have been addressed by increasing community expectations, sharing information and providing a meeting place. However, allied to this, the training programme contributes to local communities bringing about real changes in their health by strengthening the community members' capacity to access employment in health services.

Another example of community development for health within an ethnic minority community is the Somali Community Health Project. It was established in response to the concerns of the Somali refugee community in Sheffield, that the Somali Community Health Project was established (Somali Community Health Project, 1996). This was 3 year project based on a community development approach, which employed a part-time project worker. The Somali community had experienced many hardships that impacted on their health due to the suffering created by forced migration from their country. On arrival in Sheffield, issues related to their refugee status, poverty, communication problems, racism and access to health and social services further affected their health. The aims and objectives of this project were to develop a comprehensive strategy to improve the health and well-being of the Somali communities in Sheffield as listed in Box 11.2.

BOX 11.2	*Aims of the Somali Community Health Project*

- To enable the Somali communities to participate in the identification of their health and social needs
- To influence the planning of health and social care services
- To work directly with service providers to make services appropriate and responsive to the needs of the Somali community
- To use a community development approach to facilitate the empowerment of the Somali communities to have greater control over and improve their health

Initiatives have included: (1) workshops for women and children at which health issues such as diet and nutrition, stress, etc. were explored, (2) the provision of women-only swimming sessions and (3) a women's health bus run in collaboration with the Recreation department of the local council, which provided information about services and access to health professions with interpreters.

In addition to the above, further funding was acquired for an information project. This was a community participative initiative, resulting in the development of appropriate and accessible information on health access and health issues. The Somali community was involved in identifying information needs, developing, producing and disseminating their resources. They also participated in the evaluation of the pack.

With reference to Beattie's Model of Community Development for Health, the project can be described as taking a community empowerment approach, where the worker engendered a spirit of self-help. After the success of the Somali Community Health Project, the community itself developed and acquired funding for the Somali Mental Health Project. This was set up in response to the community's own concerns about mental health and aims to improve access to better mental health care provision by acting as a bridge between the health services and the community. If this project goes beyond self-help and results in change in service provision, the processes of enablement and empowerment set in motion during the original Somali Community Health Project will have facilitated the community into community action.

In summary, community development for health with ethnic minority communities is concerned with a holistic approach to health rather than one that focuses on disease. Needs are identified by the people and emphasis is placed on issues pertinent to the whole community rather than on individual concerns. Through participation, communities work on actions to overcome the identified needs. Workers 'develop' communities by facilitating access to political structures and organisations that affect their lives, by increasing people's expectations, developing skills and providing practical support (Sidell, 1997). This process facilitates the enablement of individuals and builds the capacity of a community to bring about small local changes to enhance health. Raising awareness of the 'reality' of the social context of health in ethnic minority communities and enabling communities to take action is part of the process of empowerment.

HEALTHY ALLIANCES

This section explores the issue of healthy alliances, relating this kind of working to the field of ethnic minority heath promotion. Two types of alliance will be outlined, the first of these is alliances with communities themselves. Healthy alliances and collaborative working between agencies will then be explored. Examples of these two types of alliances in the field of ethnic minority health will be provided and discussed.

The modern day concept of healthy alliances has its roots in the World Health Organisation's *Health for All in Europe by the Year 2000* (WHO, 1985). This is discussed in some depth in Chapter 2 and so will not be explored here. However, it should be pointed out that the principle of joint working espoused by the *Health for All* philosophy is also illustrated in British health policy of the 1990s. *The Health of the Nation* (DoH, 1992) was the country's first national health strategy which aimed to bring about significant improvements in the population's health. The then government emphasised the need for collaborative working in order to bring about these improvements. Their document *Working Together for Better Health* (DoH, 1993) laid out the advantages of healthy alliances as listed in Box 11.3.

BOX 11.3	*Advantages of Healthy Alliances*

- Ensures more effective use of resources
- Breaks down barriers between organisations and improves knowledge
- Exchanges information between partners
- Develops local health strategies
- Generates networks
- Develops 'seamless' services

Speller, Funnell and Friedli (1994) list the main types of organisation involved in healthy alliances. These are local authorities, the education sector, voluntary groups, the NHS, businesses and employers, employees, trade unions, workplaces and the media.

Local partnerships have been emphasised again by the Labour Government, in their White and Green Papers *The New NHS* and *Our Healthier Nation*, respectively (DoH, 1998a,b). They call for the wide range of local agencies and organisations, which can influence the health of the local people to work together closely with the health authority in selecting local priorities for action. These are to be implemented via the health improvement programme and the health action zone frameworks to address the causes of ill health and reduce inequalities.

Alliances with community groups

Jones and Siddell (1997) suggest that these alliances can be divided into two categories based on whether they were initiated by communities themselves or by particular agencies. This standpoint has obvious similarities with the view of Beattie (1986) outlined earlier. The first of these are referred to as 'bottom-up' alliances. Community groups form alliances with organisations when some of the work they want to carry out is dependent on the cooperation of those groups.

An example of such an alliance is the Oldham African-Caribbean Mental Health Drop-in Sessions (Community Links, 1997). These sessions are organised and staffed by an African–Caribbean community worker who is employed by a community organisation. They are held at a local community centre and provide an opportunity for individuals who have either been diagnosed with a mental health problem or are experiencing difficulty coping to get advice and support. The community worker acts in an advice-giving capacity, providing information and assistance with welfare rights, housing etc. At the request of users of these drop-in sessions, a range of activities is provided. These include outings, outside speakers and the regular attendance of social workers at the sessions. This alliance, initiated by the community itself, provides a service that has been developed in response to the voiced needs of its users.

Top-down alliances between agencies and community groups are those which are initiated by an agency or agencies. As the introductory section of this chapter argued, the publication of the Local Voices (NHS Management Executive, 1992) document and the purchaser–provider split in the health service has led to pressure to involve local groups in the decision-making process. This is further emphasised in the recent White and Green Papers *The New NHS* and *Our Healthier Nation*, respectively. This involvement can result in one-off consultations often with only the most vocal members of a community or group. This kind of exercise, in which community members are, in effect, asked solely to rubber stamp existing plans are both tokenistic and disempowering. There is a need for ongoing dialogue in which the views of individuals will contribute to the overall planning process.

There are a number of examples of top-down alliances in the field of ethnic minority health. Many health authorities across the country have set up ethnic minority advisory groups. These function very differently between health authorities with varying levels of involvement in the actual decision-making process. Examples of issues covered by these groups are provision of a range of menus catering to various cultural/religious requirements in hospitals and the provision and use of interpreter facilities for health services.

An example of a top-down alliance in the area of ethnic minority health is the Chinese subgroup of the Tameside Ethnic Health Forum. The Tameside Ethnic Health Forum, itself a top-down alliance, is a group of community members with an interest in health issues who meet quarterly with health authority representatives and interested professionals from the local authority and health services. The group was initiated by the district health authority and is chaired by the Director of Public Health. The Forum identified the health of the Chinese population as one which needed additional attention and the Chinese subgroup was formed. It included representation from the local health trusts, the health and local authorities and the community itself. The group functioned for a limited time span, but during its activity was involved in a range of initiatives as detailed in Box 10.4.

BOX 11.4	*Initiatives involving the Chinese Subgroup*

- The setting up of a Chinese interpreter service by training community members and employing them on a sessional basis
- The production of a Chinese language leaflet outlining health services available and their functions
- The setting up of a weekly drop-in health visitor session at a local library used extensively by the Chinese community

In addition to the issue of tokenism, another potential pitfall of top-down alliances with communities concerns the issue of representation. It should always be remembered that those individuals who become involved in consultation groups are probably not representative of a community as a whole. They are likely to be the most 'easy to reach', educated and confident members of that community, and may have very different attitudes and perceptions from less well-educated, less confident individuals. This is not to negate the use of such methods in groups altogether. However, they should be just one method in a repertoire of obtaining community views. Others should take into account the 'harder to reach groups' and attempt to gather their views also. There are arguably more challenges associated with accessing 'hard to reach' members of non-English-speaking ethnic minority communities. It is therefore perhaps of particular importance that a range of consultation and involvement techniques are employed, including those which do not rely on language skills.

The preceding discussion concerned the formation of alliances between agencies and communities. Bottom-up and top-down categories of alliance were described and examples from the field of ethnic minority health provided. One further point to be made about joint working between ethnic minority groups and organisations concerns the roles of any professionals from these communities who may be involved. It is very important to be clear about the capacity in which an individual is involved in an alliance. A member of a particular community who attends the alliance in their professional capacity should be viewed as such. This individual should not be expected to speak from a community rather than a professional perspective in this scenario as it may present conflict of interest.

Interagency collaboration

Interagency collaboration for health refers to a situation in which two or more organisations work together to address a health issue or issues. Powell (1992) in Health Promotion Wales (1994) describes on alliance of this sort as:

'... a partnership for health gain that goes beyond health care. It attempts collectively to change social and environmental circumstances which affect health.'

(p10)

This definition provides an indication of one of the most important reasons for collaborative working. Health is a consequence of far more than health services. Much more important are the social and economic conditions within which individuals live. It has already been suggested elsewhere in this chapter that effects of these broad issues are arguably especially important when considering the health of ethnic minority communities. Many live in poorer housing, with higher levels of unemployment than the population as a whole (Modood et al, 1997). The introductory section of this chapter argued that these conditions, in combination with racism, both direct and indirect experienced by some members of ethnic minority communities impacts negatively on health. Agencies with a responsibility for addressing these sorts of issues must therefore be involved in serious attempts to promote health in its broadest sense within ethnic minority populations.

The Ashton Asian Health Development Project, discussed earlier, is an example of an ethnic minority health promotion initiative using interagency collaboration. This initiative was set up to promote the health and well-being of local Asian communities. Funded from the Tameside Single Regeneration Budget, it is the result of joint working between agencies including Tameside Metropolitan Borough Council, West Pennine Health Authority, Tameside Community and Priority Services and the NHS Ethnic Health Unit. The project is managed by a steering committee whose role is to set targets for the work undertaken and monitor progress.

This section of the chapter has discussed two categories of healthy alliances and provided real examples from the field of ethnic minority health. The importance of avoiding disempowering practice and tokenism in the area of alliances with community groups and members has been emphasised. The final section of the chapter builds on earlier discussions on the importance of contextualising ethnic minority health and the need for community development and healthy alliance building to be part of a broad strategy addressing the health needs of ethnic minority groups.

STRATEGIES AND CONCLUSIONS

The social and economic context of people's lives is closely bound up with their health experience. For many of Britain's ethnic minority populations, this includes higher levels of poverty than the population at large and the experience of discrimination. As these are issues concerning the distribution of power within society, efforts to improve health should aim to shift power towards these communities.

Communities should not be viewed as passive victims of their circumstance, unable to increase control over issues affecting their health. In fact, people's control of their health is the central tenant of health promotion underpinned by the *Health For All* philosophy. An important part of shifting power towards communities themselves is to involve them in decisions about issues to be addressed. As a result, their own 'reality' will be taken into account and initiatives will address issues that they view as important. Individuals and communities should be involved at all stages of an initiative, including making decisions about planning, implementation and evaluation. This process is, by its very nature, empowering.

Surveys of ethnic minority communities indicate that health concerns tend to focus on issues such as housing and experience of racism (HEA, 1994). Agencies able to influence these factors should therefore be involved in initiatives. Healthy alliances with a range of agencies will best be able to tackle issues and concerns raised by communities. In order to redistribute some power for decision making, healthy alliances should include community representation in some form. It is important that this is more than just tokenistic consultation. Active participation at all levels should be the aim.

The method of choice with which to promote the health of ethnic minority communities is community development. Community development is largely practised within disenfranchised and disempowered communities. The community development process, through enablement and empowerment, aims to shift power towards communities. It incorporates but moves beyond information sharing and skills development, and addresses felt need and self-defined community priorities. This process of community development will enable communities to take effective action to bring about change.

REFERENCES

Adams, L. (1986) Community Development and Health Education. *Radical Health Promotion*, Winter, 23–26

Ahmad, W.I.U. (1993) *'Race' and Health in Contemporary Britain*. Buckingham: Open University.

Asian Health Development Project (1996) *Actioning the Needs of Asian Communities in Ashton: Health Needs Assessment Report*.

Beattie, A. (1986) Community Development for Health: From Practice to Theory. *Radical Health Promotion*, Summer, 12–18.

Bhopal, R. & White, M. (1993) Health Promotion for Ethnic Minorities: Past, Present and Future. In *'Race' and Health in Contemporary Britain*. Ahmad, W.I.U. Buckingham: Open University.

Bunton, R. & White, M. (1993) *The Sociology of Health Promotion*. London: Routledge.

Carley, J. (1991) The Influence of Paulo Freire's Ideas on Theories of Social Change. In *Roots and Branches*. Paper from OU/HEA 1990 Winter School on Community Development and Health. Milton Keynes: Open University.

Community Links (1997) *Ideas Annual '97: A Guide to Good Ideas in Community Development and Health*. Sheffield: Community Links.

Curtice, J. (1991) Can Participation Achieve Changes in Health? In *Roots and Branches*. Paper from OU/HEA 1990 Winter School on Community Development and Health. Milton Keynes: Open University.

Cranidge, EAL. (1996) *Training Manual, Oldham NHS Community Development Service*. Oldham: Oldham NHS Trust.

Department of Health (DoH) (1989) *Working for Patients*. London: HMSO.

Department of Health (DoH) (1991) *The Patient's Charter*. London: HMSO.

Department of Health (DoH) (1993) *Working Together for Better Health*. London: HMSO.

Department of Health (DoH) (1998a) *The New NHS*. London: HMSO.

Department of Health (DoH) (1998b) *Our Healthier Nation*. London: HMSO.

Douglas, J. (1991) Influences on the Community Development and Health Movements – A Personal View. In *Roots and Branches*. Paper from OU/HEA 1990 Winter School on Community Development and Health. Milton Keynes: Open University.

Douglas, J (1995) Developing Anti-Racist Health Promotion Strategies. In eds Bunton et al

Harris, V. (1994) *Community Work Skills Manual*. Association of Community Workers.

Health Education Authority (HEA) (1994) *Black and Ethnic Minority Groups in England: Health and Lifestyles*. London: HEA.

Health Promotion Wales (1994) *Communities for Better Health: Proceedings of a Seminar 'Building Healthy Alliances'*. Cardiff: Health Promotion Wales.

Henley, A. (1983) *Caring for Sikhs and their Families*. London: DHSS/King Edward's Hospital Fund.

Jamadagni, (1996) *Purchasing for Black Population*. London: King's Fund.

Jones, L. & Sidell, M. (1997) *The Challenge of Promoting Health: Exploration and Action*. Oxford: Oxford University Press.

Modood, T., Berthoud, R., Lakey, J. et al (1997) *Ethnic Minorities in Britain: Diversity and Disadvantage*. London: Policy Studies Institute.

Nazroo, J.Y. (1997) *Health and Health Services*. In Modood, T. et al (1997) *Ethnic Minorities in Britain: Diversity and Disadvantage*. London: Policy Studies Institute.

NHS Management Executive (1992) *Local Voices: The Views of Local People in Purchasing for Health*. London: NHSME.

Popple, K. (1995) *Analysing Community Work: Its Theory and Practice*. Oxford: Oxford University.

Rathwell, T. (1991) The NHS Reforms and Britain's Ethnic Communities. *Ethnic Minorities Health: A Current Awareness Bulletin*, 3(1): 1–3.

Sidell, M. (1997) Partnerships and Collaborations: the Promise of Participation In *The Challenge of Promoting Health Exploration and Action*. eds Jones, L. & Sidell, M. Oxford: Oxford University.

Skinner, S. (1997). *Building Community Strengths: A Resource Book on Capacity Building*. Community Development Foundation.

Smaje, C. (1995) *Health, 'Race' and Ethnicity: Making Sense of the Evidence*. London: King's Fund Institute and Share.

Somali Community Health Project (1996) *Working Together for Health in Sheffield*. Project Report, Autumn 1994–1996. Sheffield: Somali Community Health Project Steering Group.

Speller, V., Funnell, R. & Freidli, L. (1994) *Towards Evaluating Healthy Alliances*. Wincester: Institute of Public Health Medicine.

Stubbs, P. (1993) 'Ethnically Sensitive' or 'Anti-Racist'? Models for Health Service Research and Delivery. In *'Race' and Health in Contemporary Britain*. Ahmad, W.I.U. Buckingham: Open University.

Webster, G. (1991) Community Development: The radical interaction of theory and practice – a personal view. In *Roots and Branches*. Papers from the OU/HEA 1990 Winter School on Community Development and Health. Milton Keynes: Open University.

World Health Organisation (WHO) (1985) *Health For All in Europe by the Year 2000, Regional Targets*. Copenhagen: WHO.

FURTHER READING

Ahmad, W.I.U. (1993) *'Race' and Health in Contemporary Britain*. Buckingham: Open University.

A collection of chapters exploring the political and sociological context of ethnic minority health. There is an interesting chapter critiquing research about ethnic minority health.

Nazroo, J.Y. (1997) *The Health of Britain's Ethnic Minorities*. London: Policy Studies Institute.

The write up of a national survey carried out by the Policy Studies Institute. Includes sections of the health status of ethnic minority groups, the impor-

tance of socio-economic factors in health and the use and experience of health services by ethnic minority groups.

Jones, L. & Sidell, M. (1997) *The Challenge of Promoting Health: Exploration and Action.* Oxford: Oxford University.

Katz, J. & Reberdy, A. (1997) *Promoting Health: Knowledge and Practice.*

A general introductory text to health promotion theory and practice. Includes chapters outlining the principles and practice of community development for health and partnerships.

12 'Queer health': health promotion the hard way

Tony Russell-Pattison (formerly Harrison)

KEY ISSUES

- Importance of language
- Self-help community responses
- Professionalisation of the voluntary section
- Politics and voluntary sector responses
- Unusual alliances
- Outreach work. Native or naïve?
- De-gaying and Re-gaying the human immunodeficiency virus (HIV) pandemic
- Sexual health vs HIV prevention

'I belong to a community which has faced, collectively and individually, the social challenges presented by HIV. In that community, people with HIV have not been ostracised; they have not had their autonomy threatened by calls from the uninfected majority for coercive measures to protect them. Members of that community have volunteered in their thousands to provide financial, practical and emotional support to those infected ... And as a result I, and many other people with HIV, have been able to achieve our own personal and private victories against this disease.'

(Grimshaw 1989, p217)

INTRODUCTION

This chapter will address a number of quite fundamental issues. First and most importantly, it will define the terminology to be used. The chapter will then examine the historical context of HIV within the 'community' of gay men and lesbian women (within the context of the larger population). The communal responses in terms of health promotion for these groups of people (infected, affected and disinterested) will be examined and finally, the work to date in the hope of gaining insights for the work required in the future will be evaluated.

The HIV epidemic in the UK provides for those who wish to see (and not everyone does) an encapsulated 15-year period of significant responses to one of the most devastating diseases of this century. HIV, the virus which causes acquired immune deficiency syndrome (AIDS) is a threat to health on two specific fronts. As Treichler (1987) puts it: 'the AIDS epidemic with its genuine potential for global devastation is simultaneously an epidemic of transmissible lethal disease and an epidemic of meanings and signification' (p2634).

HIV has devastated populations physically within the UK, most notably the population of gay men. The significances attributed to the disease have further eroded the social and mental well-being of both those infected and affected by HIV. This is a disease not only of the body physical. In many respects it is also a disease of the bodies politic and social. The current author, like Grimshaw, is part of the community about which he writes. This is advantageous in that it brings with it the insights of a health professional whose personal and professional worlds seem, at times, to be at the heart of this epidemic. Advantageous again (although some may justifiably see it as a disadvantage in terms of bias) in that this study and opinion is fuelled with a passion which hopes to see this area of health promotion have real effects for those close to the author. The current author declares his vested interest in promoting health so that no one need ever be inflicted with this disease again and also that those infected already might have their health enhanced by empowerment and by choice.

Uniquely in the modern era the snapshot of UK HIV infection provides examples of tragedies, mistakes, victories and, above all, lessons which can and will be utilised for other populations and other threats. The current author acknowledges the shared tragedy of HIV by heterosexuals, both children and adults, but here looks at the queer world where health promotion has been achieved the hard way, by necessity, in order to help stop the death of those who we know. Grief as a motivator to behaviour change is powerful if not always universally positive. It is, however, always hard!

DEFINITIONS THE IMPORTANCE OF LANGUAGE

'Words are chameleons, which reflect the colour of their environment.'
(Hand 1948)

Precision in the use of language is sometimes viewed as pedantry but in this particular case should be viewed as a desire for accuracy.

As Hand observed, words can have several or no actual meaning depending on who uses and hears them.

This chapter is entitled 'queer health'. Many words have, and are, used to describe the population in question. Homosexuality, with its medical overtones comes from the era when being gay was both not only seen as a medical disorder but was also criminal. This term was largely abandoned by those to whom it applied after the decriminalisation and demedicalisation of our sexuality. The next emerging self-identification term was 'gay', which some say is an abbreviation of 'good as you'. This petulant sounding label arguably belonged to a period of assimilation politics and the foundation of the gay liberation movement which, while accomplishing significant victories and certainly enhancing the lives of gay men and women everywhere, did, to a degree, emphasise the 'sameness' of all regardless of sexual orientation. Latterly the term 'queer' has gained currency although the degree to which any given term is adopted by the group concerned is somewhat hotly contested.

Neal and Davies (1996, p6) for example, suggest that comparatively few gay people choose terms which were previously pejorative in nature. The term 'queer' seems mostly to be used by radical lesbians and gay men who wish to emphasise the difference as opposed to the sameness. Assimilation politics has, therefore, given way to acceptance politics. In this mindset, queers are not the same, they are different – different but equal. 'Queer' encompasses both men and women and is gender neutral; the process gains much of its impetus from the civil rights movement in the USA, where the word 'nigger' was appropriated by the radical black communities who stole the insult and turned it into a term of pride (Patton, 1990), Such definitions are not only essential to understanding the focus of this chapter but are also essential for understanding the many facets of the queer world, especially when addressing health promotion issues within this population. For the purposes of this chapter, the word 'queer' will be used as a term with which the author feels most comfortable.

The opening quote used the term 'community', a primary focus of this text. The gay/queer/homosexual community is however not one but many communities, as indeed is the heterosexual 'community'.

Patton (1990) in looking at how communities affected by HIV overlap, discusses the move towards describing the gay community as the gay communities. However, she does go on to argue that this is still an inadequate way to describe the diversity of the group. Interestingly the term 'heterosexual community', Patton argues, first appeared around 1985 as a method of differentiating the heterosexual world from the gay community and most notably (and interestingly) specifically when discussing health promotion in relation to HIV.

Such terminologies are essential to both review and direct health promotion initiatives. Communities are defined, often as a matter of convenience, but essentially are noted as being groups of people who share some significant facet of their lives. This might be colour, gender, experience, prejudice or, as some would argue, disease. Paton's use of plurals, discussed earlier, would suggest that, in fact, communities are frequently highly complex and overlapping of numerous subcommunities. Thus the gay community may be subdivided further into those who categorise themselves in certain ways. This may be by sexual proclivities, age, fashion or politics. This self-definition is, it could be argued, reflected in the terminology chosen by such groups to label themselves. This brings us back to self-determining labels. Queers, gays and homosexuals, puffs, fags et al, while all having at least one common factor may actually be so radically different as to make shared health promotion approaches somewhat nonsensical.

 Why is it important when considering health promotion to understand the language which the target clients/population use to describe themselves?

The idea of a gay community, Paton would argue is actually derived from a civil rights lobby approach used by many gay North Americans to demonstrate support for those who are HIV positive and to campaign for services for them. The canvassing of the wider community of those who shared not only the political will but also the sexual orientation was made simpler by the shear scale of the tragedy. With so many gay North Americans actually knowing someone with HIV disease, the ranks of the politically motivated were consequently swelled by those who were physically or emotionally affected. However, it remains dubious, to the current author at least, whether such a ground swell of support actually constructs or construes that a wider community actually existed or whether what happened was that temporary and sometimes rather ill-fitting alliances were made. This model of politicisation, augmented by a form of grief recruitment was not without price in terms of the newly co-opted members (see 'survivor guilt', the experience of negative emotions in relation to surviving HIV (Odets, 1995). This created an 'ephemeral community', i.e. a community rallied for a cause which temporarily swelled the originally affected community; health promotion flowed between the two.

This communal enlargement and construction was mirrored in the UK. However, the water gets more muddied and certainly more complex the more subdivisions are added. The community constructs, i.e. how definitions are applied to delineate a community by those who are seeking to promote health, can be either self-identified by the group concerned or identified by an agenda set by the health promoter.

Scott (1995) makes this point eloquently when he disputes whether health promoters should be focusing on communities constructed by their own political correctness. He argues, with some justification, that the deaf gay community is probably less of a priority than the community of gay men, who are actually more significant in terms of numbers, such as those who share the characteristic of not being self-assured enough to have sex unless bolstered by drugs and/or alcohol. This does not of course negate the needs of deaf gay men but restructures them in terms of priority.

In this example, the definition of the community has rested with the health promoter not with the community concerned, but of course this may also be the case in the scenario set by Scott. It is very unlikely that those who share the characteristics of being both gay and dependent on drugs for sexual confidence are going to feel any solidarity with those others who share the latter characteristic. It is possible that the health promoter in this scenario must work to empower those individuals to recognise their common characteristics in order to feel less isolated and so start on the road to establishing a power base from where they can seek to promote their own health.

The difference, although subtle is important in that in this case the empowerment is to bring about recognition of a shared problem. In the former example, it is about selecting a group on the basis of a liberal/pragmatic agenda on the part of the health promoter. Pragmatic in that the group chosen may be encapsulated and an easily evaluatable group. This sometimes is done to secure funding from sources which share such political agendas, i.e. it must be evaluatable and politically correct.

History, like language can be both constructed and interpreted in different ways. Berridge (1996) in her excellent historical research reiterates this point. For example, she differentiates between those histories which choose as their focus the medical model or place history within the context of past epidemics such as Fee and Fox (1992) and what she terms 'journalistic histories' such as the now famous Shiltz (1987) text (her book coming too early to include the UK equivalent by Garfield 1994). Berridge focuses on history as it affects public policy making between 1981 and 1994. She divides this period into four distinct phases dependent on policy response at the time. Such histories provide for us a convenient starting point to examine the recent history of this pandemic.

The detective story which is the story of the discovery of the virus is now part of history. While it was a time of intense scientific discovery and in consequence a time of much complication, this factual history is actually the 'simple' past when the issue under consideration is present day health promotion strategies. Nonetheless, without the detailed scientific 'who dunnit', which eventually unearthed the culprit, we would have little ability to prevent the disease. The scientific story, at least in the developed world, began in the queer world, although the current author would suggest that such an assertion tragically negates the history of 'Slim' (the name AIDS is given in central Africa). This still remains a largely unrecounted history because the resources required to both prove and recount it were never available.

Pratt (1992) now in itself an historical document, recounts in epidemic terms the beginnings. In early 1981 five young men were admitted to Los Angeles hospitals with a disease called Pneumocystis carinii pneumonia (PCP). Normally PCP was only seen in transplant patients who were made immuno-supressed by their treatment. These five young men alerted the medical world with their bizarre disorder. They had however one thing in common. They were all queer. The Centre for Disease Control in Atlanta, Georgia, USA, the monitoring body for infectious disease in the USA, duly noted this strange occurrence and reported it. Soon other cases were noted in other areas such as New York and reports of Kaposi's sarcoma, a rare skin cancer, started to appear. The common denominator in nearly all cases was the sexual orientation of the individuals concerned. Nearly all were queer.

The history of the discovery of the causative organism of AIDS, the HIV virus. The sad discovery that it could be spread to anyone via blood routes, predominantly during sexual intercourse, regardless of the orientation of the individual concerned and its massive spread throughout the USA are all documented points of history which readers are encouraged to investigate but which space does not allow for in this chapter.

 Read *The End of Innocence* (Garfield, 1994). Using this text try to determine the pivotal role of queer individuals and the queer communities in developing prevention services for their own communities.

The sheer scale of the US problem is difficult to comprehend for anyone who was not or is not a member of the communities most affected. Odets (1995) sums this up well:

'The San Francisco Mayor's office has said that by 1990 more San Franciscans had died of AIDS than all the San Franciscans who died in the four great wars of the twentieth century, combined and quadrupled.'

(p14)

'... The first decade of the epidemic alone has made certain that all gay men now live or will live with loss that is unimaginable to most Americans.'

(p63)

As our focus is on the UK, I now return to Berridge's time slots in order to discuss the community responses to the UK epidemic. The response of the USA queer communities to the HIV crisis, while within a different cultural ethos, provided not only a model but also a source of inspiration, support and impetus for the responses of the UK queer communities to the emerging epidemic. The international queer community, at least within the developed world, became linked in order to support members in other countries. Such transatlantic influences in terms of health promotion were as significant as similar influences had been on gay liberation and gay culture prior to the advent of HIV. Whether by cultural quirk or simply through the power of the US marketing machine, the UK gay scene had, to some extent, mirrored or at least taken as its fantasy a distinctly North American flavour.

This author would argue that it was this link that was to be fortuitous in alerting the communities of this country to the oncoming danger and allow for some early responses.

Berridge titles her first section 'AIDS Missionaries: Self help and the Initial Response to AIDS' and covers the years 1981–1985. This was a period of great uncertainty and an even greater lack of knowledge. She describes this time segment as being characterised by a bottom-up approach to policy.

As previously mentioned, the voluntarist interventions within this period commenced almost immediately the danger was alerted. Gay men who had travelled to the USA, came back to the UK armed with sketchy information but with a considerable amount of anxiety about the new 'gay compromise syndrome,' which in the very early days was referred to as the 'gay cancer'.

The nature and role of these front line alerters is important from a community health promotion perspective. These men had the financial status which permitted such travel, they were predominantly white and for the most part they were well educated. I would argue that these characteristics greatly increased their effectiveness as information couriers to a society which valued such characteristics. It is possible to conjecture that around the same time, or maybe even earlier people acquainted with the African tragedy of Slim had returned to the UK, but their personal attributes, i.e. colour, made them less efficient couriers to a country which remains to some extent somewhat racist. These two distinct sets of couriers also delivered their message to different communities, one predominantly white, affluent and well placed, the other not. The information brought back to the UK by these two distinct groups of couriers encapsulated, almost perfectly, a practical example of one of Tannahills (1985) domains, namely health education/disease prevention. It also demonstrates that this information best travels along socially powerful routes.

A gay man by the name of Terry Higgins died at St Thomas' Hospital in London in 1982. His death was undignified and within the then climate of fear he received extremely poor care.

In November of the same year, the Terry Higgins Trust (THT) was set up by a group of his friends. Berridge notes that many histories of this period concentrate on the THT as the epitome of response although in fact, it was only one of several community-based responses. Initially the group was created from within the gay disco community in order to raise funds to support medical research into the cause of AIDS. Health promotion was seen as being a much lesser priority. This initial response, however, contains some germs for analysis within the context of this text, which will be considered before moving on to look at other developments.

The Terrence Higgins Trust (note Terrence. not 'Terry' – the name change came later, which Berridge correctly identifies as a major turning point for the new organisation) formed and coalesced around two features: the grief of bereaved friends and the outrage regarding the care given by the professionals. As alluded to earlier, grief can be a powerful generator of energy which can be harnessed to generate community activism. Although it may sound callous, at a pragmatic level it may be beneficial not only for those on whom such energy is expended but also for those suffering grief and outrage in gaining a powerful sense of being able to do something positive. The opportunities are considerable for the health promoter in particular, who may encounter individuals bereaved or stigmatised, to both support the grieving and direct them to resolution activities. However, it must be considered that the professionals involved in supporting individuals during any bereavement must also be aware that activism, particularly in this field, can perpetuate grief and on many occasions may even exacerbate it, plugging that individual into the traumas of others. It is incumbent on the professionals as advocates to make clients aware of this so that they can make informed decisions as to whether they become activists or not.

As a health promoter, how would you analyse the grief response of individuals or groups to ascertain whether activism would be positive or detrimental to them?

As Berridge points out, THT was not the only self-help organisation to respond to the fear of AIDS in those early days. The Lesbian and Gay Switchboard, set up in 1974, began to respond to many health-related calls, particularly when televised HIV-related stories started to appear. This was not unusual, as the switchboard had previously responded to requests for information regarding hepatitis, etc. What was different, however, was the scale. Again, in terms of our chosen topic of community health promotion and empowerment, there are interesting comparisons to be made between these two organisations and their subsequent responses. The two organisations are diverse in nature. The characteristics of each are detailed in Box 12.1.

BOX 12.1	*Characteristics of the original THT and The Lesbian and Gay Switchboard*

THT
- Built and based on a medical condition and the need to do something about it
- Approach is disease prevention and treatment

The Gay and Lesbian Switchoard
- Set up: to inform the queer community on all aspects of gay life
  - Recreation venues
  - Coming out (the process of declaration of your sexuality to others) matters
  - Health matters
- Holistic in nature
- Approach is health education/promotion

The focus of The Gay and Lesbian Switchboard could be seen as being more holistic, although whether this affected the type of health advice (health education) it gave is somewhat of an unknown quantity. It is tempting to characterise the potential approaches of the two organisations as the THT is one of disease prevention, while the Switchboard is one of health education/promotion from within a holistic sexual health model and sees equilibrium with one's sexuality as a prerequisite for behaviour which will in turn protect one from HIV disease.

The professional, seeking to benefit from this analysis of events should however note that there is room for both models. The current holistic ethos of health care and health promotion sometimes negates the focused disease prevention model, which, for those gay men who are perfectly at ease with their sexual orientation might be far more suitable.

This model however does require factual knowledge, such as the answers to the following questions:

- What sort of sex passes the virus?
- Is oral sex of low, medium or high risk?
- How can a person change that risk rating?

A Rogerian focus which seeks to get the client into equilibrium with their orientation requires different skills. It also requires few facts. Both skills and facts are required if clients at both an individual and communal level are to be offered a wide range of health promotion alternatives in order to meet their needs and desires.

In 1983 the THT re-grouped under new volunteers, and its aim widened from fundraising to include health education, media coverage, and medical and social support. These new members were a different breed from the original founding members and believed that political power could achieve what, to date, social power had eluded.

The communal response from the now emerging groups could now be classified as those that supported linking with the political power of the day (i.e. Margaret Thatcher's government) and those who would view any such an alliance as selling the gay liberation fight down the river and climbing into bed with a government many thought to be uncaring and antagonistic to gay people in general. This tension within and between alliances would prove to be pivotal and would determine the change in response of the queer community in the coming years. But first there were other alliances which were of a different calibre.

ALLIANCES: HEALTHY OR OTHERWISE?

The medical world, like the queer world (particularly where the two overlapped) was also grappling with this new disease. Most AIDS histories recount the valiant attempts of the medical pioneers in AIDS care in the UK. (Anthony Pinching, Professor Adler and many many others) and in so doing note their evolving alliances with the other most knowledgeable group with regard to this disease, namely gay men themselves.

The UK AIDS epidemic saw in many of its earliest victims an almost stereo-type of the gay male – white, middle class, educated and articulate – attributes stereotypical of individuals in other groups, especially those in the field of medicine. While the totality of the queer community was, and is, as diverse as any other, representing both the affluent and the poor, the white and non-white, one of its important subgroups seemed even more stereotypical. Users of the global gay scene commercial venues – discos, bath houses, saunas and the like – needed almost by definition to be affluent. Those who attended these venues transatlantically were most certainly within this bracket of substereotype.

This had some notable effects. As discussed earlier, it meant that health-related information crossed the continents, particularly between the USA and UK on very articulate wings. Second, it provided the scientific/medical community with a client group for both treatment and research purposes which was articulate and indeed similar in constitution to the medical professionals themselves. Added to this, there were of course those white articulate, well-educated gay men who where themselves medical professionals and some of these queer individuals became the communities insider heroes in those early days. These individuals were also able to articulate and point to the inequality implicit, at the time, by the UK government and establishment who seemed not to acknowledge the possibility of the epidemic to come.

While it is not at all unusual for medical staff to encounter articulate, middle-class clients, and while not all conditions and diseases favour the poor (although disproportionately more do – ironically this is also true of HIV disease in most areas of the world). What was unusual in this situation, however, was the time, the number and the newness of the condition, which required the cooperation of the clients as research subjects. This ultimately evolved into a different relationship between the medical professionals and those affected by HIV disease. This relationship became notable in that it was more collegiate than any other previously formed en mass between medical professionals and those for whom they provide treatment and care. This is of more than simply historical interest. It is notable as it became almost a new way of working. It delineated a group whose view of health was that they were the major stakeholders in that health and this ownership of a concept of health was translated into action in terms of its validation by the medical world. Its continuation by some clients became critical to the empowerment of those who were already infected, but who required empowerment as individuals and groups to promote their own health by avoiding potential pathogens and boosting their immune responses and holistic sense of well-being. The fact that previously those who were actually already infected had been largely ignored by those responsible for health promotion is a tragedy. The sea change occurred in that HIV-positive clients were seen as having a right to health promotion to enhance both the quality and extent of their life. The failure of bodies dealing with health promotion to address these needs merely gives credence to the suspicion that the focus of health promotion is in fact on preventing spread (à la Tannahill's disease prevention domain), i.e. protecting the uninfected majority from the infectious minority. To many this all seemed to refute the oft touted claim of health promotion that its approach is holistic and developmentally enhancing. While prioritisation is understandable in some cases, the sort of absence of health promotion intervention at a community level which has been evident until recently seems a clear indication of an abandonment approach. These suspicions in terms of community empowerment are also detrimental to preventative approaches in terms of HIV spread. The community which lives in intimate closeness with its infected members and is almost universally affected is likely to view with healthy scepticism bodies and individuals purporting to promote health when those within that community at most risk of immediate and physical ill health, much of which could be prevented by health promotion, are not included on the agenda.

Berridge, moves on within the same time period, to the growing realisation of transmission via blood and its products. This realisation of the threat to the wider population as a whole, produced one of the most remarkable liberal consensus of a right-wing bureaucracy ever known. The wheels of the national government moved towards recognising and doing something about the threat that was HIV disease, albeit a little too little and a lot too late for many in the queer community who saw their health needs disregarded until the threat reached to a wider heterosexual community. In some ways, it might be argued, this perceived overt prejudice may indeed have strengthened the community response. Those discriminated against can feel a bond which is evident in many minorities who experience shared prejudice. This bond may have strengthened the resolve of the queer community to deal with issues which the wider community felt unimportant. This however is a view in hindsight and hardly a strategy which should ever be repeated. The queer community showed its communal willingness to act to benefit the community as a whole in its readiness to give up being donators of blood once this was identified as a risk. This is frequently ignored in terms of the histories of responses to HIV disease or seen as being insignificant, but for many it was very significant indeed. The queer community responded further by lesbians offering their blood, given, that at the time this section of the community was perceived to be at the lowest risk of HIV. This part of the queer community is still regarded, by many as being at low risk of infection (although high risk of affection given that many women support queer men with HIV disease and so are intimately affected by the epidemic). The blood services looked with some disdain on this offer giving rise to accusations of prejudicial rather than scientific responses. This low-risk status metamorphasised into a no risk status for many women. Health promoters failed to address the significant health promotion needs of this subgroup and sadly this extended to some of the communal responses of the queer community itself who joined the silence. Lack of information and divisions between queer men and women allowed a situation in which some members of the community are ignored in terms of HIV prevention programmes. Numerical statistics cannot solely justify this exclusion of queer women when protection from infection was the aim.

The period from 1986–1987 is what Berridge calls 'the wartime years'. This period is exemplified by action from the Government in terms of funding predominantly gay organisations such as the THT and culminates in the delivery of the HIV leaflet 'Don't Die of Ignorance' in 1987.

This period, as Scott (1995) notes, is also characterised by the de-gaying of HIV and AIDS. This phenomena involved the perpetuation of the belief of shared and equal risk. Everyone all of a sudden was equally at risk of HIV infection, although this was not supported by the medical evidence available. The mid 1980s were notable in that many erstwhile queer bodies and organisations re-focused their HIV-related work on a wider community model (i.e. the straight communities). They were, in fact, de-gayed. Scott hypothesises several possible reasons for this which are summarised in Box 12.2.

BOX 12.2	*The de-gaying of HIV infection and AIDS disease*

Altruism: Gay men, having experienced the devastation of HIV move towards preventing a replication in other groups of individuals

Media and social hostility: The media in particular had attributed blame to the queer world for the epidemic. The fact that anyone could get infected may have been seen as a godsend for queer groups trying to deflect prejudice

Social responsibility: In response to such blame approaches, the community overemphasised its success in encouraging safer sex, implying the problem for the queer community was now resolved

Heterosexual denial: The perceived need to deal with this denial may have led to an overstatement of risk. Statistics were manipulated to prove a point, which was in turn over-made

Exclusion of protestors: There were radical queers who disagreed with spreading sparse resources across many diverse groups when, in fact, most cases at that time remained within the queer community and were made to feel unwelcome within their organisations and so left

Reproduced from *Purchasing HIV Prevention. A No Nonsense Guide for Working with Gay and Bisexual Men*, Scott, P., 1995, with permission.

Although much of this re-focusing was done in the name of equal opportunities, it enshrined the dogma of de-gaying given that only those who agreed with it remained!

The truth both then and now is of course that all sexually active and blood recipient individuals are at some risk of HIV but *not* equally so. Those who select partners from a community with higher infection rates have a higher risk of encountering a partner with HIV disease, although their risk is then dependent on the type of sex in which they indulge. The different sexual mores of the queer community may also have contributed to the de-gaying of the epidemic as Scott (1995) and SIGMA (see Weatherburn et al, 1992 further reading) note queer sexual activities are not necessarily (nor is there any indication that they should be) the same as their heterosexual counterparts. Both authors and others note higher partner exchange, polygamy, friends as sexual partners and a variety of relationship types for both queer men and women which may have no equivalent with heterosexual communities. De-gaying, it could be argued allowed for such diversity. Some however found this embarrassing or even a bar to assimilation within the wider community, to be swept under the carpet. In some respects the rise of queer politics and the move away from assimilation liberation to an acknowledgement of diversity has mirrored the re-gaying of HIV which has occurred over the last few years.

Acknowledgement of such diverse social and sexual networks is essential for promoting health to those uninfected. Once understood and when strategies have been developed which value such networks, it can provide access to the huge informal communication routes which are the grapevine of the queer community.

These routes can be formal, through the gay scene (i.e. gay pubs, clubs, saunas, businesses, cafes etc.) or informa through word of mouth and social networks. Arguably an understanding of the diversity of gay relationships is also vital when promoting health to those who are already infected. Support and love are undoubtedly the key to empowering individuals to maintain and improve their health when they are HIV positive. Support from the empowered community will in most cases allow the individual concerned more control and assistance outside the medical model. Such support then could be seen as the single most empowering health promotion measure for this particular client group. Only if this is fully understood can support be fully appreciated and harnessed.

One could argue, that regardless of the causes of de-gaying, the effect was to make available official support and finance which sceptical or realistic individuals (depending on the perspective) might claim would not have been forthcoming if a general threat to the population had not been perceived and broadcast.

Whatever the rationale, funding and support to combat the menace of HIV was channelled through organisations whose main ethos was queer. Unfortunately the usurping of statistics, the overemphasis of risk to the general population as a whole and the political game play to keep HIV in the spotlight was to rebound.

In the 1990s it became apparent that although risk was not equal between queer and straight individuals, allocation of resources regarding health promotion and indeed services were being applied equally. The net result was that the groups most at risk, i.e. the queer community received insufficient support for its health promotion initiatives while resources were targeted at those with little or moderate risk. So began the long road of re-gaying HIV and AIDS.

This de-gaying, re-gaying merry-go-round is important in planning future health promotion for this group of individuals, because it highlights how reckless use of statistics to scare money out of funders can backfire. It is understandable, given the tragedy of HIV within the queer community, that individuals and organisations might see means justifying ends. In this case however the long-term effect was actually to achieve a reduction in funding for the group in question. In addition, the backlash from the media and public could arguably be viewed as damaging to the cause as a whole.

This period in the UK epidemic mirrored a period in the history of USA HIV response which occurred in the mid-1980s and was described fetchingly by Paton (1990) as 'from Grassroots to Business Suites'. This was a move from community-generated health promotion and services to a more professionalised approach. This was partly necessitated by the partnerships discussed earlier, principally with governments and medicine. Such bed fellows required, and in many cases demanded, professional approaches, measurable criteria, models of practice and accountability which introduced a new dimension to the HIV-prevention effort. Queer-orientated groups such as the THT started to beureaucricise themselves in order to achieve their objectives.

This sea change had far-reaching effects. On the one hand it enabled those organisations which undertook the process to access the establishment bodies, and in doing so was able to utilise their funds, expertise and processes. At a different level and discussed by Paton (p10), divisions began to grow between organisations which could loosely be labelled as 'self-help' or 'other helping'. Body Positive in the UK personified the self-help, community empowerment model which saw clients with HIV helping themselves and others because of their feeling of ownership of the problem at hand. On the other hand the more professionalised helping bodies were also motivated by a community spirit but now had a wider outlook.

In terms of health promotion the situation was further complicated by the fact that health promotion was focusing on prevention of infection. The self-help groups were largely comprised of those already infected and to some degree had formed as a response to dissatisfaction with other organisations whose main aim seemed to be to prevent infection but whose commitment to those already infected was seen as in some way deficient. There then followed a period of accusation and recrimination. The HIV 'gravy train' had arrived amidst much steam and hot air. The infected accused those who took up posts in the newly professionalised helping industry as cashing in on the epidemic for personal reasons of ambition. Undoubtedly, in some cases, the accusation did indeed have merit but overall this period was indicative of a fracturing of the community response under the pressure of de-gaying and under the perceived necessity to alter in order to achieve funding and recognition.

The HIV 'gravy train', to the extent that it existed, peaked in the early 1990s when ring fenced funds for both services and prevention work began to dwindle, eventually to be lost altogether. De-gaying had reached its zenith and achieved its aim. HIV services became genericised (a process which continues) and in particular health promotion took on a more generic approach perhaps most personified by the advent of the expression 'sexual health'.

The publication of *The Health of The Nation* strategy (DoH, 1992) encompassed HIV prevention within the broader heading of sexual health. Many would argue that effectively this reduced its priority to a fraction of what it was by subsuming it within an overall strategy.

The queer community, now suffused with professionalised workers in relation to HIV moved slowly towards a health promotion model that was sexual health focused. This move was and is influenced by the evolving philosophies of the establishment bodies which were set up to 'assist' with queer community initiatives to prevent HIV infection.

In tandem with the idea of sexual health has come the proposition that, in terms of the community in question, it must be decided who would be the best person/group to facilitate health promotion initiatives in this area. The rather simplistic answer was that a member of the community in question would be. Feminism suggested that women had a right to be treated and supported by other women. Racial equality gave rise to similar assumptions regarding the black community, i.e. that it would be best served by a member of that community. Work with queer communities seems to have followed a similar model, ably abetted by eminent figures like Scott, who would suggest that there is a wealth of untapped expertise within the community itself.

The premise that queers best empower other queers is based on one central assumption: that being a member of a given group provides the basic understanding on which health promotion skills can be built and then adapted to the community in question. While this is undoubtedly true in some cases it is certainly not in others. A favoured means of empowering these communities has been the use of outreach workers to facilitate change. This person (normally singular) is, à la, the above assumption, generally a gay man. His job is to work with the community to generate owned and self-powering initiatives within that community. Generally, sexual health rather than HIV prevention is his remit and he is launched into a community which although generically queer, is populated by individual members who he will have absolutely nothing in common with and he is encouraged to change the world. Some hope (Harrison, 1995).

While the premise that an in-depth knowledge of a community is important for a person to have to enable them to work with it is not in dispute. What this author would dispute is the assumption that membership of a community actually bestows this depth of knowledge on a person automatically. Given that it has been already argued that the queer community is in fact several communities, it must follow that membership of one section of this community does not necessarily give insights into the rest of it. Mixed with this premise is the idea that queer men will respond best to other queer men, lesbian women to lesbian women etc. This would seem to be a premise borrowed from feminism and accepted as a universal truth without much confirmation.

On an individual and communal level, the assumption that the queer community will benefit from having 'native guides', i.e. that the natives will respond best to one of their own seems to have been accepted out of hand. It could be suggested that, for example, gay men would respond more easily and with more comfort to a woman health promotion worker given that there would be little sexual possibility between the two. This factor in turn would make the topic of discussing sex and sexual health far easier, and would run counter to such an argument. While the current author is not suggesting that this is conclusively proven, i.e. gay men responding better to women, he would argue that the current premise that they respond better to other gay men has not been tested let alone proven.

COMMUNITY PARTICIPATION OR MANIPULATION?

This does not, of course, negate the excellent and innovative projects undertaken by many queer men and women (for example the work of Healthy Gay Manchester – see Trueman and Gudgin, 1996 and Gay Men Fighting AIDS – see Corrigan 1996 as two of many possible examples). Indeed one could argue that some of the most empowering communal health promotion approaches with regard to HIV prevention have been those self-generated and carried out by the communities themselves. This is however not the issue. An actual difference exists between what might be categorised as 'self-help' initiatives and those which are professionally engineered. The professional queer working with the communities may indeed stimulate self-help approaches within the communities and may indeed be efficacious. What is being questioned however is how much this is attributable to that individual's sexual orientation and how much is attributable to other skills. The answer is almost certainly a mix of the two. The current author would contend that growing up with what might be described as an 'alternate' (to the majority of society) sexual orientation makes of that individual a quite different persona to one who has developed within the majority and that this may indeed produce attributes, not to mention knowledge and skills which may assist health promotion but equally may not. The issue is one of equipping all such workers with the requisite skills and not relying solely on a presumed expertise in the name of political correctness.

Much has been reviewed in relation to empowerment and health promotion with this group in respect of HIV prevention. Much of this has focused on both the initiatives stimulated within professional or semi-professional (i.e. voluntary sectors adopting professional approaches) sectors and those carried out in large conurbation centres. It may be that this approach has been inevitable given that such professional approaches *by their nature* have evaluative formulations which translate well into print. Moreover, large cities have sample groups and interventions based on the actual number of individuals who are registered as infected, from which the risk of others gaining the infection is extrapolated. It does however neglect both rural or non-capital endeavours and those which are solely based within the community (a surprise given the current en vogue status of qualitative research approaches). The problem with evaluation strategies in HIV prevention in general is that they focus on the formal and ignore the informal. The professional (or semi-professional) intervention has evaluation built in or funding never comes; the informal grapevine of the gay communities does not lend itself to the largely quantitative criteria of evaluation much beloved of most funding and professional bodies. This however does not mean that it doesn't happen or isn't effective.

If this is the case how do we evaluate or value such informal community-generated health promotion work?

HIV prevention and health promotion to those who are already infected are vast areas of endeavour. The aim of this chapter has not been to attempt to review them all but rather to raise questions which may bring the reader to explore in more depth assumptions and discourses surrounding work with these communities which have arisen in the last decade and in so doing lead to a greater understanding of the actual issues.

One could be accused of having laid into such assumptions critically without providing many alternatives but would suggest that exploration and debate leads the reader to hypothesise different approaches based on the questions raised. The following issues have been examined.

- Language and definition
- Role of the international queer community
- Nature of health promotion messengers within the communities in question
- Grief as a motivator to change and assist others to change
- Holism vs AIDS prevention
- Effect of political agendas on health promotion and how the community mobilises itself
- Actual shameful neglect regarding health promotion for those actually infected
- De-gaying, re-gaying debate and the work of native guides regarding sexual health.

Some of the lessons learned from this discourse by this author could be summarised in a mnemonic (not, please note, a model – mnemonics are not models unless philosophy, approach, evaluation and methodologies are included). This author, utilises another motivator – humour (sadly neglected in academic circles but gaining credence in clinical ones) would suggest the nemonic CESPIT (Box 12.3).

BOX 12.3	*Meaning of CESPIT*
C	Communities in question
E	Education – type, style, content
S	Subgroup of the community in question
P	Participation of that subgroup
I	Implementation
T	Time to reflect and evaluate

Such an approach is by no means novel and could be seen as a little torturous, however returning to our opening discourse involving language and the queer philosophy of usurping pejorative terms and making them ones of pride, it seems appropriate to usurp the famous James Anderton quote that homosexuals are swirling around in a CESPIT of their own making.

REFERENCES

Berridge, V. (1996) *AIDS in the UK. The Making of Policy 1981–1994*. Oxford: Oxford University Press.

Corrigan, N. (1996) Sometimes quick and always dirty: volunteers at gay men fighting AIDS as researchers. In *Building Bridges: Linking Research and Primary HIV Prevention*. Conference report. ed. Deverell, K. London: Nam.

Davies, D. & Neal, C. (1996) *Pink Therapy. A Guide for Counsellors and Therapists Working with Lesbian, Gay and Bisexual Clients*. Buckingham: Open University Press.

Department of Health (DoH) (1992) *The Health of the Nation*. London: HMSO.

Fee, E. & Fox, D.M. (1992) *AIDS: The Making of a Chronic Disease*. Berkeley.

Garfield, S. (1994) *The End of Innocence. Britain in the Time of AIDS*. London: Faber and Faber.

Grimshaw, J. (1989) The individual challenge. AIDS and cultural politics. In *Taking Liberties. Ecstatic antibodies*. eds Carter, E. & Watney, S. London: Rivers Oram Press.

Hand, L. (1948) Commissioner V National Carbide Corporation. In *The Oxford Dictionary of Humorous*. ed. Sherrin, N. (1995) New York: Oxford University Press.

Harrison, T. (1995). Gay men and sexual health. *Agenda* (March-May). Manchester: George House Trust.

Odets, W. (1995) *Living in the Shadow of the Epidemic*. London: Cassell.

Paton, C. (1990) *Inventing AIDS*. London: Routledge.

Pratt, R.J. (1992) *AIDS A Strategy for Nursing Care*. London: Edward Arnold.

Scott, P. (1995) *Purchasing HIV Prevention. A No Nonsense Guide for Working with Gay and Bisexual Men*. London: HEA.

Shiltz, R. (1987) *And the Band Played on: Politics, People and the AIDS Epidemic*. New York: Penguin.

Tannahill, A. (1985) What is Health Promotion? *Health Education Journal*, 44(4): p 167–168.

Treichler, P. A. (1987) AIDS, homophobia and bio-medical discourse. An epidemic of signification. *Cultural Studies*, 1(3) Cited in *Ecstatic Antibodies*. Boffin, T. & Gupta, S. (1990) London: Rivers Oram Press.

Trueman, C. & Gudgion, G. (1996) Community Based Needs Assessment: A View from the Bridge In *Building Bridges: Linking Research and Primary HIV Prevention*. (conference report) ed. Deverell, K. Nam.

FURTHER READING

Evans, B., Sandberg, S. & Watson S. Eds (1992) *Working where the Risks Are: Issues in HIV Prevention.* London: HEA.

An overview of many issues pertaining or relevant to gay men's health promotion in relation to HIV.

Kramer, L. (1995) *Reports from the Holocaust.* London: Cassell.

Larry Kramer is one of the most well known gay activists in the field of HIV/AIDS – while he is not always a majority voice this text details the strategies and realities of gay men working together in the fight against AIDS.

Scott, P. (1995) *Purchasing HIV Prevention. A No Nonsense Guide for Working with Gay and Bisexual Men.* London: HEA.

A singularly unprissy, pragmatic and sensible approach to arranging gay men's health services within the frameworks of the purchaser/provider split.

Weatherburn, P., Hunt, A.J., Hickson, F.C.I. & Davies, P.M. (1992) *The Sexual Lifestyles of Gay and Bisexual Men in England and Wales.* London: Project Sigma.

The research data on gay men's views of their own sexual acts and intrigues as gathered by Project SIGMA from a huge sample group.

13 Health promotion for older people

Gordon Evans

KEY ISSUES
- Demographic trends
- Health-related legislation and older people
- Older people as health consumers
- Primary Care Groups and their influences upon older people
- Health screening in old age
- Pressure groups
- Education initiatives
- Strategies for specific health issues

This chapter focuses upon the importance of health promotion for older people. Those over retirement age are in an age band that is rapidly increasing within our society, many with both years and life left to enjoy (OPCS, 1995). The dynamic concept of health promotion will be explored as it relates to older people with health being viewed as an expansion of the consciousness encompassing the elements of mind, body and social context. Whilst there are a numerous examples of positive practice, ageism and inequitable practices are highlighted and challenged. This provides a focus for the reader to reflect upon their own areas of influence and care provision. Whilst the debate is focused around the issue of either integrating older people into mainstream health promotion or whether to have a specialism for older people. It is clearly never too late to implement health promotion strategies and investment in both human and financial resources can only be beneficial.

INTRODUCTION

The popular stereotype of older people as possibly ill, lonely and confused is far from true. Over three-quarters of people over 65 years of age report that they see themselves as in good health, with ill health tending to be more prevalent in those over the age of 85 years. The view of the young old (those over retirement age) and the older old (those over 75 years of age) is being developed. However, there may be some decline in health and independence due to a reduction in physical abilities as we get into old age (Carnegie, 1992). The concept of health has many meanings and many expectations to all sorts of people. It is important to start from a focused philosophical base point, where health and the older person is considered a determinant of the individual and the individual is considered as an active agent involved in their own surroundings. The approach to the philosophy may colour the way that the the

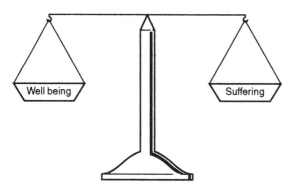

Figure 13.1 Health in old age

paradigm is viewed. The importance and effects upon taking a holistic approach to meeting the needs of older people are profound (Ewles and Simnett, 1995).

The cries of adding years to life and life to years should be made a reality for older people. Where younger age groups would not only expect but demand such an approach, many older people may still view health promotion as an unwelcome intrusion into their lives or at best a leaflet distribution exercise. It is breaking such perceptions in older people and pushing back the ageist barriers that exist both in health and social care professionals as well as strategist that are the real challenges. The concept of health in old age is often centred around accepted levels of independence with older people and the health and social care agencies accepting that the focus needs to be put upon balancing interactions between the states of suffering and well-being experienced by older people. This often leads to a state of adapted independence (Fig. 13.1) though at times the older person may feel that the suffering they are experiencing is an inevitable consequence of old age, a myth to be challenged.

Older people and health care professionals may have differing perspectives of health, particularly as it relates to old age. A list of differing perspectives is given in Box 13.1. Health has a number of facets which for some includes goals and targets to achieve. Governments establish targets as an approach to managing and monitoring services. Investment may be directed towards reducing an identified disease process, though at the same time accepting that individuals with other equally important ill-health episodes may not be receiving the same attention through government-funded initiatives. For some, health is seen as an absence of illness; whilst this may be possible in old age, a reduced level of function may be noticed. Importantly the focus should be upon quality of life coupled with the older person's perception of a positive old age. This is an area where at times the older person's personal expectations may need to be raised.

BOX 13.1	*Perspective of health*
■ *Goal/target* ■ *Oblivian of illness* ■ *Quality of life*	■ *Investment* ■ *Absence of disease*

CONTEXT

Demographic trends

The population of the UK is projected to rise to 61.3 million by the year 2011. The proportion of those over 65 years of age among the total population is expected to continue to rise and to approach 20% by the year 2011 (McGlone, 1992). A rapid rise in the proportion of those aged 85 and over will occur when the large groups born before and just after World War One reach this age. Relatively few people were born in the late 1920s and 1930s, so much smaller increases are expected in the proportion of young pensioners by the year 2011. By the years 2020–2030, those born during the 1960s baby boom will re-enter the dependency part of the population as pensioners and the dependency ratio is expected to rise sharply (OPCS, 1995). All of these factors make this a very important group of people within the population to include when planning health promotion initiatives.

Health-related legislation and older people

The Patient's Charter includes a commitment to establish general services that may be of both interest and benefit to older people. Where the Charter makes a clear commitment to individuals with acute ill-health episodes, the additional support for those with chronic conditions is very limited and often left to individual interpretation of service provision at a local level. Improved services could improve the quality of life in general for older people. *Caring for People* (DoH, 1989) and part three of the National Health Service and Community Care Act include some additional aspects of care provision which can improve the health of older people. Emotional health could improve as many older people would wish to remain supported in their own homes rather than to be admitted into continuing care establishments. A model of health in old age that is emerging centres around the concepts that underpin the World Health Organization's Ottowa Charter (1986) including:

- Absence of disease
- Optimal functional status
- Adequate system of social support

Despite extensive debate highlighting the importance of promoting the health of older people, it remains unclear at a national level the true commitment to such a concept. This was highlighted by Harvey and Fralick (1997), who reviewed the implementation of *The Health of the Nation* targets and found there were 26 national targets which were set in five key areas and some had not been accepted at a local level. Over half of the responding trusts indicated that they either had not accepted the targets or had made modifications. Such actions throws into question the effectiveness of a national strategy; it also has profound implications for health promotion activities at a local level. It is hoped that the more recent *Our Healthier Nation* targets are found to benefit older people more favourably. *The Health of the Nation* targets that were reported as not being actioned in all areas, which have implications for older people are those listed in Box 13.2

BOX 13.2	*The Health of the Nation targets affecting older people*

- Reduce the death rate for stroke in people aged 65–74 years of age by 40% by the year 2000
- Reduce the death rate from coronary heart disease in people 65–74 years of age by 30% by the year 2000

(DoH, 1992)

It is to be hoped that *Our Healthier Nation* (DoH, 1998) principles are given much more support and do in fact underpin an emerging national strategy. It is outlined how good health is to be treasured; such a foundation will underpin improvements in both the country's health and its economy. Inequalities in health are again highlighted, along with socio-economic factors as contributors to poor health. The government's two key aims are listed in Box 13.3.

BOX 13.3	*Aims of Our Healthier Nation*

1. To improve the health of the population as a whole by increasing the length of people's lives and the number of years people spend free from illness
2. To improve the health of the people who are worst off in society and to narrow the health gap

(DoH, 1998)

The extent to which health promotion is mobilised is influenced by basic economics coupled with powerful economic and political influencing lobbies from commerce, manufacturing industries and tobacco industries. All of these factors exert a strong influence over the lifestyle and environment of older people (Holland, 1992). It is often left to local groups to integrate or initiate new health promotion practices. Health professionals can work to identify measures to improve the public's health. However, they cannot select public health priorities alone – this must be done in collaboration with the public and key organisations. Both factors are central to the new primary care groups. The discussions that surround socio-economic inequalities are not new and their existence has been noted though they are not accepted by some. These implications for older people are quite notable. In 1977, the Research Working Group on *Inequalities in Health* – The Black Report was convened. Its findings were not welcomed by the government of the day when it was published in 1980; copies though in short supply were read with interest on both sides of the Atlantic (DoH, 1980). Promoting health in people at all ages should be viewed as an investment, particularly for those of old age. However as old age and retirement might in some instances encompass half a century, such a group should not be excluded from initiatives (Smith, Bartley and Blane, 1990). Whilst some commentators describe the existence of a two-tiered health system (Kammering and Kinnear, 1996), a strong case continues to be made that all health provision including health promotion should be provided with equity based upon need. A key contribution of the Black Report has been the importance of differentiating between the quality of life experienced by an individual and the extension of life measured in years. Both are central to the discussion relating to health promotion and older people. Hunt (1997) describes Britain's middle classes as holding the key to improving the health of the poorest people in society. Real opportunities exist to promote health in the community, particularly directed towards older people. Whilst the targets proposed in *Our Healthier Nation* (DoH, 1998) clearly do not directly affect elderly people, they will prepare future generations to enter old age in a much healthier condition. Where some of the declared four targets do focus upon the under 65 year olds, the last of the three setting of contracts for health action must be turned to for innovation and dynamism. Healthy neighbourhoods focusing upon older people will be areas in which local alliances will be formed that may include commerce. Health inequalities continue to be fashionable to discuss, which is often due to the middle classes not feeling threatened about their own state of health. This it is hoped will encourage people from all ranks to speak for the nation's health. Making health promotion a national platform and local issue within the primary care groups will promote health and remove health inequalities.

Older people as health consumers

'Onwards and upwards,' the cry of many unions in the 1980s, is still alive today. As we move to a stance of empowerment of citizens including older people, providing real choices and equity is of paramount importance. At the inception of the National Health Service (NHS), the key question was 'can I be cured'? Today the focus of patients' enquiries is different. Clearly they expect more, are better informed and wish to know what their choices are. Ideally placed to discuss such options are health care practitioners. Regrettably though extensive debate exists around the issue of care rationing, at times directed primarily at older people. Viewing them as major users of both health and social care resources, viewed at times as a drain upon the existing resources. Such issues are not new. However, recent changes in the marketplace of care has meant that this as an issue has come to the fore (Harrison and Hunter, 1993). Seen as frustrating with the more recent surge of interest in care rationing is that cost effectiveness and high quality of care are polarised at extremes of the same scale. Great emphasis should be made that high-quality care can be cost effective. The idea of rationing health care would seem to contradict the principles upon which the NHS was established; it also appears to conflict with medical ethics which hold doctors duty bound to do the very best for their patients.

Rationing is inevitable in any health care system where services are not directly charged to the patient, but are paid for through a third person in this case central government. In this system, consumer demands will be increased around services that are free and what consumers perceive as good. Providers may be driven in their decisions of what range of care to provide by anticipated long-term overall benefits to society as a whole. General practitioners (GPs) are expressing concern over health care rationing. The new era rationing is being carried out by GPs by either establishing their own waiting lists or waiting to block book patients for procedures, thus taking benefit of a marketplace economy to receive discounted costs for block contracts (Ayres, 1996). It is against this backcloth that it is vital that promoting health is in the range of care choices. The processes of psycho-neuroimmunology are well recognised, though not necessarily well respected by all. This is where positive thoughts and body images are portrayed upon the mind which in turn influence the body's immune system. When applying those principles to older people, it is very relevant to encourage an older person to think positively in order to promote a healthy immune system (Evans, 1991). This ability of being in a state of readiness for their bodies to be able fight opportunistic infections and other health challenges is desirable to both the individual and the country at large.

It is important to remember that most older people live in their own homes within the community. It has been found that 95% of all those over retirement age live in their own homes either alone or supported by family and friends, whilst the remaining 5% live in continuing care settings such as nursing homes/residential homes and hospital wards (OPCS, 1995). Arithrodynamics, a concept to outline the location of older people based upon where they live and the inference that they may at times of ill-health and social crisis move from being community based to living, albeit in the short term, in a continuing care setting, highlights the need for community-based older people to retain their health as inadequate numbers of continuing care placements exist. Older individuals have been found to adapt to disabilities in order to retain their independence. A state of learnt independence is seen as desirable where possible, where resources to provide health and social care are limited. It is clear that health promotion for older people is not only about primary interventions, but also is at a secondary and tertiary level of helping the individual to live within the limitations that illness and disability may have produced.

Primary Care Groups and their effects upon older people

Hanlon (1990) emphasises the need for having a structured approach to the provision of health promotion. Whilst there is a place for opportunistic interventions, a strong case exists for the formulation of strategies. It is also important to encourage older people to view health promotion as a treatment option. Where blame is not attached to being ill, more should be directed to an opportunity and responsibility of the individual to move where possible to an improved state of health. There is a strong case to move away from a model of medicalistion and cure, at times this is the only acceptable approach for some service consumers. Health promotion has a fundamental part to play in assisting older people with chronic disabilities to develop a state of adjusted independence. With the introduction of GP fundholding and payment schedules for health promotion clinics (Le Touse, 1996), in some areas there was a clear indication made that such sessions were only for younger age groups. 'Too late and too expensive' might have been the claims made when considering the provision of health promotion for older people (Killoran, 1993). Coupled with the view expressed by some GPs that if an illness or disability came to light, the older person might be both encouraged and motivated to attend the GP surgery more often and expect treatment, though this was clearly found not to be the case. Where older people were predicted to be the new unpopular patient based upon the unfounded view that they are a drain of resources, it was soon realised that the middle-aged individual with a chronic illness quickly was assigned this role. GPs have claimed that in the past they have found themselves in a situation where they were financially encouraged and rewarded to provide health screening and health promotion sessions but with no additional revenue to meet the care costs of illness detection. The role of primary care teams and more specifically that of GPs should not be overlooked. Therefore they should be viewed as pivotal to the decision process of both care and health promotion to their practice population. In theory it would mean giving GPs regular updated information on the recent health promotion material and an analysis of how it might influence commissioning. Salter's (1991) earlier work that urged GPs to review their focus for health promotion strategies, with the initiative to establish primary care groups is even more pertinent. Such groups will initiate health improvement programmes for their own local community that will run on a 3-year basis. It is envisaged that the GPs will chair such groups and have majority influence, though nurses and other professionals allied to medicine should along with their medical colleagues direct attention to wide issues and not lose sight of those of particular marginalised groups. These groups could include clients who are mentally ill have learning disabilities or are elderly. We must also not lose sight of older people themselves and the views that they might offer on the adequacy and appropriateness of health promotion if approached as service users. Evaluation of service users is central to the monitoring of the activities of primary care teams.

Health screening in old age

When screening was introduced for older people from the age of 75 years, having an integrated service regardless of age that these client can attend along with individuals from other age groups may go some way to remove ageist practices that are often evident. Brown and Groom (1995) found that where the general practice was smaller with fewer patients, a more personal service was perceived to be provided to older people. This was often coupled with a higher than average uptake of health checks in such a client group. Such increased levels of involvement with services provides a greater opportunity to introduce health promotion activities. It might also be the case that those who attend health screening sessions are the healthy people whose lifestyle needs very little attention. A key issue is how to attract the older person who does not attend, without promoting a victim-blaming approach. They may feel that such sessions do not apply or are not relevant to them. Similar parallels can be drawn to the pregnant mother – the challenge is to attract those who are reluctant to attend. In both arenas the individual is not only denying themselves the opportunity for health check-ups but also the linked opportunity for access to health promotion initiatives and advice. Initiatives such as mobile day hospitals and care centres that visit different geographical locations such as seen in North Yorkshire, take services to the older people at home and may go some way to increasing the uptake of health promotion initiatives. However it was felt that the introduction of an increased capitation fee for older people on the General Practice lists may go some way for the GP to encourage involvement with the over 75 year olds.

Initiatives such as improving the nutritional status of older people was highlighted by the joint working party of the English National Board (ENB) and the Department of Health (DoH), which worked to produce benchmarks to identify

This activity is intended to encourage individuals to critically review health promotion activities that may influence their lives and determine the relevance and appropriateness to older people.

Visit your local health centre and from your observations address the following points:

1. From the health promotion literature available in the waiting area, decide the potential relevance and appropriateness to older people.
2. A wide range of health promotion activities are now available at health centres. From the displays available, determine which if any are either deliberately targeted at older people or might be used by such an age group.
3. If older people were to attend the health centre, particularly those with mobility problems, how easily accessible is the building where activities take place?

good practices (Watson, 1993). This related both to the content of educational courses and the work/care environment. Moves were then made at local levels to highlight the real energies and motivators behind such developments.

Hancock (1993) made clear the case for nurses to be partners in the primary care setting and as such would play a major part in care provision and the health promotion activities (RCN, 1993). The older person might be viewed by some as the new unpopular patient, being old with many years of potential life left, also being articulate and knowing their rights however in some cases having a multiple pathology.

Sidell (1995) describes the myth that such a drain on resources occurs, going on to highlight differing approaches adopted by older people to cope with experiences of ill-health. This all leads to a potential drain of health and social care resources. It is not suprising that often a conscious decision is made by both the service provider and older person to promote a state of adjusted independence.

COMMUNITY DEVELOPMENTS AND PARTICIPATION

There is a need to focus health care initiatives at three distinct levels:

1. To consider the current literature and research that relates specifically to the chosen area,
2. To analyse and interpret such information, highlighting threads and themes that may inform practice or guide further research activities.
3. To translate such work into everyday practice.

All three levels of engagement are important and supplement and support each other, although the value is in the latter level. Emphasis should be placed upon the older people's expectations of health events. It might be that advice, support and attempts to refocus the older person's philosophy of health are needed (Box 13.4).

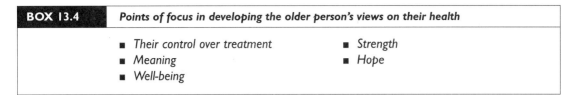

BOX 13.4 | *Points of focus in developing the older person's views on their health*

- *Their control over treatment*
- *Meaning*
- *Well-being*

- *Strength*
- *Hope*

The patient's needs should be the focus throughout a during health care professional/client interaction. The nursing focus can be developed with emphasis on the following issues:

- *Helping*
- *Life-saving initiatives*
- *Interpersonal activities*
- *Activities of daily living-based skills*
- *Sensitivity to the patient/client and themselves*
- *Advocacy for promoting health needs.*

Accidents in old age

More than 300 000 individuals over 65 years of age attend Accident and Emergency (A&E) departments each year in England and Wales as a result of accidents in the home, the majority of which are falls (Bowling, 1992). It has been estimated that between 5–10% of falls result in injury, the most common of which are fractures. These injuries account for 40% of the deaths in this age group (Nuffield Institute, 1996). Falls in old age are a major cause of morbidity and may lead to reduced independence. Such is the extent of the problem that reducing falls in vulnerable groups of individuals such as the young and old were a focus in *The Health of the Nation* targets. Community surveys suggest that about one-third of elderly people experience a fall during a 12-month period. Whilst a whole range of factors may have contributed to an individual's fall, clear regard has been paid to reviewing risk factors that may exist in the environment.

Bowling (1992) highlights how little research-based evidence exists on potential medical causes of falls in old age. Health promotion initiatives are wide and varied, including the improvement of the uptake of eye testing. The health promotion practitioners armoury of potential actions are wide and varied, and relate to this issue. There is some evidence to suggest that improving an individual's body posture is effective in reducing the risk of falls in older people. The introduction of Tai Chi classes for older people at some day centres is hoped will strengthen joints and develop balance in older people (Effective Health Care, 1996). Such interventions play a part in improving balance as well as reducing what might appear to some as an accelerated bone loss. GPs would need to be convinced of the benefits and possibly the cost-effectiveness of such activities before they might prescribe such activities to their patients for therapeutic benefit.

A range of health promotion interventions exist, the most appropriate one is tailored to the older individual (Box 13.5). The aim of reducing falls in old age highlights the range of options available to both health care professionals and older people. It allows the development of a model underpinned by the event

BOX 13.5	*Health promotion options to reduce falls in old age*
■ Home assessments ■ High-dose vitamin D ■ Fitting shoes ■ Stopping and talking	■ Protector pads ■ Balance training ■ Carers' first aid skills

of a risk assessment. This is then followed by the formulation of care plans that are supported by wide-ranging research. Current literature highlights practices that are based upon basic issues such as ensuring that older people are wearing well fitting footwear. Interestingly, it has been found that the most stable shoe for older people is not the commonly worn trainer but the thinner-soled footwear with a firmer middle arch (Robbins et al, 1992). There is growing interest, though it is not put actively into practice, in the padding of joints that are vulnerable to fractures if older people fall. Traditional medical-based interventions are not ignored, such as the provision of a high-dose vitamin D supplement diet. Dietary advice is of particular importance during winter months and in the housebound, low levels of vitamin D are found, which leads to a lowering of bone densities (Gloth, Gundberg and Hollis, 1995). One interesting development are the local projects where older people have been trained to carry out home assessments on other older people. The advantages of this programme are a low running cost and a high acceptance by older people both assessing and being assessed. The participants visit an older person's home to carry out a risk assessment relating to potential risk of falls and then provide practical and realistic advice (North Yorkshire Specialist Health Promotion Service, 1997).

Exercise to aid mobility

Opportunities exist for all health care staff involved at the interface with older people to promote exercise and educate older people and their carers in a range of activities that will promote health. The benefits of such actions are wide ranging and include the easing of arthritic joints and reducing falls in old age. Improved body posture through Thai Chi and yoga can improve individuals' balance. When considering health in the wider context, the ability to mobilise in order to bring about social interaction through mobility is of paramount importance. Advice, clear leaflets and a stressed importance of foot care can be the basis of achieving such targets. With an increasing incidence of diabetes in old age, sound foot care practices are vital. MacKinnon (1993) makes a strong case that health promotion underpins all diabetic care (see Box 13.6).

BOX 13.6	*Health promotion for diabetics*
■ Foot care ■ Wash feet ■ Skin care ■ Information on diabetis ■ Effects upon lifestyle ■ Regular check-ups	■ Eye care ■ Prevent falls ■ Prevent infection ■ Remove fears ■ Clothing issues ■ Early detection of circulation deterioration

Sexual health in old age

This is an area that is fast gathering interest amongst those who care for older people. Extensive debate continues around the notion of sexual health, where at one end of the continuum is the focus on effective sexual intercourse, with all aspects of the physical process working in harmony. At the other end of the continuum are attempts to describe sexuality in terms of a holistic inner feeling associated with the mind and recognition as an individual. Sexual health as a concept is often avoided when care is provided for older people and is not included in health promotion interventions for individuals in this age group. Over recent years, the development of well-men clinics in addition to the already well-established women-related health clinics have focused the attention upon positive health in this age group as an investment for the future. The emergence of human immunodeficiency virus (HIV) has made major contributions to pushing back the boundaries of sexuality and sexual health in old age. Nokes (1996) highlights how 10% of all those known to be infected with HIV in this country are over 55 years of age, whilst many more are affected by the virus, having to come to terms with either their own children or grandchildren being infected (Butler, 1993).

Older people at times may indulge in sexual activities that would lead them to being viewed as engaging in a high-risk lifestyle. A large proportion of current health promotion literature does not reflect the older person as being the focus of such targets. There is a clear need to review the information available and the points of access to both services and information on HIV and other related sexually transmitted diseases. Traditional models depicting the elements of health have now had to be reframed and now include sexual health (Naidoo and Wills, 1994) (see Fig 13.2).

Older people are often viewed at retirement age as developing a state of asexuality, a myth that must be removed. It is often viewed as not important to include health promotion issues in the hospital discharge advice of patients from this age group. Such views are often reflected in the absence from care planning of such necessary actions or even in some instances the removal of sexual health from the care plan format. What is documented in the care plan highlights much more about the author's attitudes to sexual health than often

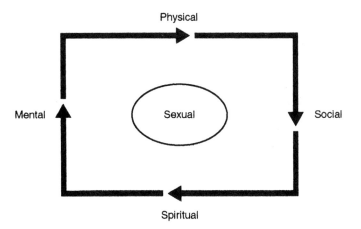

Figure 13.2 Health model

the individual to whom they relate. It is a combination of the British culture of not talking openly about sexual health and the way in which professionals have been developed as part of their ongoing training that leads to what is one of the last taboos in health care and in the wider population to be addressed. Older people today often come from an era where such issues were not openly addressed. This in itself is a barrier to health care staff attempting to promote sexual health. It is particularly problematic where the older individuals accept and promote a negative ageist view about their own health and the relevance of health promotion initiatives to themselves and others in their age band. This is seen where continued attempts are made to impress upon older people the value of safer sexual practices. On occasions it is seen by some older people to indicate that safer sex is not applicable as older women can no longer become pregnant. Though they lose sight that such safer practices can offer a degree of protection from unwelcome infections that would necessitate care by a genitourinary medicine service. This issue necessitates nursing interventions that not only challenge such false beliefs but also inform older people (Hinkle, 1991). Health promotion advice is important at all ages, particularly so in old age. Age Concern England (Age Well, 1997) has mounted extensive campaigns to highlight the cost of human life from not extending routine recalls to mammography screening and cervical screening for all women over retirement age.

A screening service has always been available if requested specifically by the older individual. For others, this has only recently been resolved in some areas as a result of extensive lobbying, where the system of routine recalls after testing has been introduced. It was found that significant improvements were found when screening was offered to women aged 65–74 rather than to individuals in younger age groups. This was thought in part to be attributed to a higher incidence of abnormalities in the older age group.

Similarly, older people who undergo gynaecological surgical procedures should not be denied health promotion advice offered to younger people, simply because of their age. Advice about the effects on sexual activity following some surgical procedures should not be denied because it is viewed as irrelevant because the individual is past retirement age and therefore assumed asexual (Booth, 1990). Similar access to advice should also be made available to older men who undergo surgery for prostate cancer.

Focus upon an older person in your area of practice or local community who has diabetes mellitus or a similar health problem. From the available literature, identify potential problem areas where the individual with diabetes might benefit from health promotion interventions, including:

1. Identify the areas, providing a synopsis of why the individual might be regarded as a health problem.
2. Outline actions that you might take to heighten the individual's health awareness for each issue identified.
3. Relate your proposed interventions to models of health described earlier.

Your responses relating to a diabetic patient might include:-

1. Health problems:
   ■ Reductions in eye sight

- Poor healing of skin lesions
- Falls
- Dietary inadequacies
- Impotence
- Problems with warmth
- Sore areas on feet
- Reduction in social activities.

2. Various information:
- Information leaflets
- Joining local diabetic groups
- Access to appropriate health care agency
  — Podiatrist
  — Specialist clinics.
- Telephone contact points for information
- Meeting other individuals with diabetes.

3. Assessment:
- Group identified problems and interventions under physical/mental/social/spiritual/sexual categories.

The development of exercise is also of benefit in attempts to reduce the progression of osteoporosis in older people. The message is beginning to be understood that such actions can be both enjoyable and develop a positive health benefit. In the ideal world, success might be measured in terms of years rather than months. It has been found that our bone structures are laid down during the teenage years. Where this has not been carried out effectively, it is not until many years later that decay and depletion of the bones' calcium levels are found to cause degenerative problems. Attempts to promote health in old age clearly on this occasion cross many age barriers, beginning with the promotion of a social climate that actively encourages exercise during school years. This is then followed in the mid-life years with bone density scanning to determine those most at risk, due to poor bone formations, of developing osteoporosis at an early age. This can then be used as the rationale for guiding health strategies for early selective interventions. However, current debates, which are quite mixed, have understandably lead to individuals approaching the early introduction of hormone replacement therapy (HRT) with caution. The decision might be to postpone the use of HRT as long as possible because of the suggestions of a potential link with their use and breast cancer, though it does leave the individual very prone to bone degeneration (Compston, 1996). The action in later life, though it is contentious, might be to promote safety in the home situation and teach carers first aid skills. A realistic approach might be to equip carers with the skills necessary to meet common emergencies that they may encounter if the older person falls and has brittle bone structures. Ruddlesden (1994) highlights how care staff in all continuing care settings have a role to play in promoting exercise and mobility not least to prevent mental boredom and develop carer-induced dementia. The latter is a vegetative state brought about by a lack of stimulation and an active desire by care staff to systemise all that is taking place in such settings. The older people are reduced to little more than being fed and watered. This could be said to actively dehumanise elderly people.

Promoting stroke care

It is well accepted that the incidence of stroke increases with age. Stroke is the third most common cause of death in the Western world, with a prediction that 100 000 people will suffer their first stroke this year (Utting, 1995). In addition, it will also lead to serious disability, resulting in premature death in 1 out of 11 individuals in the 65–75 year age group. Current care accounts for 5% of the total NHS expenditure (DoH, 1991; 1995), with 25 000 people dying each year from strokes, heart diseases and related illnesses (DoH, 1998). With an anticipated increased prevalence in stroke of 30% this will remain a major health care and health promotion challenge for many years. It is clear that the focus of health promotion interventions in this arena currently lies with preventative work. One area to explore is the support and guidance of those living with stroke and their carers. Tertiary interventions are often not viewed as ideal, but do assist individuals to live a reasonably independent lives with what can only be described as a learnt dependence.

INFORMAL ELDERLY CARERS

A growing number of areas now have support groups for carers with a focus on support, respite and education. Another important benefit gained by elderly carers is the reduction of their stress levels, as their mood can be affected by the one they support, and pressures of the relationship can be quite tense at times. Efforts need to be made to identify hallmarks of good practice when carer support is considered. Purchasers of services must adopt a position of benchmarking to emphasise service parameters and what can be expected.

One area to review is the preparation of carers for their role as hands-on carers. It is not adequate to leave such a group to develop their care skills on an ad hoc, experimental basis. Such programmes should be developed that reflect the identified needs of carers to enable them to face their challenges and include aspects of a preventative nature that reduce the chance of ill-health developing both for the carer and the cared for. In the current health and social care climate where funded resources are limited, it is important and in everyone's interest to ensure that what are described as the 'silent army of elderly carers' do not reduce in number or lose their momentum. There is an importance to further develop collaborative links between agencies, which include the voluntary and private sector to demonstrate the need for agencies to work together more effectively.

Mr Wilson, who is 80 years old is due home from hospital next week after having experienced a stroke. When planning his care to be implemented on his return home, you decide to determine the needs of his wife who will take on the role of principle carer. His wife is younger than he is (69 years old), though reasonably fit. He is of heavy build and she is described as 'slight', though very willing and feels duty bound to be his carer. She describes her duties as 'part of the marriage vows – for better or for worse'. Outline what could be implemented to prepare her to care for her husband on a day-to-day basis.

Focus particularly on advising her regarding care and support interventions based on the activities of daily living (Roper, Logan and Tierney, 1983).

You should include in your answer:

1. Support for Mrs Wilson
   - Link to caring for carers group, e.g. Crossroads
   - Provide contact point for local stroke support group
   - Advise her of the national stroke support network
   - Details of your contact point
   - Take time to listen to her views and worries.
2. Preparation for care role
   - Techniques for moving and handling her husband
   - Approaches to communication where this is a challenge
   - Meeting dietary needs where this is going to be different from usual
   - Assisting with dressing her husband
   - Self-management to avoid stress and burnout
   - Social Security benefits and how to access the system
     — Negotiation of health and social care support.

Positive aspects of mental health

Pender (1987) describes the importance of attempting to ensure that older people along with people of other age bands are able to cope and adjust to the life crises they will meet. Their strength is that they have experience of making such adjustments in their own lives.

In addition, the older person may have come through life with a predisposition to responding in a negative manner to life's challenges and the way they cope in old age is no different to earlier life. On attaining old age, individuals can be left with feelings of low self-worth, loss of purpose in life and at times a lack of drive. It is not a surprise that depression and suicide are seen commonly. It has been stated by Blazer et al (1994) that one in 20 individuals experience depression and as much as 20% of all suicides in the UK are by people over retirement age (Blazer, 1994). Health screening should be already established prior to retirement age and at set intervals afterwards, and should always be seen as an opportunity to review the individual's mental state.

Gearing, Johnson and Heller (1988) highlight the range of mental phenomena presented in old age. It is at times difficult to determine what is normal and to what extent ill health is presented to the point where intervention is required at any age. However, it is clear that at times life crises and the environment in which the individual lives plays a part in the development of mental health deterioration. When the older person is often subjected to an institutional routine that removes their need to think or participate in the decision-making processes, they become dehumanised and at times reduced to a state of an object that is merely fed and watered. In instances such as this, it is important for those with authority to act promptly and initiate changes. The long-term benefits of health promotion in this instance is for the benefit of developing a positive quality of life for the older person, whilst the initial target of intervention need to be clearly directed at the carers (Phair and Good, 1995).

Norman and Redfern (1995) considers the need for developing mechanisms to audit and monitor nursing care to such vulnerable groups as older people. Indirect benefit is to be gained by raising the awareness of care staff to the holistic needs of older people and how they might be met; the barriers to the range of options to enriching the older person's life is often the limitation of the care staff's minds. A strong case can be made for shaking off the medical model and going down the route of promoting a social model that will underpin care. The latter is more likely in the majority of cases to promote the activities of the mind, develop a feeling of worth in the older person and reduce dependency on others.

Promoting activities that stimulate the care staff as well as the older individual into engaging in activities and reducing the introduction of a routine will in turn benefit the mental health of the older person. This might include participation in team meetings, education opportunities or simply a health promotion theme for the month. However, we must not lose sight of this rising incidence of older people who experience bouts of clinical depression. They in the main come from an era that is supportive of the medical model and in turn are very cautious where medical interventions are not offered. Medication by many is viewed as much more beneficial than the skilled intervention of psycho-therapeutic techniques. This coupled with the 'stiff upper lip syndrome,' which dictates that episodes of mental illness should not be expressed to others for fear of being classed as 'weak' and a 'social outcast' makes intervention at times difficult (McKeon, 1986). Clare (1994) goes on to highlight how it will take time to address the cultural issue and attitudes, and to encourage a situation where it is accepted to voice feeling about an individual's own feelings of mental health. Some of the hallmarks to promoting mental health in the older person include ensuring acceptable noise levels to the older person, taking time to talk with someone that they trust and to be heard, though prevention of boredom and the positive promotion of social interaction should be an initial prerequisite. At times a major barrier to the promotion of health including that of mental health is the older person themselves. They may see retirement as an excuse not to get involved and support the view that they should become passive observers of life.

HEALTHY ALLIANCES

Current developments in practice are towards collaboration between differing agencies. This can be seen in such schemes as Manchester's Crucial Crew Scheme that addresses accident prevention. Developments around elder abuse illustrate the effectiveness of collaboration and can be used as a template to illustrate the effectiveness of collaboration. It also makes the case for a clear national strategy that can be a driving force for local groups. It is becoming clear that no one organisation is able to promote health in an effective manner. To have a global perspective, making use of the many resources both physical and human that exist is a positive proactive strategy. A failing of many health promotion initiatives that are of special benefit to older people is that they are not at times brought together as part of a wider network. There is also a clear need to highlight and publicise examples of good practice to a wide range of people in both the statutory and voluntary sectors, with a view to developing a system of benchmarking. These would then be the baseline standards and aims built into commissioning contracts.

Enormous interest is now being generated into issues that relate to elder abuse, a topic that has existed for at least the last decade but has only recently achieved standing on individual, local and national agendas. As an issue it encompasses the elements of health in that abuse in any form has the potential to diminish the health of the individual who is abused. Additionally, the dynamics within the family unit where this is taking place can be expected to be strained and this in turn may cause health deficit for the carer, who may also be the perpetrator of such abusive actions (Ogg and Bennett 1992). Action on Elder Abuse have brought together many agencies both from the voluntary and statutory sectors to address these problems.

Whilst there is a growing realisation that elder abuse both exists and has been present in this country for some years, a clear reluctance is demonstrated to accepting the well-developed work on this topic from the USA. The earlier framework developed by Eastman (1984) and more recently updated (Eastman, 1996), continues to underpin the operational framework both in this country and the USA.

The work over recent years highlights all that is positive and possible when addressing a health issue; the model that is emerging is one that can be applied to a number of other health issues that might be seen as benefiting from health promotion at all levels. Initial work is focused upon raising the level of consciousness to the ramifications of elder abuse, the effects upon the individual and the carer which may affect their health. Action on Elder Abuse is a national agency in its own right which took on the lead role in highlighting this as an issue and brought together many interested individuals and organisations. From the outset a combination of information provision and support of a behavioural change model was adopted in an attempt to make inroads into reviewing care practices. The core issues of elder abuse raise much more debate about the quality of life of older people. It is not sufficient to enable older people to maximise their life potential – there is a need to review the quality of those additional years.

Current debate is focused on removing the notion that elder abuse is a medical label for a social phenomena that is influenced by people and various situations encountered. With demedicalisation, society at large might take a much heightened interest and a move would be witnessed that is proactive compared to today's scenario, which is mainly reactionary.

Jenkins (1993) does question whether the Health and Social Care agencies are geared up to face such challenges of a raised awareness to elder abuse and the potential increased reporting of such events. National lobbies can have an influence on legislation and the resulting health-relating interventions. Action on Elder Abuse took the lead role in guiding and supporting the development of a framework that might be used to develop education programmes at a post-graduate level by the health care professionals. In addition, they acted as a catalyst for the development of education support material to meet the outcomes of elder abuse to be addressed by those working to achieve the outcome statements for National Vocational Awards. Such interventions provide care givers the opportunity to review the care delivered and the environment of care, hopefully resulting in a reduction of mental health stressors. Developments at a local level require individual organisations to collaborate, initially for the purposes of formulating joint strategy documents. Ongoing evaluation of such work from a strategy formulation stage to that of implementation needs to be carried out.

Where there are already numerous studies that are service/incidence orientated, little work exists that focuses upon an evaluation from the users perspective. Addressing behavioural approaches of promoting health takes considerably longer, though the benefits are greater and ongoing. The approach to raising public levels of knowledge and ownership of issues encourages a sustained campaign and continuation of the venture.

Mr Wilson and his wife live at home and have support from the community nursing team, who visit daily and attend to dressings on Mrs Wilson's leg ulcers. When you visit as a family friend, you notice that over a period of 3 weeks you are aware of mixed bruising appearing on her arms and legs. You have a suspicion that Mrs Wilson is being abused. On one of your visits, she was found to be upset and withdrawn. On discussion with Mrs Wilson, she confides in you that she is being abused but doesn't wish any action to be taken.

1. What action might be taken in this situation? Check that your planned actions are harmonious with your local policies if you work within a voluntary or statutory agency.
2. Because Mrs Wilson stated that she does not wish you to take any direct action, consider how her health might be placed at risk and outline the action that you might take.

Your answer might include:

1. arranging shorter but more frequent visits
2. organising with Mrs Wilson's agreement for other social agencies to visit as this might lesson the tensions and chances of further abuse
3. taking extra time to talk in general with Mrs Wilson
4. informing Mrs Wilson of help that might be available for specialist help:
    ■ Action on Elder Abuse
    ■ Age Concern
    ■ Samaritans
    ■ Marriage guidance
    ■ Local priests, if appropriate

Another high profile group who have a leading part to play in informing the provision of services and the development of health promotion is MIND. Their area of focus is mental health care, with particular reference to carers and the ongoing support of those who have experienced mental health problems. Where services are being developed, they have a key role to play in guiding care providers. In addition, they develop information packs relating to hospital admission that are viewed as user friendly. A development appearing over recent years is the provision of education events that guide those who have mental health problems (such as stress), and their carers.

STRATEGIES AND EVALUATION

Community nurses are well placed to have an influence over individuals in the community. A major change in role is needed for both district nurses and health visitors to take on fresh challenges of health promotion and to maximise such individual's specialist skills. Health visitors have been acknowledged for their acclaimed interest from the cradle to the grave. District nurses' skills are better utilised, not just as hands-on care givers but as supervisors, advisors and assessors of need. This will give time for the needs of carers and untrained staff to be identified and developed. With the aim to develop the care skills in others, health promotion plays a very important role in such situations. Aspects of positive living along with the reduction of health deficits would feature centrally in such innovations. Formulating networks of carers and supporters would act as a focus for passing out new health promotion messages and campaigns. Despite extensive attempts to elevate the debates about health promotion in the older diabetic client, major areas for further development still exist. Regrettably it was not identified as a *Health of the Nation* (DoH, 1992) or more recently *Our Healthier Nation* (DoH, 1998) target. However, serious health issues exist that can benefit from health promotion. They should include a 'look after your feet' emphasis, as it is predicted that many early problems with circulation initially present themselves in the feet of diabetics. Education to care for the feet of diabetic individuals is vital, including advice about shoes and observations of the feet. Accessibility of health promotion service provision is important for older people. Discussions in other health arenas have included the establishment of health shops. These are both information and advice centres, situated at central locations to include shopping malls, libraries, and local age-specific voluntary groups. Where this is not viewed as practicable or desirable, health promotion therefore needs to be integrated into all specialisms without ageist barriers. The need to revisit health promotion as a condition of continued practice for nurses has never been greater.

Additionally, the need to review how health promotion is intertwinned in pre-registration courses has never been greater.

CONCLUSIONS

Health promotion is everyone's business. A strong case can be made for it to be integrated into all aspects of health care. It can be seen that resources in the arena of health and social care are limited and great benefits can be achieved in encouraging individuals to adopt a healthy lifestyle, though older people like people in other age groups may not wish to go down this road. The concept of health has many facets, all of which clearly apply to this age group. To ignore or exclude any aspect of health promotion in such an age group is perilous. Health promotion for older people is most effective as part of a multi-agency approach that involves national directives and local application. This is currently being seen in the moves both centrally and locally to bring about, for example, the introduction of automatic recall for women over retirement age for breast screening. The provision of health promotion for older people should be initiated where possible early in life. This is characterised with the proposal to return to free school milk and compulsory exercise in an attempt to reduce osteoporosis in later life. However, efforts directed toward people at any age are beneficial. At a time of financial constraints placed upon health and social care provision, there is a need to turn the concept of 'a value for money service' on its head and refocus our efforts upon *a service that we value*. Cost cutting coupled with ignoring a large proportion of our population is not to be promoted as a wise move; health promotion can be performed in an effective manner but the delusion that it is cheap clearly must be challenged. An indication of civilisation is seen in the way a society cares and values its elders. Health promotion should be seen as a right in old age and an indicator of how we value those individuals in this age group.

REFERENCES

Age Well (1993) *Planning and Ideas Pack*. London: Age Concern England.

Ayres, P. (1996) Rationing health care – views from general practice. *Social Science and Medicine*, **42**(7): 1021–1025.

Blazer, D., Kessler, R., Mc Gonagle, K. & Swartz, M. (1994) The prevalence and distribution of major depression in a national community sample: The national comorbidity survey. *American Journal of Psychiatry*, **151**: 979–986.

Booth, B. (1990) Does it really matter at that age? *Nursing Times*, **86**(3): 50–52.

Bowling, A. (1992) Accidents in elderly care: a randomised controlled trial. *Nursing Standard*, **6**(29): 28–31.

Brown, K. and Groom, L. (1995) General practice health checks of elderly people: a county wide survey. *Health Trends*, **27**(3): 89–91.

Butler, R. N. (1993) AIDS: older people are not immune. *Geriatrics*, **48**(3): 9–10.

Carnegie Inquiry into the Third Age (1992) *Health abilities and well being in the third age*. Research Paper 9. London: The Carnegie Trust.

Clare, A. (1994) *Depression and how to survive*. Arrow.

Compston, J. (1996) *Osteoporosis; new perspectives on causes*. London: Royal College of Physicians.

Department of Health and Social Security (1980) *Inequalities in health. Report of a research working group*. London: DHSS.

Department of Health (DoH) (1989) *Caring for People*. London: HMSO.

Department of Health (DoH) (1991) *Health of the Nation*. London: DoH.

Department of Health (DoH) (1992) *The Health of the Nation: A strategy for England and Wales*. London: HMSO.

Department of Health (DoH) (1995) The Health of the Nation. *Assessing the options CHD/Stroke*. Leeds: NHS Executive.

Department of Health (DoH) (1998) *Our Healthier Nation*. London: HMSO.

Eastman, M. (1986) *Elder abuse*. London: Age Concern England.

Eastman, M. (1996) *Old Age Abuse*. London: Chapman Hall.

Effective Health Care (1996) *Preventing falls and subsequent injury in older people*. 2(4). London: Churchill Livingstone.

Evans, G. (1991) A wider perspective in symptom relief. *Nursing Standard*, **6**(1): 50–51.

Ewles, L & Simnett I. (1995) *Promoting Health: A Practical Guide*. 3rd edn. London: Scutari.

Gearing, B., Johnson, M. & Heller, T. (1988) *Mental health problems in old age*. Chichester: John Wiley.

Gloth, F., Gundberg, C. & Hollis, B. (1995) Vitamin deficiency in homebound elderly persons. *Journal of the American Medical Association*, **274**: P1683–P1686.

Hancock, C. (1993) Rationing; a dangerous game. *Nursing Times*, **93**(38): 27–28.

Hancock, C. (1993) Brave new world. *Health Service Journal*, 25 March: 19.

Hanlon, P., (1990) Health promotion under the new contract. *British Journal of General Practice*, August: 349.

Harrison, S. & Hunter, D. (1993) *Rationing Health Care*. London: IPPR.

Harvey, J. & Fralick, E. (1997) Targeting neglect. *The Health Service Journal*, **107**(5564): 26–27.

Hinkle, K.L. (1991) A literature review; HIV seropositivity in the elderly. *Journal of Gerontological nursing*, October (10): 12–17.

Holland, W. (1992) In sickness and in health. *Health Service Journal*, 19 September: 21.

Hunt, P. (1997) Health inequalities are a middle class issue. *Healthlines Issue*, **40**: March: 5.

Jenkins, G. (1993) Accidents will happen. *Health Service Journal*, 7 October: 31.

Kammering, R. & Kinnear, A. (1996) The extent of the two tier service for fundholders. *British Medical Journal*, 312(7069): 1399–1401.

Killoran, A. (1993) Pacemaker. *Health Service Journal* 18 February: 23–27.

Le Touze, Calnan, M. (1996) The banding scheme for health promotion in general practice. *Health Trends*, 28(3): 100–105.

McGlone, F. (1992) Disability and dependancy – a demographic and social audit. In *Long Term Care Data Pack (1997)* Swiss Re UK.

McKeon, P. (1986) *Coping with depression and elation*. Sheldon.

MacKinnon, M. (1993) *Providing diabetic care in general practice*. London: Class.

Naidoo, J. and Wills, J. (1994) *Health promotion foundations for practice*. London: Baillière Tindall.

Nokes, K. (1996) *HIV/AIDS and the older adult*. Bristol: Taylor and Francis.

Norman, I. & Redfern, S. (1995) The quality of nursing. *Nursing Times*, 89(27): 40–43.

North Yorkshire Health Promotion Service (1997) *Falls pevention programme*. NYHPService.

Nuffield Institute (1996) Preventing falls and subsequent injury in older people. *Effective Health Care*, 2(4).

Ogg, J. & Bennett, G. (1992) Elder abuse in Britain. *British Medical Journal*, 305: 24 October, 998–999.

Office of Population Censuses and Surveys (OPCS) (1995) *Population Trends*. London: HMSO.

Pender, N. (1987) *Health promotion in*

nursing practice. California: Appleton & Lange.

Phair, L. & Good V. (1995) *Dementia: a positive approach*. London: Scutari.

Robbins, S., Gouw, G. & McClaren, J. (1992) Shoe sole thickness and hardness influences balance in older men. *Journal of the American Geriatric Society*, 40: 1089–1094

Roper, N. Logan, W. & Tierney, A. (1983) *Using a model for nursing*. Edinburgh: Churchill Livingstone.

Royal College of Nursing (RCN) (1993) *Powerhouse for change*. Report on the taskforce on community nursing. London: RCN.

Ruddlesden, M. (1994) *You can do it! exercises for older people*. London: Hawkser.

Salter, B. (1991) Demand and fallacy. *Health Service Journal*, 5 December: 19.

Sidell, M. (1995) *Health in old age, myth, mystery and management*. Buckingham: Open University.

Smith, G., Bartley, M. & Blane, D. (1990) The Black report on socioeconomic inequalities in health 10 years on. *British Medical Journal*, 301: 18–25 August: 373–376.

Utting, D. (1995) *Positive steps, a progress report on district stroke services*. London: Stroke Association.

Watson, J. (1993) Why we should take sanctions. *Monitor Weekly*, 6 October: 14.

World Health Organisation (WHO) (1986) *The Ottowa Charter*. Geneva: WHO.

FURTHER READING

Bond, J., Coleman, P. & Peace, S. (1993) *Ageing in Society*. London: Sage.

An interesting overview that provides a clear picture of older people within society. Considers very much the issues of adjusting to life's crises in old age.

Naidoo, J. & Wills, J. (1994) *Health Promotion – Foundations for Practice*. London: Baillière Tindall.

Provides an interactive approach to the underpinning issues of health promotion. Whilst issues are in places not explored in depth, it is a sound introduction to some of the concepts and principles of this topic.

Niven, N. (1989) *Health psychology*. Edinburgh: Churchill Livingstone.

Considers the range of approaches to changing individuals' behaviour.

McClymont, M,, Thomas, S. & Denham, M. (1991) *Health Visiting and Elderly People*. Edinburgh: Churchill Livingstone.

Chapter 8 looks broadly at some of the wider issues of health promotion that relate to old age. Appendix 3 contains a well-focused summary of models that guide the application of health promotion.

Kaufmann, T. (1995) *HIV/AIDS and older people*. London: Age Concern England.

An interesting text with special reference to older people both infected and affected by the virus.

14 Health promotion and community care: the neighbourhood health strategy

Julia Mitchell

KEY ISSUES

- Context
- Community development
- Multi-agency alliances
- Links between public health and health promotion
- Empowering communities

INTRODUCTION

A neighbourhood health strategy project is a community health project which aims to develop multi-agency alliances within neighbourhoods, to develop stronger links between public health and health promotion, and to empower the community of a given neighbourhood to initiate and develop activities which have a positive impact on the health of that community. This chapter focusses on a neighbourhood strategy project which was the first of its kind and which was implemented in the borough of Stockport in the north west of England. This chapter will present:

- A description of the project including planning processes (strategic) and implementation processes (operational)
- Perspectives of health care professionals working within the neighbourhood communities including challenges faced, strategies for overcoming problems, and positive features with this type of innovative project
- Issues for evaluation of this type of project.

BACKGROUND TO THE STOCKPORT NEIGHBOURHOOD HEALTH STRATEGY

The Neighbourhood Health Strategy Project arose as the result of a number of changes in the National Health Service (NHS) including the delivery of health promotion in the primary care setting and changes in local priorities driven by *The Health of the Nation* (DoH, 1992).

Discussions at the start of 1993 between Stockport Health Commission (the purchaser) and Stockport Healthcare Trust (the provider) led to the inception of the project in October of that year. The Health Commission funded the project from monies available to implement *The Health of the Nation*. The funding consisted of:

■ Four half-time public health nurses
■ Part-time coordinator posts for each neighbourhood
■ One half-time health promotion advisor
■ A budget for each neighbourhood to implement the strategy which varied depending on population size and deprivation ratings.

Neighbourhoods

The Stockport borough was divided into 16 neighbourhoods, each of which developed and implemented its own health strategy facilitated by a public health nurse and neighbourhood strategy coordinators. The neighbourhoods were covered in four waves with the four public health nurses spending 6 months in each neighbourhood. Thus the strategy development for all 16 neighbourhoods was completed after 2 years.

The neighbourhoods are geographical units drawn so as to ensure that:

■ most people would know without consulting a map which neighbourhood they belong to
■ all councillors would be able to say 'most of my ward is in neighbourhood X'
■ most of the general practitioners (GPs) and schools would be able to say that most of their patients/pupils came from that neighbourhood.

Recognising neighbourhoods was seen to be important for a number of reasons:

1. To enable the health strategy to be put into place
2. To enable general practices to be brought into public health work;
3. To provide a basis on which the commissioning of preventive services could be devolved.

Nature of a neighbourhood health strategy

The main concept driving the neighbourhood health strategy relates to the notion of agencies working together, pooling resources and sharing information towards population health gains. It is assumed that within individuals and agencies there already exists a considerable degree of awareness of the locality and the needs that exist within it. Healthy alliances at a local level were thus perceived as having an impact on achieving health targets identified in *The Health of the Nation* and in the local level document, *Stockport Health Promise* in addition to achieving the targets in the Neighbourhood Health Strategy (DoH, 1992; DoH, 1993; Stockport Health Commission, 1994).

The overall aim of the project was thus to develop strategies to promote the health of the population of Stockport at a neighbourhood level. The work would be driven by key principles: the '*five Cs*' (Box 14.1). These were seen as a means by which agencies could work together and contribute to the strategy.

BOX 14.1	*The five Cs of Stockport Neighourhood Health Strategy*

1. **Coordination**

   Evidence suggests that health promotion interventions tend to be less effective when undertaken in isolation. What tends to be more effective is the interaction of similar and related interventions from different sources. So if the health promotion work arising from one agency is coordinated with those of others, they will tend to be increasingly effective. Through the co-ordinator of the neighbourhood health strategy this end point can be more effectively achieved.

   Example

   No smoking day: the coordinator obtains information and delivers displays to GP surgeries, clinics, library, schools, pharmacists, and any other interested agency so that at information centres the public see the same message at the same time all over the neighbourhood.

2. **Cooperation**

   This concept goes beyond coordination, wherein different agencies actively help each other.

   Example

   Gathering information. School nurses may be able to gather medical information on teenagers which could be of benefit to GP practices. Ten blood pressure readings at age 15 years will contribute to GP band 3 health promotion programmes.

3. **Collaboration**

   Going a step further, this entails one agency providing a service with or on behalf of another agency, thus freeing them to take the lead in providing other services.

   Example

   The youth service runs groups for young women and covers topics including parenting skills and mental health issues. This allows health agencies to target other groups.

4. **Community action**

   Environments affect health; the strategy addressess environmental/public health issues and promotes the development of a community spirit. Some agencies may want to be involved in this.

   Example

   Health visitors and a school staff backing local mothers request for more provision for the under 5s.

5. **Community development**

   This goes beyond community action by helping to empower the population of each neighbourhood to help solve their own problems.

> *Example*
> Community development workers are already employed by Stockport Healthcare and Social Services to work with the populations in certain disadvantaged neighbourhoods. Various initiatives have been developed in these areas including food cooperatives and credit unions.

Organisation

Each of the 16 neighbourhood health strategies attempts to address health issues of most relevance to that particular neighbourhood. The public health nurse attached to the neighbourhood spends 6 months in that locality, networking with the people and agencies who provide a health promoting service. Using the information obtained, areas of need are identified and collated into a draft strategy which is then discussed in forum with the aforementioned agencies. From this a 'final' strategy is agreed. The Public Health Nurse then identifies a coordinator and local implementation group and disseminates the final strategy. The strategy is implemented by co-ordinators from the health visiting service who facilitate the health promotion activities outlined in the strategy, convene and coordinate the local implementation group (a multi-agency group consisting of anyone who wishes to be involved in the strategy's implementation and known as an IMPACT (Implementation and Action Group), and manage the strategy budget for that neighbourhood.

PRE-PROJECT PLANNING

Concept

The idea for the neighbourhood health strategy had a number of antecedents. Discussions around locality commissioning and changes in the delivery of health care had been taking place previously within Stockport Health Commission. Issues around GP banding were also being discussed within Stockport Health Commission at this time and a decision was made that the commission would regard it as appropriate for GP practices to look at the determinants of health in their area when promoting the health of their practice population. A review of primary care nursing was going on at this time with a subgroup looking at health promotion and links into primary care and the concept of the neighbourhood health strategy in its present form came from the director of public health and this group.

Planning processes

A business case for the project which included a bid for funding was put forward by the lead director of the project (director of public health) to the chief executive of Stockport Health Commission which the commission's board agreed in principle. It was felt that a small group was needed to move the idea forward in practice, so a project management team was formed and began meeting regularly to plan the implementation of the project. It was felt that health visitors would be the best occupational group to work on the project and discussions took place with the head of community nursing, who was included on the project management team around changing practice and moving health visitors into a new 'public health nursing' role.

A job description for the public health nurse posts was written and the clinical nurse manager gave presentations about the role to all health visitors on health strategy days to get interest from health visitors. The interview process included applicants giving a presentation about how they thought the job could be done. A half-time, project advisor post was also created to help with coordination of the project and to support the project workers.

There were a range of positive features associated with these early processes. The work of the project management team on this project, in parallel with work on *The Stockport Health Promise* laid the basis for an integrated public health network rather than a fragmented purchaser/provider relationship. Setting up a team of people to develop the concept enabled issues to be fully discussed and developed collaboratively.

Those involved in the project management team shared a commitment to community ownership and *Health For All* principles and a commitment to each other for support and motivation.

The inclusion of the public health nurses on the project management team provided them with a supportive forum for their 'fieldwork' input.

There were also some problems associated with these processes. Initial information about the project was not formally recorded or disseminated. This led to problems in that the GPs, who were key stakeholders, were not given enough information about the project so that when the public health nurses initially went out to practices they encountered a general lack of awareness about the project and therefore a degree of hostility.

There was a feeling that the public health nurses were appointed too early in the general timescale of the project; this was 6 months before the project advisor was in post. It was also felt that they were starting from different levels in terms of knowledge of health promotion theory and extent of community development experience. They began their work before they had had any training and while the process of defining the neighbourhoods was still going on. However, it was recognised that their training needs were difficult to define in advance, as the role was a new and developmental one.

How could these issues have been addressed?

- *A clearer strategic vision for the project should be defined at an early stage*
- *The aims of the project need to be made explicit and made available to relevant stakeholders at an early stage*
- *GPs in particular should be involved at an early stage*
- *Initial planning needs to be completed and a clear framework for workers' roles defined before they begin their work.*

Organisation

These initial planning stages then had to evolve into working practice. The four public health nurses were responsible for developing local strategies in consultation with key individuals and agencies in each neighbourhood (e.g. GPs, local authorities, schools, community groups etc.).

Health visitors from each neighbourhood were then needed to coordinate the strategies in each neighbourhood. To promote awareness amongst health visitors, to describe the coordinator role and to raise interest in the project in general, awareness-raising days were held at the beginning of each new wave for the health visitors, run by the project management team. Health visitors came forward for coordinator roles as a result of these days. The coordinators had regular meetings with the senior nurse manager and project adviser every 4–6 weeks for feedback and support. The senior nurse manager and the public health nurses fed back to the project management team.

Project management team

From initial discussions of the concept of a neighbourhood health strategy between the director of public health (project director), the commission's health strategy project manager (project lead), the head of community nursing and the director of health promotion, other people who would have key roles in the project were identified. These were the senior nurse manager, who would be responsible for the day-to-day management of the public health nurses and coordinators and the primary health care manager, who would be the link for GPs with the project. After the public health nurses and the project advisor were appointed, they too joined the project management team.

Funding

The funding for the project came from Stockport Health Commission development monies which is received each year from central government via region. An amount £100 000 is ring-fenced each year for *The Health of the Nation* initiatives and out of this the Neighbourhood Health Strategy Project received approximately £65 000 from an initial bid of £70 000. This money was used for the neighbourhood budgets, for the half-time project advisor post, and for some central administrative support.

In addition to this new funding, the neighbourhood coordinators resource came from the public health nursing time of health visitors, this allocation being part of a review of how health visiting time was used. Stockport Health Commission and Stockport Community Health Care Trust each contributed two extra health visitors to make up the deficit, a decision which came about as a result of discussions between GPs and the trust. The decision to invest two health visitor posts in public health nursing work was taken by the head of community nursing.

The project management team decided on the allocation of neighbourhood budgets. Initially, the intention was that these budgets would be 16 equal amounts. However, after discussion it was realised that differential amounts were needed and the director of public health worked out a formula based on population size and a deprivation index. There were a number of positive features connected with the allocation of funding, however, there were also some problems as listed in Box 14.2.

BOX 14.2	*Advantages and disadvantages of fund allocation for the Stockport Neighbourhood Head Strategy*

Advantages
- The fact that the money was available from the Commission for what was an untested, innovative project
- The fact that commission money budgets can be devolved to health trust employees at health visitor level to manage was also considered to be advantageous in breaking down purchaser–provider barriers
- The funding arrangements associated with the project were seen as a major step towards putting budgets out into neighbourhoods and back into primary health care
- Neighbourhoods all had a sum of money to help with initiatives

Disadvantages
- The coordinators had problems accessing the budget. Systems for accessing money direct from the Commission are in place but the coordinators had no initial training and finance procedures proved lengthy
- Deciding on the budget allocations to neighbourhoods caused some difficulties but these were resolved through discussion
- No attention was paid to funding secretarial support
- Specific money was not kept back for 'extras', e.g. newsletter production. This meant going back to the neighbourhoods to ask for some money back from the budget

How could these issues have been addressed?
- The issue of accessing neighbourhood budgets should be sorted out at an early stage of the project
- The funding of secretarial support should be costed into the budget at an early stage
- A sum of money should be kept back for extras which involve all the neighbourhoods such as, for example, newsletters.

Staff development

During the initial planning processes, thought was given to staff development but not in a structured way. Areas in which staff might need training were voiced but no explicit action plan for staff development was put into place. Thought was given to the fact that public health nurses and the coordinators would be working in ways less structured than they had previously been used to with their normal case loads and would need training in the following areas:

- Public health advocacy
- Profiling
- Health needs assessment
- Budget management
- Managing meetings etc. However, no analysis of training needs was actually done in advance of workers starting their roles and it was left to the public health nurses to identify their own training needs and find appropriate courses. The project management team encouraged the public health nurses to access courses and money was available for this purpose. However, the nature of the work was such that much of the skills development was through process learning on the job. Training courses can provide some background but essentially cannot fulfil a definitive 'acquisition of skills'.

Training on public health advocacy was given by members of the project management team.

The public health nurses received support and supervision from the senior nurse manager, with whom they had regular contact and from whom they got good quality support and supervision. Some support also came from the project advisor and the project management team.

Peer support was also envisaged by the project management team, although this was left up to the public health nurses to arrange. In practice, it was felt that it was very much a system of 'self support' for the public health nurses. The coordinators had regular support meetings with the senior nurse manager every 4–6 weeks and also had a training session on profiling, health needs assessment and public health advocacy.

A number of positive features and problematic issues were identified in relation to staff development (Box 14.3).

BOX 13.2   *Advantages and disadvantages*

Advantages
- The project management team were receptive to training needs identified by the public health nurses and funding was readily made available for courses
- The networking that took place on courses was felt to be useful by the public health nurses
- There has been much personal and professional development for the staff involved
- The commitment of the public health nurses, the senior nurse manager and the coordinators has been a very positive factor

Disadvantages
- Practical provision to ensure that training needs would be met was not in place before the workers began their new roles. It was only when workers ran into difficulties due partly to this lack of training that this issue was addressed
- Owing to this lack of training and feedback, it was perceived by some of the project management team that some of the earlier strategies did not place enough emphasis on issues such as coronary heart disease and environmental issues, which were things that the project management team saw as major

issues. As the phases have progressed however the strategies have also progressed in this respect

How could these issues have been addressed?

■ Training and support needs could be analysed in advance of workers starting and a strategy for training and support developed. This should be adaptable to meet new training needs as they arise during the progress of the project
■ Peer support is a useful tool but it should not be assumed that workers will use it. A more structured peer support mechanism with appropriate resourcing would be beneficial
■ It is important that staff are able to go on relevant courses, particularly in the early stages of the project
■ Training on the production of a strategy including research, content and writing, should be given before public health nurses begin this work.

Neighbourhoods

The 16 neighbourhoods were decided based on carefully worked out criteria and carefully considered data analysis. Different data sets were examined, including analysis of GP practice population distributions, trying out different boundaries in draft to see how they impacted on congruence for GP practice populations, acorn analysis, work done by the community unit on what people regarded as natural communities, and even looking at streets and asking 'where does that belong?' Initial work on localities had been done previously by locality managers, the predecessors to health strategy managers and ward boundaries were also taken into account.

For the neighbourhoods, at least 75% concordance with general practice populations was aimed for, i.e. if 75% of the locality population lived and had a GP practice within the boundary of the neighbourhood. Similarly, high concordance with school catchments and with council wards was aimed for. In addition, capturing 'natural' communities was also an important factor. To fulfil these criteria involved creating and adjusting boundaries to achieve the maximum concordance possible. There was no fixed number of neighbourhoods decided before this process started. However, it was recognised that there was only funding for a set number of coordinators, thus, there had to be a manageable number of neighbourhoods in this respect, and that neighbourhoods should not be so large that people could not identify with them. The team therefore had an idea from the beginning that the number of neighbourhoods would be somewhere between 12 and 20.

The aim to achieve 75% concordance with GP populations was achieved. In fact, a level of 78% concordance was attained. The majority of the neighbourhoods do align well and this reflects the amount of care which was put into drawing the neighbourhoods at the start of the project.

The recognition of the alliances that work within neighbourhoods can be seen as a positive aspect of this process, however, there were also some problems. With any work of this nature, i.e. deciding boundaries, there are likely to be some difficulties involved. Neighbourhoods do not always fall naturally; sometimes an area which might be defined as a neighbourhood was unwieldy in terms of strategy development and implementation, and some areas that were grouped together as a neighbourhood did not align well together.

In some neighbourhoods, the two levels – the level at which natural communities exist and the level at which congruence can be obtained with primary care and with other institutions – was different. To resolve this, a system where both levels were recognised was adopted. This consisted of a single IMPACT team with different coordinators for the different 'natural' communities.

Communication

During the pre-project planning process, there was little thought given to communicating information to major stakeholders. There was no formal plan for communication of information about the project and it was only when the Stockport Health Commission had requested a communication plan that this issue was addressed. Rather, as the project developed, information was communicated but in a largely ad hoc way:

- Project aims and objectives were recorded
- The director of public health and the director of health services development wrote to GPs
- Health visitors were given information about the project at a health visitors' strategy day. When the public health nurses and coordinators were in post, a network was set up from the beginning which involved regular meetings where project feedback was discussed. Health strategy evenings were held to present the draft strategies for feedback and a play about the project was performed at a conference put on by the Commission to inform staff and the public about work taking place.

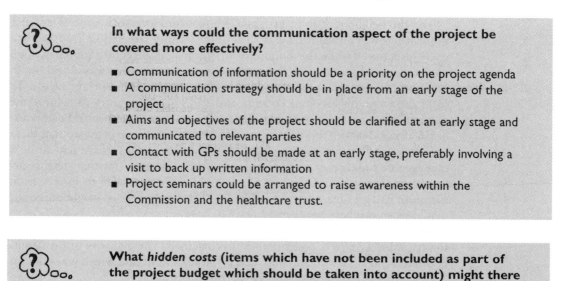

In what ways could the communication aspect of the project be covered more effectively?

- Communication of information should be a priority on the project agenda
- A communication strategy should be in place from an early stage of the project
- Aims and objectives of the project should be clarified at an early stage and communicated to relevant parties
- Contact with GPs should be made at an early stage, preferably involving a visit to back up written information
- Project seminars could be arranged to raise awareness within the Commission and the healthcare trust.

What *hidden costs* (items which have not been included as part of the project budget which should be taken into account) might there be with a project of this nature?

- Additional secretarial and clerical support; an item which needs to be resolved in advance of workers beginning their roles
- Photocopying – both materials and, without clerical support, this would include public health nurse time
- Telephone calls
- Postage
- Relief cover for staff involved in training activity
- Time of stakeholders spent attending project-related meetings, e.g. GPs, teachers, local authority workers.

PROJECT IMPLEMENTATION

Developing a neighbourhood strategy: the role and perspectives of the public health nurses.

The process

The public health nurses all followed a similar framework for developing each neighbourhood strategy, which evolved progressively from the first wave. This involved the following activities, which will each be discussed in turn:

1. Getting to know the neighbourhood
2. Collecting data for the neighbourhood
3. Networking in the neighbourhood
4. Drafting the strategy
5. Strategy evening (meeting to discuss the draft strategy with interested people from the neighbourhood)
6. Producing the final strategy.

Getting to know the neighbourhood

Using the defined boundaries for the neighbourhood, the public health nurses familiarised themselves with the area by 'walking it'. From this they gained an impression of the nature of the area, e.g. whether it was mainly residential/commercial, affluent/deprived etc.

Collecting data for the neighbourhood

The next step after familiarisation with the area was to collect data about the area and its population. A variety of data sources were used by the public health nurses. These include:

- Public health reports for the area
- Office of Population Census and Surveys (OPCS) data
- Mortality and morbidity data
- GP profiles which include vaccination rates and smear rates

- *The Health of the Nation* documents for national/local comparisons;
- Accident data
- Housing data
- Relevant reports from other agencies, e.g. Youth Service, drugs services etc.

The public health nurses accessed this data via the Stockport Health Commission information officer (who translated the data to neighbourhood level), through library research, from GPs and from local authority contacts. Although they did not always know what data was available, through networking with contacts, public health nurses had access to a sufficiently wide and detailed database.

From this core of data collected initially, the public health nurses selected appropriate data for the strategy. If particular issues arose, they collected more detailed data around it, for example alcohol consumption. They then simplified the data to make it accessible to a wide range of people.

Networking in the neighbourhood

The public health nurses liaised with a range of agencies in a neighbourhood. This occurred at two levels: first, via borough-wide agencies, i.e. those serving the whole of Stockport, and then subsequently through local agencies, i.e. those serving a particular local community. The public health nurses used a list of key people at both levels (produced as a result of a 'brainstorm' by the project management team) as a basis for contacts. As they began networking with people, they found out about other relevant contacts in a neighbourhood and the list grew. Contacts would include those listed in Box 14.4.

BOX 14.4	*Key contacts for public health nurses*

- GPs
- District nurses
- Community psychiatric nurses
- School heads or representatives
- Community development workers
- Councillors
- Church leaders
- Community drugs team

- Health visitors
- Practice nurses
- School nurses
- Social workers
- Pharmacists
- Community police
- Voluntary services

As the project gained more credibility and people became more aware of it, the attitudes of people in the field became more positive and networking became easier.

Networking proceeded along the following framework:

1. Initial telephone contact to arrange a first meeting
2. Meeting with an individual or group to explain the project to them, to find out about their agency, and to find out about issues which they felt should be included in the strategy for that neighbourhood. This step also involved inviting them to the strategy evening and explaining the IMPACT group function and structure
3. With each meeting, the public health nurses have to ascertain how much interest the agency has in the strategy and how much time they will give to

the meeting. In each case the public health nurse has to explain the project, trying to sell the idea, whilst achieving a balance between offering ideas and examples of initiatives from other neighbourhoods so that the agency/worker gets a feel for the project and eliciting ideas from the agency/worker which are relevant to that particular neighbourhood.

This initial networking is important because unless agencies feel interest in the project, a sense of ownership, and a sense that it will benefit their work in the community, they will not have the motivation for further input. Thus, it is the responsibility of the public health nurse to present the project in a positive and enthusiastic way in order to motivate as many agencies as possible to become involved. This was not always an easy task as the amount of input that a worker/agency is prepared to give is also dependent on other variables such as the personality of the worker and the constraints under which they are working, e.g. time, existing workload, job remit.

Drafting the strategy

After collecting information about the area, the public health nurses then prepare a draft strategy for the neighbourhood. In order to get credibility in an area, the ideas of people working in that area have to be taken up, but also the relevant statitical data, *The Health of the Nation* and *Stockport Health Promise* have to be incorporated into the strategy. Thus, the strategy is a combination of issues which the neighbourhood workers have cited and health statistics for that neighbourhood.

Strategy evening

An evening meeting to discuss the draft strategy is held in each neighbourhood. To these are invited all those who provided information and ideas and other workers in the neighbourhood who have an interest in the strategy, including the health visitors who will be the coodinators for each neighbourhood strategy. At these meetings further discussion around the issues which have been identified in the first draft takes place and people are recruited to form the IMPACT group, the group in each neighbourhood which will have a key role in developing initiatives from the strategy.

Producing the final strategy

From these evenings the public health nurses get the feedback necessary to write up a full strategy for the neighbourhood. This is then distributed to all interested parties.

Perspectives on the process

The public health nurses had a generally positive perspective of the neighbourhood health strategy in terms of its development, operation and sustainability. Although there had been problems during the strategy development phase, particularly at the beginning with the first wave strategies, it was felt that these were part of the learning process. As the project was a new one which was not based on any established model, with hindsight it was thought that many of the problems encountered were inevitable. Overall, the public health nurses felt that they had benefitted in terms of professional and personal development from the project as a whole.

The issues which were raised are as follows:

- Training
- Support around GPs
- Issues around networking
- Issues around coordinators
- Secretarial and clerical support
- Neighbourhoods assigned

These problematic issues that impacted upon strategy development are considered in more detail later.

Training and support

Although the public health nurses were able to go on training courses which they identified as relevant to their new role, it was still felt that there were gaps in training. A basic requirement was training around what the role involved before starting in it. For the first wave strategy there was a feeling that they did not fully understand the role and would have had more confidence if they had been able to fully understand it and explain it clearly to the professionals they networked with, rather than going in 'cold'.

Another aspect of training which they felt would have been valuable involved actually writing a neighbourhood strategy. Although they had had some previous training on community profiling, this was not felt to be sufficient for the demands of writing a full strategy. In addition it was felt that there was not enough direction from the project management team about what the strategies should include before they were started, and not enough constructive feedback during the writing process. All of the public health nurses would have welcomed constructive comments on the strategies, particularly the first strategy. There was a sense of not knowing if they were doing what was wanted as well as a certain amount of frustration that they wanted to improve on what they had written but without fuller feedback could not.

The public health nurses were unsure of what was wanted from them at first so had much discussion to try to clarify what was wanted and to give each other support. Thus on issues of training and support it was felt that there had to be self-identification of training needs and self-support. This was also seen positively in terms of personal and professional development.

Support around GPs

Another area which the public health nurses saw as an issue was that of working with GPs. Initial contact had been made either by visit or by letter from the director of public health, the health strategy manager or the primary health care manager. However, the public health nurses found that from this the

GPs had only gained a vague idea of what the project involved. Despite participation in the neighbourhood health strategy being linked to GP banding, they encountered a high degree of cynicism from GPs with only a minority thinking that the neighbourhood health strategy was a good idea. Thus they felt as if they were going in cold to GPs, trying to sell an idea that GPs did not know enough about or did not actually believe in.

The public health nurses found that GPs tended to focus on their own patients and did not look at the wider neighbourhood. In some cases, apathy or hostility towards the project from GPs made it difficult for the public health nurses to elicit any involvement. This tendency for GPs to lack a broad public health perspective is clearly a common occurrence and impacts directly on the development and implementation of the neighbourhood strategy. There was however a degree of optimism involved. It was felt that understanding this different way of working and realising the concept behind the neighbourhood health strategy would take time to communicate and it was felt that if GPs began to see the benefits of the neighbourhood health strategy for their patients they might get more involved.

Issues around networking

Networking and the new alliances being formed between agencies were seen very much as a positive part of the project but as the project involves working with many agencies, all of whom have their own health agendas, there could be difficulty keeping the strategy focused. Other agencies do not necessarily share the same concept and view of health and naturally enough all think that their agenda is the most relevant and important.

Because the public health nurses are not directing other people's work, they can only offer suggestions and as a result the final strategies cannot be as focused as people may want them to be. What can be offered is an overview that tries to cover everything that has been discussed so that those people working in the area can try to pick up on those things they see as important. Sometimes, inevitably, workers will also have agendas other than a health agenda and in some cases may try to use the strategy as a vehicle for this, e.g. internal politics within an organisation.

Issues around coordinators

The public health nurses felt that if they had been able to work with coordinators during the development stage of the strategies, the coordinators would have had more motivation during the implementation process. It was perceived that the coordinators had not had time freed and had not taken on their roles at a sufficiently early stage. Within the alloted time, the public health nurses were moving on to the next neighbourhoods and thus were less accessible for support.

In addition, it was felt that because of the demands of their health visitor role, coordinators had often been sucked into a more traditional medical model as opposed to the broader social model of health that was demanded by the values of the neighbourhood strategy. As such, it was felt that they had stayed largely within a 'task-oriented' mode of practice. Their role as health visitors had not previously allowed them to be proactive but the coordinator role expected them to broaden their perspectives and practices.

One positive progression for the fourth wave strategies is that the public health nurses who write the strategies go on to become the coordinators for the neighbourhood that they have been working in. This is seen as the ideal, as it provides continuity between strategy creation and implementation.

Secretarial support

Money was allocated for secretarial and clerical support at the start of the project but no mechanisms were put into place to utilise it. The public health nurses felt that this should have been built into the project from the start for both themselves and the coordinators. This issue was a source of frustration throughout the project. The public health nurses have spent time doing clerical tasks such as photocopying or experienced delays in getting their finished strategies typed up.

Neighbourhoods assigned

As a deliberate strategy for the first wave, the public health nurses were sent to areas that they were not familiar with in order to eliminate any preconceived ideas about the neighbourhood. However, there was a feeling that it would have been more appropriate if they had been familiar with the area. In general, the public health nurses did not consider knowing an area as being detrimental to developing the strategy for that neighbourhood.

Definitions of success

The public health nurses identified a number of factors to ensure the success of the neighbourhood health strategy project (Box 14.5).

BOX 14.5	*Criteria for success of the neighbourhood health strategy project*
	1. Putting public health into health visiting 2. Achieving 16 written strategies 3. Number of initiatives undertaken during a year 4. Number of people using the service 5. Alliances formed between agencies 6. Awareness of community health issues raised 7. GP interest 8. Sustainability

The public health nurses had positive feelings about the success of the project. It was felt that health visitors were now looking at a broad range of public health and a broad range of age groups.

In the 2 years of the project the following goals were realised:

- The whole of Stockport was covered and networks have been built up
- Initiatives arising from the strategy are up and running
- Working alliances have been formed and there is now the opportunity to build on those relationships
- The knowledge base of agencies is now much greater
- Workers in a neighbourhood feel valued because they are consulted and included
- Groups in a neighbourhood now have a forum, through co-ordinators and IMPACT group, for publicising initiatives in that neighbourhood
- People's awareness of public health and health promotion has been raised and they are more aware of their community.
- The strategies have been a good catalyst for discussion and networking.

In terms of professional and personal development, the public health nurses felt that they had been able to greatly extend their knowledge and skill base. They had had the opportunity to have time out to attend conferences and meetings, to read, and to think about the concept of the neighbourhood health strategy and the whole ethos of public health. From this they were able to see that there is a ground swell of people who want to challenge the medical intervention model and who recognise that creative and innovative methods of health promotion are worthwhile.

Box 14.6 contains an example of a strategy for one of the 16 neighbourhoods.

BOX 14.6   *Example of a neighbourhood health strategy*

Life cycle group: 0–5 years
Parenting
- Identify those families 'at risk' by using input from midwives, health visitors, GPs, teachers and clinic staff
- Set up groups in the community aimed at dealing with their problems, e.g.:
  — young (under 18) mother and baby groups
  — unsupported mother and baby groups
  — weaning groups
- Use locations and workers who are non-threatening (non-professionals can reduce the perceived threat of authority). Other projects which have proved successful elsewhere in the country have used local people who have suitable skills and knowledge, e.g. community mothers, buddy schemes

Breastfeeding and infant nutrition
- Offer more support for mothers in both the antenatal and postnatal period who wish to breastfeed
- Offer a more community-based approach to breastfeeding, with more facilities being made available for breastfeeding mothers
- Raise awareness amongst the community that 'breast is best'
- Introduce concept of healthy eating and home cooking into social events of mother and toddler groups, young women's groups etc.

Working mothers
- Set up 'out of hours' services for babies and young children of working mothers

Life cycle group: 5–18 years

Home alone children

■ Develop more after school and holiday care along the lines of that already running

Diet

■ Schools to continue to pass on the message of the importance of healthy diets
■ Leisure services to make links with schools to offer advice and information on diet and exercise

Exercise

■ Provide adequately supervised safe routes to school
■ Make exercise opportunities available to this age group more attractive
■ Develop joint ventures between education, leisure and health

Teenagers

■ Develop counselling facilities aimed specifically at local young people
■ Organise a young people's forum
■ Increase the outreach work done by the detached youth service to reach those teenagers least likely to attend more formal groups. Use the mobile resource if appropriate

Life cycle group: 18–65 years

Diet

■ Set up a community cafe offering cheap, healthy foods and cook and taste sessions

Exercise

■ Develop a database of all exercise opportunities in the area
■ Develop more crèche facilities at exercise venues
■ Introduce exercise on prescription to the area

Alcohol and smoking

■ Support the development of non-smoking areas in public places
■ Develop 'drop ins' in the area with crèche facilities that young mothers could use, as they often smoke as a coping strategy and more social support facilities can provide alternative coping strategies

Cancers

■ Coordinate a multi-agency approach, e.g. yearly campaigns on skin cancer

Mental Health

■ Increase the provision for under 5s and 'pop in' facilities for young mothers
■ Provide more community-based counselling
■ Raise awareness of mental health issues within the community
■ Set up a structured group facilitated by professionals, aimed at the needs of carers. Group to be run at the clinic if possible and carers to be offered respite care so they can attend regularly.

Life cycle group: 65+ years

Isolation

■ Set up a good neighbours' scheme

Transport and inaccessibility of services
- Extend the 'ring and ride' service

Diet and exercise
- Increase opportunities at home and in the community for gentle exercise

Heating
- Coordinate a campaign before winter, e.g. in October throughout the neighbourhood by all agencies to highlight problem and solutions available

Information
- Run regular 'healthy forums' aimed at this age group, where people can get advice and help

Accidents
- All agencies that undertake home visiting to the elderly to use a 'safety in the home for older people checklist' as produced by a joint working party including representatives from police, fire service, Age Concern and Housing and Environmental Health

- Identify those households which do not have a smoke alarm and the supplying and fitting of alarms if desired

INITIATIVES UNDERWAY AS A RESULT OF STRATEGY RECOMMENDATIONS

The strategy is intended to be an ongoing, sustainable programme of work in the neighbourhood, thus laying foundations, building links and empowerment within the community is of prime importance. The process of developing initiatives is therefore as important as the number of initiatives. The following are examples of initiatives which address strategy recommendations to give the reader an idea of the type of work which is possible within the remit of the neighbourhood health strategy:

1. A community week was held to examine all community groups in Hazel Grove; this week coincided with a child safety week. The neighbourhood strategy was promoted at this event.
2. Cards about the Information and Advice Centre, which is run from the Hazel Grove Civic Hall, were printed and distributed throughout the neighbourhood to raise awareness of the service The service deals with such issues as welfare rights, housing, employment, local groups and activities, form filling and other issues such as bereavement, retirement etc. and provides confidential, professional advice from trained staff employed by Stockport Borough Council. The service was already running before the introduction of the neighbourhood health strategy but it is felt by all of the workers involved that the strategy has given a new impetus to the service, has increased awareness in the community, and has increased working links.
3. The Information and Advice Centre promotes the use of smoke alarms in collaboration with the fire service and undertakes the distribution and

monitoring of the alarms. It also provides hearing aid batteries for 5.5 days a week, whereas previously people in need would have to go to the audiology clinic, which would only supply on 2.5 days each week.

4. A notice board displays information about community events and local group activities and is updated every 2 weeks. This service addresses a whole range of the recommendations in the Hazel Grove strategy and is an ongoing and sustainable community programme.

5. There is a link up between Neighbourhood Strategy and the Young Women's group run by Youth and Social Services for young women aged 16–25. The strategy funds the crèche and some activities for example assertiveness training, aromatherapy etc.

6. Strategy monies will fund respite care for carers to attend a planned carers' group at the clinic. This is intended to provide some time off for carers, to enable them to meet other carers and to support each other, and to provide fun and relaxing activities such as aromatherapy. It is intended that Social Services will be involved in this initiative.

7. A keep fit for the over 50s club has been started up and is run in the local civic hall.

SUMMARY

The initiatives that have been advanced are wide ranging rather than specific to any particular topic or issue. This is compatible with the philosophy of 'holistic' health, seeing health as a combination of physical, psychological, social and environmental factors and not as factors in isolation. The strategies have clearly raised awareness in the community of holistic health promotion and it was felt that they are going some way towards enabling people in the community to take responsibility for and ownership of initiatives. They also appear to have catalysed the development of links between agencies within communities, potentially reinforcing the concept of holistic health, proving more effective in the use of resources and avoiding the duplication of work.

EVALUATION

With a project of this nature, evaluation has to focus on qualitative aspects in the main. Thus the evaluation centred on an interactive relationship between the researcher and those being researched using a range of methods such as semi-structured questionnaires, one-to-one interviews, focus groups and analysis of initiatives which started as a result of the project. The different groups of people involved in the project all need to be researched, including:

- Project management team
- Public health nurses
- Neighbourhood coordinators
- Workers from statutory, voluntary and community groups
- Service users.

Evaluation occurs on three levels: (1)process, (2)impact and (3)outcome, which will be discussed in turn.

Process

Process evaluation looks at the way the project is set up and implemented from its initial inception, through subsequent stages. Process evaluation considers both the positive aspects and problems encountered and considers ways of overcoming problems. Part of the aim of an evaluation for a project like the neighbourhood health strategy is to identify a model of good working practice and to highlight what has been learnt through the process.

Impact

Impact evaluation examines the system that has been set up and implemented as a result of the neighbourhood health strategy. It considers the short-term effects of the project in terms of the actual initiatives in a neighbourhood, the effect on the work of those involved in the project and the effect on the community.

Outcome

Outcome evaluation looks at whether strategy initiatives are sustainable over time and at the health gain to the community in the longer term. As the neighbourhood health strategy has been brought in as a rolling programme, this part of the evaluation needs to be ongoing.

In addition to the whole project evaluation, the neighbourhood coordinators also need to evaluate specific initiatives in neighbourhoods on an ongoing basis through setting initial aims and objectives and reporting on the costs and benefits of each initiative.

CONCLUSION

There is a need to evaluate a project such as the neighbourhood health strategy as encompassing both the evaluation of individual neighbourhood initiatives as well as the concept and operation of the project as a whole. Evaluation can begin to address questions about the ongoing enthusiasm and commitment to such a project and whether individual neighbourhoods feel more empowered to express and resolve their own health needs as a result of the neighbourhood health strategy.

ACKNOWLEDGEMENTS

Sincere thanks are due to Stockport Health Commission for their kind permission to use some of the material contained in this chapter.

REFERENCES

Department of Health (DoH) (1992) *The Health of the Nation*. London: HMSO.

Department of Health (DoH) (1993) *Working Together for Better Health*. London: HMSO.

Stockport Health Commission (1994) *The Stockport Health Promise*. Stockport: Stockport Health Authority.

FURTHER READING

Tones, K. & Tilford, S. (1994) *Health Education. Effectiveness, Efficiency and Equity*. 2nd edn. London: Chapman and Hall.

Contains chapters on evaluation and community health promotion which will give more in-depth information on issues raised to this chapter.

Ashton, J. & Seymour H. (1988) *The New Public Health*. Milton Keynes: Open University.

Includes perspectives on the shift in emphasis for public health from disease orientated to a recognition of social determinants of health.

Benzeval, M., Judge, K. & Whitehead, M. *Tackling Inequalities in Health. An agenda for action*. London: King's Fund.

Offers perspectives on determinants of health and policy responses, community development, and the role of the NHS in tackling inequalities in health.

Department of Health (DoH) (1998) *Our Healthier Nation*. A contract for health. London: HMSO.

An overview of current government policy on health.

Index

Abandonment approach, 253–254
Abuse
    homelessness, 159, 163
    of older people, 279–280
    see also Domestic violence
Accident and Emergency departments
    homeless people, 164
    older people, 271
Accidents, 118
    children, 104–105
        targets to reduce, 116
    gender differences, 211, 214
    old age, 271–272, 303 (Box)
    private sector rented housing, 161
Action for Sick Children, 118
Action on Elder Abuse, 279
Action on Pre-Eclampsia, 69
Activists
    grief, 251
    'professional participators', 17, 38
    representation by, 240
    see also Advocates
Adolescence (process), childbearing, 57,
    85–86
Adolescent Social Action Program (New
    Mexico), 144–145, 146
Advice Centre (Hazel Grove), 303–304
Advocates
    HIV epidemic and grief, 251
    mental health care, 199, 200
Africa, 'slim' (AIDS), 249, 250
African–Caribbean Mental Health Drop-in
    Sessions (Oldham), 239
Age, maternal, 56–57
Age Concern, on screening, 274
Age of consent, and teenage pregnancy, 86
Ageing *see* Old age
Ageing in society (Bond et al), 283
Agendas
    pre-identified, 236
    setting, 38
Aggleton, P., *Health Promotion and young
    people*, 154
Ahmad, W.I.U, *'Race' and health in
    contemporary Britain*, 243
AIDS *see* HIV
AIMS (Association for Improvements in the
    Maternity Service), 68
Air pollution, intersectoral collaboration
    example, 15
Alcohol
    accidents, 214
    children, 133 (Box)

gay men, 220
    men's health, 211, 213, 222 (Box)
    and pregnancy, 54, 55–56
Alexandria (Scotland), Teenage Health Club,
    151
Alienation, 40
Allergic conditions, 118
Alliances *see* Healthy alliances; Interagency
    collaboration
Alma Ata declaration, 18, 171
    primary health care, 21, 22
Amniocentesis, pressures on women, 73
And the band played on (Shiltz), 248
Anderton, J. (police chief), 260
Anencephaly, 53
Animosity, primary care staff, 166
Antenatal care
    poor information, 75
    postnatal depression prevention, 192
    teenage pregnancy, 88, 89, 90–94
Antidepressants, prescriptions, 196
Anti-racism, 232
APEC (Action on Pre-Eclampsia), 69
Arithrodynamics, 268
Arnstein, S., ladder of participation, 17, 18
    (Box)
Ashton and Seymour, *The new public health*,
    13–22, 23, 306
Ashton Asian Health Development Project,
    236, 241
Asian women, suicide rates, 187
Assimilation
    ethnic minority groups, 230
    'queer' community, 247
Association for Improvements in the
    Maternity Service, 68
Association of Radical Midwives, 69–70
Asthma, self-management, 118–119
Autonomy
    and mental health, 198
    see also Empowerment
Awakenings (Sacks), 7
Awareness-raising days (Stockport), 289, 290

Bagnall and Dilloway, on child health
    promotion, 117, 121
Barnardo's, 118
Base 51 (Nottingham), 150–151
Beattie, A., community development
    234–235, 236
Bed and breakfast accommodation, 159
    health of occupants, 160

Bed and breakfast accommodation (*contd*)
    inadequacy, 161
Behaviour, individuals, 9–11, 13, 106
Behavioural measures, mental health
    promotion, 191
Bem, S.I., sex-role inventory, 210
Benzeval, M. et al, *Tackling inequalities in
    health*, 306
Berridge, V., history of AIDS epidemic,
    248–249
'Best interests', child health, 102, 103, 130
    (Box)
Beveridge, W., 5
Big issue, The, homeless people not registered
    with GP, 164
Bines, W., on mental health and homelessness,
    160–161
Biology
    gender, 208–209
    men's health promotion, 217
    see also Medicalisation
Birth plans, 76
Birth weight, 52
Black communities (USA), health promotion,
    36
'Black pathology', 231
Black Report (1980), 11–13, 18, 266–267
Blair administration, 32
Blame culture *see* Victim blaming
Block booking, general practitioners,
    267–268
Blood donation, 'queer' community, 254
Body image
    disorders, 216
    teenage pregnancy, 86
Body Positive, 256
Body under siege, 7, 8
Bodybuilding, as disorder, 216
Bond, J. et al, *Ageing in society*, 283
Bottomley, Rt. Hon. V., quoted, 173
Bottom-up approaches, 16
    community development, 36, 44, 234–235,
        239
    HIV epidemic, 250
Bradford, N., *Men's health matters*, 227
Brady, J., on empowerment, 30
Brazil, education and empowerment, 28–29
Breast cancer
    mortality, 215
    screening, older people, 274
Breastfeeding, Stockport neighbourhood
    health strategy, 301 (Box)
Brighton, homeless people not registered with
    GP, 164
Britain
    teenage pregnancy, 83, 133 (Box)
    see also UK National Screening Committee
Bronchial cancer, 215
Bronchitis
    gender differences, 211
    men's screening, 218
Burden, older people seen as, 269, 270
Bureaucracy, and intersectoral collaboration,
    14–15
Business case, Stockport neighbourhood
    health strategy, 288–289

Calman, Sir K., *Project to strengthen public
    health function*, 12
Campaign Against Living Miserably
    (CALM), 188 (Box), 219
Canada
    Kids in Action, 144, 146
    suicide, group interventions, 195–196
Cancers
    children, 104 (Box)
    gender differences, 215
    male reproductive system, 213
    older people, screening, 274
    Stockport neighbourhood health strategy,
        302 (Box)
Capitation fees, older people, 269
Car fumes, and suicide, 187–188
Care Programme Approach (1990), mental
    health promotion, 188 (Box), 198
Carer-induced dementia, 275, 277
Carers
    first aid skills, 275
    hidden health work, 16
    mental illness in, 194–195
    older people, 276
    support meetings, 304
Caring for people (1989), older people, 265
Carroll, S., *Which? guide to men's health*, 227
Case notes
    midwifery, 76
    portable record cards, 178
Cerebrovascular accidents
    gender differences, 211
    Health of the nation targets, 266 (Box)
    informal carers, 276–277
Cervical screening, older people, 274
CESPIT (mnemonic), 259–260
Chamberlain, G., definition of pre-conception
    care, 52
Changing childbirth (Expert Maternity
    Group), 70–72, 73–74, 75, 76, 77
CHAR, on homelessness
    figures, 156
    sexual abuse, 159
Charity organisations, child health, 118
Chemicals, conception, 56
Chest X-rays, men's screening, 218
Child health in the community (NHSE),
    106–107
Child health promotion, empowerment,
    101–123
Child Poverty Action Group, 118
Childbirth, and empowerment, 65–81
Children
    caring for adults, 120
    decision making involvement, 120–121
    home alone, 302 (Box)
    knowledge on illness, 112
    loss and mental disturbance, 162–163
    responsibility for health, 112–113
    rights, 102–103, 113–115, 129–130
        Convention on the Rights of the Child
            (UN), 102, 129–130
        The Children Act (1989), 128–129, 133
    views of, 107–111, 130 (Box)
Chinese subgroup, Tameside Ethnic Health
    Forum, 239–240

Choice
  childbirth care, 73–75
  free, 10–11
  informed, childbirth care, 73–75
Chronic bronchitis *see* Bronchitis
Cities, sexual health and HIV, 259
Clerical requirements, neighbourhood health
    strategy projects, 295, 300
Client-centred health promotion, 221
Clients (term), 36
Clinical nurse manager, Stockport neighbour-
    hood health strategy, 289
Clinics, pre-conception care, 57–58
Clunis, C. (case), 198
Cocaine, pregnancy, 56
Co-habitation, and health, 213
COHSE, consumer groups, mental health
    services, 199
Collective empowerment, *vs* individual,
    34–35, 221–224
Colleges, 139–140
Colonisation, community health promotion
    as, 36
Colorectal cancer, 215
  screening, 218
Combined primary health services, homeless
    people, 173
Coming out, Gay and Lesbian Switchboard,
    251 (Box)
Commercial interests, 10–11
Commercialisation of health, 6
Commissioning, child health services, 120
Commodity, health as, 6
Communication skills
  men's health, 222–223 (Box)
  midwifery, 72
  see also Information
Communities, construction by AIDS
    epidemic, 247–248
Community action, 235, 287 (Box)
Community capacity building, 234
Community children's nurses, asthma
    management, 119
Community coordination, 235
Community development
  disadvantages, 21
  empowerment, 35–36, 224
  ethnic minority groups, 233–238, 242
  older people, 270–271
  Stockport neighbourhood health strategy,
    287–288 (Box)
  workers, 20
  young people's involvement, 144–145
Community drugs and alcohol teams, young
    people's health, 134
Community groups, 39
  alliances with, 239–240
Community Mental Health Centres (USA),
    190, 191
Community nurses
  head of community nursing (Stockport),
    289
  older people, 280, 281
  outreach work, 148
  see also Public health nurses
Community participation, 16–18

homeless women, 166–171
  older people, 270–271
  sexual health and HIV, 258–260
  young people's health, 132
Community psychiatric nurses, 187, 193
Competent childbearers (Parsons and
    Perkins), 75
Compliance, *vs* cooperation, 221
Compulsory treatment, mental illness,
    198–199
Conception, and weight, 52
Confederation of Health Service Employees,
    consumer groups, mental health
    services, 199
Confidential Enquiry into Sudden Deaths in
    Infancy, 72
Confidential Inquiry into Homicides and
    Suicides by Mentally Ill People (Royal
    College of Psychiatrists), 198
Conflict of interest, health professionals from
    communities, 240
Conformity, teenagers, 94–95
Connect 4 Health Training Programme, 236
Consciousness raising, critical
    (conscientisation), 29, 35
Consumer groups
  childbirth, 68–70
  mental health services, 199
  see also Community groups; Self-help
    groups
Contraception
  services, teenagers, 96
  sex education, 93
  see also Family planning
'Contract for health', 106
Control
  disguised as participation, 18
  with empowerment, community
    development programmes, 145 (Box)
  vs helplessness, 8
  locus of (Rotter), 9–10
  in research interviews, 170
  vs responsibility, 21
Conurbations, sexual health and HIV, 259
Convention on the Rights of the Child (UN),
    102, 129–130
Cooperation, *vs* compliance, 221
Coordinators, Stockport neighbourhood
    health strategy, 287, 288, 291 (Box),
    294, 299–300
Coping skills, mental health as, 184
Coping strategies, smoking as, 302 (Box)
Coronary heart disease *see* Ischaemic heart
    disease
Council houses, 157–158, 179
Counselling
  carers, 194–195
  men, 222–223 (Box)
Couriers, cross-cultural, information on AIDS
    epidemic, 250
Court Report, *Fit for the future*, 121
Creative Support services (Manchester), 196
Credibility, hierarchy of, 39
Crime
  vs participation, 39–40
  and poverty, 12

Critical consciousness raising, 29, 35
Cross-curricular subject, health education as, 136
Cultural critique, 7, 8
Cultural factors
  gender differences, 209–210
  mental health, 184
Cultural invasion
  Brazil, 28–29
  health promotion as, 33
Cultural minority groups *see* Ethnic minority groups
Culturalism, ethnic minority groups, 230–231
Curriculum guidance 5 (National Curriculum Council), 154

Dampness, 11–12
Data collection, Stockport neighbourhood health strategy project, 295–296
Days, for awareness-raising (Stockport), 289, 290
Deaf gay men, as community, 248
De-gaying, HIV, 254–255, 256
Dementia
  carer-induced, 275, 277
  carers for, 194
Demography, old age, 265
Department of Social Security, Health and Homelessness Unit, 160
Depression
  gay men, 220
  group interventions, 195
  mortality, 219
  older people, 277, 278
  Sweden, general practitioner education, 196
Deprivation *see* Poverty
Deprived areas, 105
Descartes, R. (1596–1650), 3
Detached approaches, young people's health promotion, 147–149
Development rights, children, 129 (Box)
Developmental monitoring, 107
Devonshire Street General Practice (Sheffield), health services for homeless people, 174 (Box)
Diabetes mellitus, 272, 274–275, 280–281
Dialogue, in community development, 35–36
Didactic methods, young people's health promotion, 143
Diet
  children's views, 110–111
  men's health, 222 (Box)
  older people, 272
  pre-conception care, 52–53
  Stockport neighbourhood health strategy project, 301 (Box), 302 (Box)
  see also Nutrition
Direct-access clinics
  homeless people, 172
  school nurses, 137
Disabilities
  babies with, support networks, 59–60
  children, 105
    rights, 130 (Box)

Discovery of HIV, 249
Discrimination, training on homelessness *vs*, 177
Disenfranchisement, 12
Dishonesty, shock horror approaches, 142
District nurses *see* Community nurses; Head of community nursing (Stockport); Public health nurses
Domestic violence, 159, 162, 178
Dominance, 7
Douglas, J., on health promotion in black communities, 36
Doyle, W., birth weight, 52
Drain on resources, older people seen as, 269, 270
Draw and write techniques, views of children, 108–110
Drop-in health clinics *see* Direct-access clinics
Drug abuse
  gay men, 220
  general *vs* specialist health services, 150
  Kids in Action programme, 144
  and participation, 39–40
  pregnancy, 56
  shock horror approach, 141–142
  young people, 133 (Box)
Dualism (Descartes), 3

Eastman, M, elder abuse, 279
Eating disorders, 216
Economic policy, 13
Education
  of carers, 276
  and empowerment, 28–29
  legislation on sex education, 92
  midwifery, 67
  pre-conception care, 54
  teenage pregnancy, 85, 86, 90–93
  universities, 139–140
  young people's health, 126–127
  see also Parents, education of
Effectiveness of mental health promotion interventions (Tilford et al), 205
Efficacy expectancy, 9
Eiser, C., children's views on health, 111–112
Elder abuse, 279–280
Elites
  medico-scientific, 31–32, 43
    journals, 44
  'professional participators', 17, 38
Emergency hostel provision, 159–160
Employers, workplace stress, 191
Empowerment, 27–47
  AIDS epidemic, 253
  asthma, 119
  child health promotion, 101–123
  and childbirth, 65–81
  of communities, 235
    gay community, 257–258
  in conception and pregnancy, 58, 60
  construction of communities, 248
  fetus, 73
  vs health promotion, 32
  meanings, 20
  men, 221–224
  misuse, 23, 28

Empowerment (*contd*)
 teenagers and sex, 93, 94–95
 young people's health, 125–154
 see also Power
Empowerment in community care (Jack), 93
Enablement, *vs* empowerment, 33, 93
End of innocence, The (Garfield), 248, 249
English National Board
 Learning from each other, 200–201
 practice benchmarks, older people, 270
Environmental factors, 11–13
 conception, 56
Epidemiology, 22, 31
Equity, community development, 18–21
Ethics
 peer education, 147 (Box)
 research interviews, 170–171
Ethnic minority advisory groups, 239–240
Ethnic minority groups, 11, 229–244
 children, 105, 120
 and participation, 38
European Network of Health Promoting
 Schools, 92, 149
Evaluation, neighbourhood health strategy
 projects, 304–305
Evans, B. et al, *Working where the risks are*,
 261
Eviction, illegal, 158–159
Evidence-based practice, mental health
 promotion, 188
Ewles and Simnett
 educational approaches, 95
 men's health, 221
 primary prevention, 59
Exercise
 children, 275, 302 (Box)
 older people, 272, 275
Exercise and mental health (MIND), 189
Exhaust emissions, and suicide, 187–188
Expert Maternity Group, *Changing childbirth*,
 70–72, 73–74, 75, 76, 77
Exploitation, 7
 in research interviews, 169–170
Expressive support (Thoits), 74

Facilitators, community development
 programmes, young people's health,
 145
Factory pollution, intersectoral collaboration
 example, 15
Fahlberg, L.L., definition of empowerment,
 28
Falls, 271–272
Families
 as carers, 194–195
 child health, 113–115
 housing policy biased to, 158
 rejection by, 157
 schizophrenia, 197
 young people's health, 134–135, 142
Family planning
 clinics, and young people, 134
 ethnic minority groups, 230
 see also Contraception
Family planning nurses, sex education, 92
Family values, New Right, 42

Fatalism (magic consciousness – Friere), 29
Feedback, Stockport neighbourhood health
 strategy project, 294
Feminism
 applied to gay community, 257, 258
 research on homelessness, 168–171
Ferguson, K., mental health promotion, 189
Fetus, rights of, 73
Finance, teenage pregnancy, 86
First aid skills, carers, 275
Fit for the future (Court Report), 121
Fitness, *vs* health, 220
Five C's, Stockport neighbourhood health
 strategy, 287–288
Folic acid supplements, 53
Foot care, 272, 280–281
Footwear, older people, 272
Foucault, M., on power, 28
Fractures, and padding, 272
Free choice, 10–11
Friere, P.
 empowerment, 233
 education and, 28–30
 praxis, 29, 132, 145
 youth health promotion programmes,
 144–145
Function, and health, 5–6
Fundholding, general practitioners, and older
 people, 268–269
Funding
 AIDS and health, 256, 257
 community development, 41–42
 midwifery initiatives, problems, 76
 Stockport neighbourhood health strategy
 project, 290–291

Garfield, S., *The end of innocence*, 248, 249
Gay, as term, 246
Gay and Lesbian Switchboard, 251–252
Gay men
 health promotion, 220
 as outreach workers, 257–258
 'queer' health, 245–261
 stereotype, 252–253
Gay Men Fighting AIDS, 258
Gender awareness, training on homelessness,
 177
Gender differences, 209–213
 cancers, 215
 suicide, 216, 219
Gender-specificity, health definition, 208
General practitioners, 21–22
 child health, 117–118
 education on depression (Sweden), 196
 and homelessness, 164, 165–166
 information for, 177
 mental health promotion, 188 (Box),
 193–194
 older people, 268–269
 rationing of health care, 267–268
 Stockport neighbourhood health strategy,
 289, 293, 298–299
 young people's health, 134
Genetic counselling, 58
Glamorisation, 'Heroin Screws You Up'
 campaign, 142

'God's power' account, 8
Government documents, 10
Grace, V., on empowerment, 33
Graham, H., on research interviewing,
    169–170
Great Chapel Street Medical Centre
    (London), 174 (Box)
Greater London, midwifery initiative, 76
Grief, 246
    activists, 251
    politicisation by, 248
Grimshaw, J., quoted, 245
Group interventions
    carers, 194–195
    depression, 195
Guidelines, maternity care, 71
Gynaecology, and sexual health advice, 274

Hall Report, child health, 107
'Handy women', 65–66
Hannover General Practice (Sheffield), health
    services for homeless people, 174
    (Box)
Harassment of tenants, 158–159
Hazel Grove, Information and Advice Centre,
    303–304
Head of community nursing (Stockport), 289
Health, 5–9, 106, 185
    children's portrayal, 108
    gender, 208
    and old age, 264
Health action zones, 32, 219, 224
Health alliances see Healthy alliances
Health and Homelessness Unit, Department
    of Social Security, 160
Health authorities
    mental health promotion, 188
    as purchasers of health care, 232–233
Health belief model, 10
Health centres, older people, 270
Health checks see Screening
Health Commission (Stockport), 286,
    288–289
Health contracts, 117
    see also 'Contract for health'
Health divide, The (Whitehead), 18
Health education, 224
    co-ordinators, 140–141
    ethnic minority groups, 230–232
    homeless women, 163
    mental health promotion, 189, 191
    and risk reduction, 35
    schools, 126–127, 135–136
    youth clubs, 138
Health education. Effectiveness, efficiency
    and equity (Tones and Tilford), 306
Health Education Authority
    health alliances, 118
    World Mental Health Day, 192–193
    with Youth Clubs UK, 139
Health fairs, 139
Health fascism (Skrabanek), 3
Health for all see Alma Ata declaration
Health for all by the year 2000 (WHO), 13,
    27
Health for all in Europe by the year 2000
    (WHO), 238

Health impact assessment, 32
Health needs assessment, 62
Health of Britain's ethnic minorities, The
    (Nazroo), 243
Health of the nation, The (1992), 10, 238
    child health, 115–116
    health-promoting schools, 130–131
    Key area handbook, mental illness
        185–186
    older people, 265–266
    sexual health and HIV, 257
    Stockport neighbourhood health strategy
        project, 286
    suicide prevention, 187
    teenage pregnancy, 84
    young people's health, 127–128, 133
Health of the young nation, The, 116, 127
Health professionals
    from communities, conflict of interest, 240
    giving sex education, 91–92
    and parents, 114
    working with schools, 136–137
Health promotion, 8
    and AIDS, 246, 255–256
    child health, 107
    construction of communities, 248
    and homelessness, 175–176
    men, 217–220
    National Health Service, 61
Health promotion – foundations for practice
    (Naidoo and Wills), 283
Health Promotion and young people
    (Aggleton), 154
Health promotion specialists, for young
    people, 140–141
Health promotion Wales (1994), on healthy
    alliances, 240–241
Health psychology (Niven), 283
Health strategy days (Stockport), 289, 290
Health strategy evenings (Stockport), 294,
    297
Health visiting and elderly people
    (McClymont et al), 283
Health visitors, 117
    older people, 280
    post-natal depression, 195
    as public health nurses (Stockport), 289,
        290
    sex education, 92
Healthcare Trust (Stockport), 286
Health-promoting schools, 130–131, 134,
    138, 149–150
    Our healthier nation (Green Paper), 117,
        128, 131
Healthy alliances
    AIDS epidemic, 252
    child health, 115–119
    ethnic minority groups, 238–241
    homeless people, 171–175
    neighbourhood health strategy projects,
        286
    older people, 278–281
    young people's health, 134–139
Healthy Gay Manchester, 258
'Healthy schools initiative', Our healthier
    nation (Green Paper), 117, 128, 131
Healthy settings work, 149–150
    see also Health-promoting schools

Hearing aid batteries, 304
Helplessness, *vs* control, 8
Heroin, pregnancy, 56
'Heroin Screws You Up' campaign, 141–142
Heterosexual community, as term, 247
Hidden health work, 16
'Hidden homeless', 156–160
Hierarchy of credibility, 39
Higgins, T., death from AIDS, 250
Hippocrates, fetal development, 52
History, 3–9
  construction, AIDS epidemic, 248–249
HIV
  de-gaying, 254–255, 256
  health promotion, 220
  older people, 273
  outreach work, 148
  re-gaying, 256
  scale of epidemic, 249
HIV/AIDS and older people (Kaufmann), 284
Hodgson, R.J. et al, on mental health promotion, 185
Holism, 7
  direct-access clinics, 172
  health fairs, 139
  HIV epidemic, 252
  Stockport neighbourhood health strategy, 304
  young people's health promotion, 143
  see also Health-promoting schools
Holland, starvation 1944–1945, 52
Home ownership, 'Right to Buy' policy, 157–158
Home tutors, teenage pregnancy, 86
Homelessness, 155–157
  health, 160–162
  see also Women, homelessness
Homes
  older people in own, 268
  see also Families
Homeworking, 12
Homicide, Confidential Inquiry (Royal College of Psychiatrists), 198
Homosexuality
  homelessness, 156–157
  'queer' health, 245–261
  see also Gay men; Lesbian women
Hormone replacement therapy, 275
Hospital patients, mental illness in, 196
Hospitalisation
  childbirth, 66
  mental illness, 193
Hostel provision, emergency, 159–160
Hostility, primary care staff, 166
House of Commons Select Committee (1997), child health, 103
Housing, 11–12
  childhood accidents, 105
  ethnic minority groups, 241
  insecurity, 156
  lobbying on, 178
  mental health, 196
  older people, 268
  Royal College of Physicians on, 178–179
Housing Act (1996), 160
Housing Projects Advisory Service, harassment cases, 159

How to look after yourself (MIND), 189
Human immunodeficiency virus *see* HIV
Humanist theories of health, 7
Hypertension, pregnancy-induced, teenage pregnancy, 88

Ideal state, health as, 5
Illich, I., on medicine, 4
Illness, children's knowledge, 112
Immune system, psycho-neuroimmunology, 268
Impact evaluation, neighbourhood health strategy projects, 305
IMPACT groups (Stockport), 288, 294
Implementation groups, local (Stockport), 288, 294
Impotence (sexual), 213–214
Incentives, 9
Income distribution, and inequalities, 19
  see also Poverty
Independence, health in old age, 264, 268
Independent midwifery practice, 77
Individualism, 8, 33
Individuals
  behaviour, 9–11, 13, 106
  empowerment, *vs* collective, 34–35, 221–224
  responsibility, 23
Inequality
  of access, 7
  in community, 18–21
  older people, 266, 267
Infectious diseases
  health promotion, 253
  see also HIV; Sexually transmitted diseases
Infertility
  male, 213
  rates, 61
  and smoking, 55
Information
  childbirth care, 73–75, 76
  children's right of access, 130 (Box)
  and community development, 41
  cross-cultural couriers, AIDS epidemic, 250
  for homeless people, 176–177 (Box)
  Somali Community Health Project, 237
  Stockport neighbourhood health strategy project, 294–296
Information and Advice Centre (Hazel Grove), 303–304
Information technology, children, 115
Injuries, children, 104–105
Insecurity, professional rivalries, 141
Institutionalisation (carer-induced dementia), 275, 277
Instrumental support (Thoits), 74
Integration, ethnic minority groups, 230–231
Intensive care, families of patients, 194
Interactive methods, young people's health promotion, 143
Interagency collaboration, 14–16, 41, 115–119, 240–241
  The Children Act (1989), 129
  in homelessness, 178
  neighbourhood health strategy projects, 286, 296, 299
  statutory requirement, 175

Interagency collaboration (*contd*)
  Stockport neighbourhood health strategy,
    287 (Box)
  see also Partnership models
Interest, conflict, health professionals from
    communities, 240
Internal market *see* Providers of health care;
    Purchasers of health care
Intersectoral collaboration *see* Interagency
    collaboration
Interviews, feminist research, 169–171
Ischaemic heart disease
  Ashton Asian Health Development Project,
    236
  gender differences, 211, 212, 214
  Health of the nation targets, 266 (Box)

Jack, R., *Empowerment in community care*,
    93
Jacobson, B., on socially excluded groups, 40
Journals, research on community
    development, 44
Justice, 19

Katz and Reberdy, *Promoting health:
    knowledge and practice*, 244
Kaufmann, T., *HIV/AIDS and older people*,
    284
*Key area handbook, mental illness, The
    health of the nation* (1992), 185–186
Kids in Action (Canada), 144, 146
King's Fund Review of Health and
    Homelessness
  on mental health and homelessness, 161
  on women and primary health care, 175
'Know your Midwife' scheme, 75
Knowledge–attitude–behaviour approach, 9
Konje, J.C., study on teenage pregnancy,
    87–88
Kramer, L., *Reports from the holocaust*, 261
Kroll, D., on midwives, 78

Labonte, R., on empowerment, 38
Ladder of participation (Arnstein), 17, 18
    (Box)
Landlords, 158–159
Language, 'queer' health, 246–252
Learning from each other (English National
    Board), 200–201
Legal action *see* Litigation
Legislation
  sex education, 92
  see also named Acts
Legitimisation of illness, 6
Lesbian and Gay Switchboard, 251–252
Lesbian women
  blood donation, 254
  homelessness, 156–157
Liaison psychiatry services, 196
Liberation
  community participation as, 42–43
  empowerment as, 28
Lifeskills (Hopson and Scally), 34–35
Lifestyle, 106

Link workers, combined primary health
    services, homeless people, 173
Litigation
  maternity care, 71
  workplace stress, 191
Liverpool, intersectoral collaboration, 15
Lobbying, 224
  on homelessness, 177–178
Local Agenda 21, 35
Local authorities
  ethnic minority advisory groups, 239–240
  health education initiatives, 127
  homelessness, 176
    figures, 156
  Housing Act (1966), 160
  rented housing, 157–158, 179
Local implementation groups, Stockport
    neighbourhood health strategy
    (IMPACT groups), 288, 294
Local voices (NHS), 233
Locality managers (Stockport), 293
Locus of control (Rotter), 9–10
London
  health services for homeless people, 174
    (Box)
  midwifery initiative, 76
Lone parent families, 105
Low paying employment, 11
Lung cancer, 215

Machine, body as, 3, 4, 7, 8
MacIntyre, P., information on childbirth, 74
Magic consciousness (Friere), 29
Magpie profession, health promotion as
    (Seedhouse), 34
Mammography, older people, 294
Manchester
  Creative Support services, 196
  health action zone, 219
  homeless people not registered with GP,
    164, 165
  suicide rates, 187, 219
  Woodhouse Park Clinic, 150
Manipulation, and peer education, 147 (Box)
Marriage, and health, 213
Masculinity, 210–211
Maternal age, 56–57
  see also Teenagers, pregnancy
Maternity
  and empowerment, 65–81
  pre-conception care, 51–64, 77
  see also Pregnancy
McClymont, M. et al, *Health visiting and
    elderly people*, 283
Medical profession
  AIDS epidemic, 250, 251, 252, 253
  mental health promotion, 190
  obstetrics, 66–67
  power, 4, 5, 6, 31
Medical records
  midwifery, 76
  portable, 178
Medicalisation, 3, 4, 6, 23
  care of older people, 278
  childbirth, 67, 74
  community development, 38

Medicalisation (*contd*)
  compliance *vs* cooperation, 221
Medicines, and suicide, 187–188
Men
  health, 207–227
  'refusing to be men', 225
  smoking, fertility, 55
  suicide rates, 187
MENCAP, 118
Men's health, readership, 220
Men's health matters (Bradford), 227
Men's health review (Royal College of
      Nursing), 227
Men's Health Trust, 210
Menstruation, early menarche, 87
Mental health, 183–205
  definitions, 184
  older people, 277–278, 281
    carer-induced dementia, 275, 277
  Oldham African–Caribbean Mental Health
      Drop-in Sessions, 239
  promotion for men, 219
  Somali Mental Health Project, 237
  Stockport neighbourhood health strategy,
      302 (Box)
  stress, 215–216
Mental Health Act (1983), 198
Mental Health Act (1995), 199
Mental Health Nursing Review Team (1994),
      190, 200–201
*Mental health promotion: paradigms and
      practice* (Tudor), 205
Mental illness
  homelessness, 160–163
  impact, 183, 186
Middle classes, health promotion and older
      people, 267
Midwifery, 65–81
Midwives
  relationships with clients, 77–78
  sex education, 92
  teenage pregnancy, 96
Midwives Institute, 66
Miller, M., study on homeless women, 167
Millstein, S. et al, *Promoting the health of
      adolescents*, 154
MIND
  booklets, 189
  consumer groups, 199
  older people, 281
Minimum intervention, mental health care,
      199
Minority groups, cultural, and participation,
      38
Minors, finance, teenage pregnancy, 86
Mnemonics, CESPIT, 259–260
Mobile facilities, for older people, 269
Morbidity
  children, 103–104
  gender differences, 211–213
Morris, J., on testicular self-examination,
      218–219
Mortality
  cancers, 215
  children, 103–104
  depression, 219
  gender differences, 211–213

homelessness, 161
male reproductive system cancers, 213
teenage mothers, 84
see also Suicide
Mortgages, and single women, 157
Mothers
  post-natal depression, 192, 195
  teenage, 89, 96
  views on childbirth, 74–75
Multi-agency alliances *see* Interagency
      collaboration
Multiple births, 104 (Box)
Multisectoral collaboration *see* Interagency
      collaboration

Naidoo and Wills, *Health promotion–
      foundations for practice*, 283
Naive consciousness (Friere), 29
National Asthma Campaign, 119
National Childbirth Trust, 51, 68
National Children's Bureau, 118
National Curriculum, health education,
      126–127
National Curriculum Council, *Curriculum
      guidance 5*, 154
National Health Service
  'doing one's best', 67
  ethnic minority groups, 232–233
  Health Advisory Service, *Suicide
      prevention: the challenge confronted*,
      205
  and homelessness, 165–166
  pre-conception care, 57–58
  see also Health authorities
National Health Service (NHS) and
      Community Care Act (1990), 61
  older people, 265
National Medical Association (USA), speech
      on violence, 40
National Union of Teachers, on sex
      education, 91
Nazroo, J.Y., *The health of Britain's ethnic
      minorities*, 243
Needs-led approach, 62
Neighbourhood health strategy projects *see*
      Stockport, neighbourhood health
      strategy project
Neighbourhoods, Stockport neighbourhood
      health strategy project, 286, 293–294,
      300
Neonatal mortality, 61, 104 (Box)
Netherlands, starvation 1944-1945, 52
Networking *see* Interagency collaboration;
      Partnership models; Support networks
Neural tube defects, 53
New Mexico, Adolescent Social Action
      Program, 144–145, 146
New NHS. Modern, dependable (White
      Paper), 16, 19, 175, 238–239
New public health, The (Ashton and
      Seymour), 13–22, 23, 306
New Right, family values, 42
New Zealand, mental health education, 190
NHS Health Advisory Service, *Suicide
      prevention: the challenge confronted*,
      205

Nigger, as term, 247
Niven, N., *Health psychology*, 283
'No smoking days', Stockport neighbourhood
    health strategy, 287 (Box)
Northern Ireland, health and youth clubs,
    139
Norwich, Under the Stars project, 148
Notice board, Stockport neighbourhood
    health strategy, 304
Nottingham
    Base 51, 150–151
    health services for homeless people, 174
        (Box)
Nurses
    mental health
        training on, 196
        views on, 200–201
    primary care, older people, 270
Nutbeam, D. et al, *Youth Health Promotion*,
    154
Nutrition
    on fetus, 52
    old age, 270
    Stockport neighbourhood health strategy,
        301 (Box), 302 (Box)
    see also Diet

Oakley, A., on research interviewing, 170
Obesity, 216
    and pregnancy, 52–53
Obstetrics
    maternal age, 57
    pressures on women, 73
    rivalry with midwifery, 66–67
    teenage pregnancy, 85, 88
Occupation
    chemicals, conception, 56
    gender differences, 209–210
    see also Workplace
Occupational health nurses, colleges, 140
Odets, W., scale of AIDS epidemic, 249
Old age, 263–284
    carers, 194
    elder abuse, 279–280
    mental health promotion, 188 (Box)
    Stockport neighbourhood health strategy,
        302–303 (Box)
    see also Elder abuse
Oldham African–Caribbean Mental Health
    Drop-in Sessions, 239
Opinion polls, on homelessness, 178
Opportunistic health promotion (Bagnall and
    Dilloway), 117
Oppression, 7
    disguised as participation, 18
Organogenesis, 53
Osteoporosis, 275, 281
Ottawa Charter for Health Promotion, 27
    empowerment, 30, 32, 35, 224
    older people, 265
Our healthier nation (Green Paper), 10, 106,
    171, 238–239
    child health, 115
    collaborative approach, 14, 116–118
    and communities, 224
    disease-based targets, 32

'healthy schools initiative', 117, 128, 131
    justice, 19
    men's health, 217
    mental health, 186, 190
    older people, 266
    young people's health promotion, 151
Outcome expectancy, 9
Outcome measurement
    and community participation, 17
    neighbourhood health strategy projects,
        305
    pre-conception care, 61–62
Outrage, activism, 251
Outreach, young people's health promotion,
    147–149
Outreach workers, to gay community,
    257–258
Overeating, 216
Overweight, 216
    and pregnancy, 52–53
Owner occupation *see* Home ownership
Ownership of health, 253

Padding, and fractures, 272
Paracetamol, 188
Parents
    asthma, 119
    education of
        Stockport neighbourhood health strategy,
            301 (Box)
        teenage pregnancy, 90
    giving sex education, 91
    groups, pre-conception care, 51
    and health professionals, 114
    sexuality of offspring, 96–97
    women categorised as, 167
    young people's health, 135
Parsons, T., definition of health, 6
Parsons, W. and E. Perkins, competent
    childbearers, 75
Participation
    community development, 36–44
    ladder of (Arnstein), 17, 18 (Box)
    mental health services, 199
    rights, children, 129 (Box)
Partnership models, child health, 113–115
Paternalism, 5
    child health, 103
    empowerment by others as, 34
Patient's charter, 233
    older people, 265
    quoted, 173
Patton, C., HIV and communities, 247
Peer educators, young people's health, 145,
    146–147
Peer pressure, teenagers, 94–95
Peer support, Stockport neighbourhood
    health strategy, 292, 293
Pejorative terms, 247, 260
Perinatal mortality, 61
Personal and social health education (PSHE),
    136
Persuasive models, health promotion, 106,
    107
Physical abuse
    homelessness, 159, 163

Physical abuse (contd)
  see also Domestic violence; Elder abuse
Physical illness, mental illness with, 196
Physique, health as, 220
Piper, S., on well-man clinics, 217–218
Pneumocystis carinii pneumonia, 249
Politicisation, by grief, 248
Politics
  community development, 20–21, 42
  and empowerment, 29–30, 34–35, 224
  HIV epidemic, 252
  see also Lobbying
Polluting factory, intersectoral collaboration
    example, 15
Population, old age, 265
Portable record cards, 178
Postmodernism, and Friere, 30
Postnatal care, poor information, 75
Postnatal depression, 192, 195
Posture, and falls, 271, 272
Poverty, 11–12
  child health, 105–106
  conception and pregnancy, 53–54
  vs participation, 39–40
  teenage pregnancy, 85, 132
  women, housing, 157–158
  young people's health, 142
Powell, on healthy alliances, 240–241
Power
  community development, 20–21
  dominance, 7
  evolution of meaning of, 27–28
  medical profession, 4, 5, 6, 31
  vs participation, 37–38
  professionals vs parents, 114
  in research interviews, 170
  see also Empowerment
Pragmatism, construction of communities,
    248
Pratt, R.J., history of AIDS, 249
Praxis (Friere), 29, 132, 145
Pre-conception care, 51–64, 77
Pregnancy
  alcohol, 54, 55–56
  cocaine, 56
  frequent, 54, 66
  heroin, 56
  as normal, 69
  smoking, 54, 55
  unsupported, 88
  see also Teenagers, pregnancy; Termination
    of pregnancy
Pregnancy-induced hypertension, teenage
    pregnancy, 88
Pre-identified agendas, 236
Prejudices, 39
Premature birth, survival, 104
Pre-natal care see Antenatal care
Pre-school children, 106–107
Prescriptions
  antidepressants, 196
  short-term, 188 (Box)
Prevention
  mental illness, 185, 189–198
  in pre conception care, 58–60
Pridmore and Bendelow, draw and write
    techniques, 108

Primary care groups, child health, 120
Primary health care, 21–22
  homelessness, 172–173
    women, 155–181
  information on homeless people, 177
  as medical service, 21
  mental health screening, 193–194
  older people, 269
    health centres, 270
  see also General practitioners
Primary health promotion, 107
Primary prevention
  mental illness, 189–193
  pre-conception care, 58–59
Primary schools
  children, 101–123
  health education, 136
Private midwifery practice, 77
Private sector, rented housing, 158–159, 161
Problem orientation
  research on homeless women, 167
  young people's health, 126, 128
Process evaluation, neighbourhood health
    strategy projects, 305
'Professional participators', 17, 38
Professional rivalries, insecurity, 141
Professionalisation, AIDS response, 256–257,
    259
Professionalism, vs community participation,
    43
  mental health services, 199–200
Professionals see Health professionals;
    Medical profession
Project advisor, Stockport neighbourhood
    health strategy, 289
Project management team, Stockport
    neighbourhood health strategy, 289,
    290
Project SIGMA, 261
Project to strengthen public health function
    (Calman), 12
Promoting good health (Scottish Health
    Education Group), 154
Promoting health: knowledge and practice
    (Katz and Reberdy), 244
'Promoting Positive Mental Health' (World
    Mental Health Day), 192–193
Promoting the health of adolescents
    (Millstein et al), 154
Prostate cancer, 213, 215
  screening, 218
  sexual health advice, 274
Protection rights, children, 129 (Box)
Protest groups, 236
Providers of health care, 232–233
  interaction with user groups, 200
  pre-conception care, 60–62
  services for homeless people, 176
PSHE (personal and social health education),
    136
Psychiatrists, and mental health promotion,
    190
Psychology, teenage pregnancy, 85–86
Psycho-neuroimmunology, 268
Public health, new movement, 13–22
Public health nurses (Stockport), 286, 288,
    292

Public health nurses (Stockport) (*contd*)
    views of, 297–303
Public participation *see* Community
        participation
Purchasers of health care
    care for homeless people, 176
    health authorities as, 232–233
    pre-conception care, 60–62
Purchasing HIV prevention (Scott), 261

Qualitative research, 169
    Stockport neighbourhood health strategy
        project, 304–305
Quantitative research
    HIV prevention, 259
    homelessness, 167–168
'Queer' health, 245–261

'Race' and health in contemporary Britain
        (Ahmad), 243
Racism, 232, 241
Rappaport, J., on contradictory solutions, 41
Rationing of health care, 267–268
Record cards, portable, 178
Rectal examination, 218
Reducing diets, and conception, 52
Reductionism, 3–4, 31
    male, 168
Refuges, domestic violence, 159, 178
Re-gaying, HIV, 256
Relaxation exercises, mental health
        promotion, 191
Religion, 3
Rented housing
    lobbying on, 178
    local authorities, 157–158, 179
    private sector, 158–159, 161
Reports from the holocaust (Kramer), 261
Representation
    top-down community development, 240
    see also Activists
Research
    community participation, 43–44
        homeless women, 166–168, 175–176,
            178
        neighbourhood health strategy projects,
            304–305
        sex education, 93
Resources
    supportive, 41
    see also Funding
Respiratory diseases
    children, 104 (Box), 105
    gender differences, 211
    men's screening, 218
Respite care, 304
Responsibility
    child health, 112–113
    vs control, 21
    individual *vs* societal, 23, 42
Rickets, 231
'Right to Buy' policy, local authority
        properties, 157–158
Rights
    of children, 102–103, 113–115, 129–130

mental health services, 199, 200
Risks
    gender differences, 209
    HIV, 254–255
Road traffic accidents, children, 105
Rogers, A., student-centred learning, 132
Rogers, C.
    communication skills, 222–223 (Box)
    focus and HIV epidemic, 252
Rooflessness, suicide rate, 161
Ropers and Boyer, quoted on research into
        homelessness, 167–168
Rothman, B.K.
    on *Changing childbirth*, 73–74
    medicalisation of childbirth, 67
Royal College of Midwives, 75
Royal College of Nursing, *Men's health
        review*, 227
Royal College of Physicians, on homelessness,
        174, 178–179
Royal College of Psychiatrists, Confidential
        Inquiry into Homicides and Suicides
        by Mentally Ill People, 198

Sabo and Gordon, men's health, 225, 227
Sacks, O.
    Awakenings, 7
    on health as commodity, 6
Safe sex
    older people, 274
    and powerlessness, 33
    sex education, 95
    see also Sexual health
Safety *see* Accidents
Samaritans, 190
Schizophrenia
    carers, 194
    homeless women, 162
    tertiary prevention, 197
School nurses, 117–118, 137
    giving sex education, 91–92
    information for general practice health
        promotion, 287 (Box)
School teachers, giving sex education, 91
Schools
    health education, 126–127, 135–136
    health-promoting, 130–131, 134, 138,
        149–150
    Our healthier nation (Green Paper), 117,
        128, 131
    teenage pregnancy, 85
    young people's health promotion, 135–138
    see also Primary schools
Science, 4
    epidemiology as, 31
    HIV
        client group, 253
        discovery, 249
Scott, P.
    on constructed communities, 248
    Purchasing HIV prevention, 261
Scottish Health Education Group, *Promoting
        good health,* 154
Screening
    child health, 107
    and homeless people, 164

Screening (contd)
    men's health, 218–219
    mental illness, 193–194
    obstetric, pressures on women, 73
    old age, 269–270, 274
    pre-conception care, 57–58, 74
Secondary health care, British primary health
        care as, 21
Secondary health promotion, 107
Secondary prevention, pre-conception care, 59
Secondary schools, health promotion, 136
Secretarial support, neighbourhood health
        strategy projects, 295, 300
Seedhouse, D., on health promotion, 34
Self-empowerment, as tautology, 34, 223–224
Self-esteem
    and empowerment, 94
    healthy settings work, 149–150
    mental health, 184
    and teenage pregnancy, 87, 90
    young people, 131, 143
Self-help groups
    AIDS epidemic, 256–257
    see also Community groups; Consumer
        groups
Self-management, childhood illnesses,
        118–119
Senior nurse manager, Stockport
        neighbourhood health strategy, 290
Sex education, 91–93
  peer education, 146
Sex-role inventory (Bem), 210
Sexual abuse, homelessness, 159, 163
Sexual health
    gay men, 220
    and HIV epidemic, 252, 257
    men, 210
    older people, 273–275
    omitted from Our healthier nation, 128
    services
        homeless women, 163
        young people's views on, 134, 150
    see also Safe sex
Sexual intercourse
    teenagers, 83–84, 87, 131
    see also Safe sex
Sexual lifestyles of gay and bisexual men in
        England and Wales (Weatherburn et al),
        261
Sexual relationships, queer community, 255
Sexually transmitted diseases, teenagers, 83
Sheffield
    health services for homeless people, 174
        (Box)
    intersectoral collaboration, 15
    Somali Community Health Project,
        236–237
Shelter, homelessness
    figures, 156
    people not registered with GP, 164
Shiltz, R, And the band played on, 248
Shock horror approaches, young people's
        health promotion, 141–142
Shoes, older people, 272
Shorthold assured tenancies, 158
Short-termism, vs community participation,
        43

Sick role, 6
Sickle Cell Anaemia Campaign, 236
Siege, body under, 7, 8
Silcock, B. (case), 198
Single Homelessness, homelessness figures,
        156
Single issue approaches
    peer education, 147 (Box)
    young people's health promotion, 142–143
Single people, homelessness, 156
Skills
    first aid, 275
    mental health as, 184
    for self-empowerment, 132
    see also Communication skills
Skinner, S., community capacity building, 234
Sleeping rough see Rooflessness
'Slim' (AIDS), Africa, 249, 250
Smoke alarms, 303
Smoking
    children, 131, 133 (Box)
        targets, 116 (Box)
    children's views, 111, 113
    gender differences, 212
    lung cancer, 215
    and pregnancy, 54, 55
    Stockport neighbourhood health strategy,
        302 (Box)
    'No smoking days', 287 (Box)
'Soap' programmes, men's health, 214
Social class
    child health, 131–132
    childhood accidents, 105
    conception and pregnancy, 53–54
    men's health, 212, 222 (Box)
    teenage pregnancy, 85, 132
Social education, youth clubs, 138–139
Social factors, 11–13
    gender differences, 209
    mental health, 190
Social function, and health, 5–6
Social justice (equity), community
        development, 18–21
Social policies, causing inequality, 19
Social Service Departments, The Children Act
        (1989), 128–129
Social support (Thoits), 74
Societal change, health promotion, 221
Somali Community Health Project (Sheffield),
        236–237
Somali Mental Health Project, 237
Specialist services
    homeless people, 172–173
    young people's health, 150–151
Spectrum of participation, 17, 37–38
Spina bifida, 53
Spiritual wholeness, 8
Staff development see Training
Stakeholders, in health, 253
Standing Committee for Community
        Development Charter, 234
Statistics, recklessness on AIDS risk, 256
Stillbirth rates, 104 (Box)
Stockport
    intersectoral collaboration, 15
    neighbourhood health strategy project,
        285–306

Stockport
  neighbourhood health strategy project *(contd)*
    successes, 300–301
Stockport Health Promise, 286
Stop Rickets campaign, 231
Stress, 10
  on conception, 56
  mental health, 215–216
  and smoking, 55
  workplace, 191–192, 215
Stress and vulnerability model, schizophrenia,
  197
Strokes *see* Cerebrovascular accidents
Structuralism, ethnic minority groups,
  231–232
Stubbs, P., anti-racism, 232
Student health services, 140
Student-centred learning (Rogers), 132
Sudden infant death syndrome, 104 (Box)
Suicide
  Confidential Inquiry (Royal College of
    Psychiatrists), 198
  gay men, 220
  gender differences, 216, 219
  group interventions (Canada), 195–196
  older people, 277
  rooflessness, 161
  targets *vs*, 185 (Box), 186, 187–188
Suicide prevention: the challenge confronted
  (NHS Health Advisory Service), 205
Support meetings
  carers, 304
  Stockport neighbourhood health strategy
    project, 292
Support networks
  and babies with disabilities, 59–60
  pregnant teenagers, 85
Supportive resources, 41
Surgery, families of patients, 194
Surveillance
  child health, 107
  see also Screening
Survival rights, children, 129 (Box)
Survivor guilt, 248
Sweden, depression, education of general
  practitioners, 196

Tackling inequalities in health (Benzeval et al),
  306
Tai Chi, 271, 272
Tameside Ethnic Health Forum, Chinese
  subgroup, 239–240
Tannahill, A., on epidemiology, 22
Tape recorders, research interviews, 170
Targets
  child health, 116
  health for homeless people, 178
  mental health, 185–186
Technology, and childhood, 115
Teenage Health Club (Alexandria, Scotland),
  151
Teenagers
  conformity, 94–95
  pregnancy, 57, 83–99
    targets, 116
Tenant harassment, 158–159

Termination of pregnancy, 60
  pressures on women, 73
Terminology, 'queer' health, 246–252
Terry Higgins Trust, 250, 251–252
Tertiary health promotion, 107
Tertiary prevention
  mental illness, 197–198
  pre-conception care, 59–60
Testicular cancer, 213
Testicular self-examination, 218–219
The Children Act (1989), 128–129, 133
Thoits, P., social support, 74
THORN course, 197–198
THT (Terry Higgins Trust), 250, 251–252
Tilford, S. et al, *Effectiveness of mental
    health promotion interventions*, 205
Tokenism, and community participation,
  17–18, 239
Tones and Tilford, *Health education.
    Effectiveness, efficiency and equity*,
  306
Tones, K., on empowerment, 35, 60, 221
Top-down approaches, 15–16
  community development, 36, 234–235,
  239–240
Training
  Connect 4 Programme, 236
  on homelessness, 173, 177
  mental health promotion, 188 (Box)
  Stockport neighbourhood health strategy
    project, 291–293, 298
'Tramp' stereotype, 165
Travelling families, 105, 120
Treichler, P.A., on AIDS epidemic, 245–246
Tuberculosis, ethnic minority groups, 230
Tudor, K., *Mental health promotion:
    paradigms and practice*, 205
Turner, B., on power, 27–28
Tutors
  colleges, 139
  home, teenage pregnancy, 86

UK National Screening Committee, on
    prostate cancer screening, 218
Under the Stars project (Norwich), 148
Unemployment, 11, 13
  ethnic minority groups, 241
  men's health, 212
  suicide, 216
United Kingdom
  teenage pregnancy, 83, 133 (Box)
  see also UK National Screening Committee
United Nations
  on community development, 19–20
  Convention on the Rights of the Child,
    102, 129–130
United States
  black communities, health promotion, 36
  Community Mental Health Centres, 190,
    191
  influence on UK queer communities, 250
  National Medical Association, speech on
    violence, 40
  professionalisation of HIV response,
    256–257
Universities, 139–140

Unpopular patients, older people seen as, 270
Urban initiatives, sexual health and HIV, 259
User groups *see* Consumer groups

Vaginal delivery, teenage pregnancy, 88
Value, of older people, 282
Value clarification, and empowerment, 94
Variability
   health-promoting schools, 149
   peer education programmes, 147 (Box)
Verbrugge, L.M., on men's health, 212
Victim blaming, 3, 33
   child health, 107
   of communities, 40
   rickets, 231
Violence (domestic), 159, 162, 178
Vitamin D, older people, 272
Voluntary agencies, child health, 118

Walker, I., APEC, 69
Walk-in clinics *see* Direct-access clinics
'Walking' of neighbourhoods, 295
Weatherburn, P. et al, *Sexual lifestyles of gay
    and bisexual men in England and
    Wales*, 261
Weight, pre-conception care, 52–53
Well-man clinics, 207, 217–218
   older people, 273
What is mental distress? (MIND), 189
Which? guide to men's health (Carroll), 227
Whistle blowing, maternity provision, 69
Whitehead, M., *The health divide*, 18
Wilkinson, R., power and health, 28
Will-power, 8
Wolch and Akita, on homelessness, 162
Women
   homelessness
      'hidden', 157–160
      mental health, 162–163
      primary health care, 155–181
   Somali Community Health Project, 237
   suicide rates, 187
   views on childbirth, 74–75

workplace stress, 192
Woodhouse Park Clinic (Manchester), 150
Words, 'queer' health, 246–252
Working for patients (White Paper), 232
Working together for better health, 238
Working where the risks are (Evans et al),
   261
Workplace
   mental health promotion, 191–192
   risks and gender, 209
   stress, 191–192, 215
   see also Occupation
World Health Organisation
   community participation, 17
   empowerment, 198
   Health for all by the year 2000, 13
   Health for all in Europe by the year 2000,
     238
   primary health care, 21–22
   schools and health promotion, 92
   see also Alma Ata declaration
World Mental Health Day, 192–193
Wytham Hall (London), health services for
    homeless people, 174 (Box)

X-rays, chest, men's screening, 218

Young people
   health concerns, 133–134
   health promotion, 125–154
   leading health promotion, 144
   see also Adolescence (process)
Young Women's group, Stockport
    neighbourhood health strategy, 304
Youth clubs, 138–139
Youth Clubs UK, with Health Education
    Authority, 139
Youth Health Promotion (Nutbeam), 154
Youth service, Stockport neighbourhood
    health strategy, 287 (Box), 304
Youth work, detached/outreach approaches,
    147–148